D1415674

Imaging of Osteoporosis

Guest Editor

GIUSEPPE GUGLIELMI, MD

RADIOLOGIC CLINICS OF NORTH AMERICA

www.radiologic.theclinics.com

Consulting Editor
FRANK H. MILLER, MD

May 2010 • Volume 48 • Number 3

SAUNDERS an imprint of ELSEVIER, Inc.

W.B. SAUNDERS COMPANY
A Division of Elsevier Inc.

1600 John F. Kennedy Boulevard • Suite 1800 • Philadelphia, Pennsylvania 19103-2899

http://www.theclinics.com

RADIOLOGIC CLINICS OF NORTH AMERICA Volume 48, Number 3
May 2010 ISSN 0033-8389, ISBN 13: 978-1-4377-1944-4

Editor: Barton Dudlick
Developmental Editor: Theresa Collier

© **2010 Elsevier Inc. All rights reserved.**

This journal and the individual contributions contained in it are protected under copyright by Elsevier, and the following terms and conditions apply to their use:

Photocopying
Single photocopies of single articles may be made for personal use as allowed by national copyright laws. Permission of the Publisher and payment of a fee is required for all other photocopying, including multiple or systematic copying, copying for advertising or promotional purposes, resale, and all forms of document delivery. Special rates are available for educational institutions that wish to make photocopies for non-profit educational classroom use. For information on how to seek permission visit www.elsevier.com/permissions or call: (+44) 1865 843830 (UK)/(+1) 215 239 3804 (USA).

Derivative Works
Subscribers may reproduce tables of contents or prepare lists of articles including abstracts for internal circulation within their institutions. Permission of the Publisher is required for resale or distribution outside the institution. Permission of the Publisher is required for all other derivative works, including compilations and translations (please consult www.elsevier.com/permissions).

Electronic Storage or Usage
Permission of the Publisher is required to store or use electronically any material contained in this journal, including any article or part of an article (please consult www.elsevier.com/permissions). Except as outlined above, no part of this publication may be reproduced, stored in a retrieval system or transmitted in any form or by any means, electronic, mechanical, photocopying, recording or otherwise, without prior written permission of the Publisher.

Notice
No responsibility is assumed by the Publisher for any injury and/or damage to persons or property as a matter of products liability, negligence or otherwise, or from any use or operation of any methods, products, instructions or ideas contained in the material herein. Because of rapid advances in the medical sciences, in particular, independent verification of diagnoses and drug dosages should be made.

Although all advertising material is expected to conform to ethical (medical) standards, inclusion in this publication does not constitute a guarantee or endorsement of the quality or value of such product or of the claims made of it by its manufacturer.

Radiologic Clinics of North America (ISSN 0033-8389) is published bimonthly by Elsevier Inc., 360 Park Avenue South, New York, NY 10010-1710. Months of issue are January, March, May, July, September, and November. Periodicals postage paid at New York, NY and additional mailing offices. Subscription prices are USD 361 per year for US individuals, USD 545 per year for US institutions, USD 176 per year for US students and residents, USD 421 per year for Canadian individuals, USD 684 per year for Canadian institutions, USD 520 per year for international individuals, USD 684 per year for international institutions, and USD 253 per year for Canadian and foreign students/residents. To receive student and resident rate, orders must be accompanied by name of affiliated institution, date of term and the signature of program/residency coordinator on institution letterhead. Orders will be billed at individual rate until proof of status is received. Foreign air speed delivery is included in all Clinics subscription prices. All prices are subject to change without notice. **POSTMASTER:** Send address changes to Radiologic Clinics of North America, Elsevier Health Sciences Division, Subscription Customer Service, 3251 Riverport Lane, Maryland Heights,MO63043. **Customer Service: Telephone: 1-800-654-2452** (U.S. and Canada); **1-314-447-8871** (outside U.S. and Canada). **Fax: 1-314-447-8029. E-mail: journalscustomerservice-usa@ elsevier.com** (for print support); **journalsonlinesupport-usa@elsevier.com** (for online support).

Reprints. For copies of 100 or more of articles in this publication, please contact the Commercial Reprints Department, Elsevier Inc., 360 Park Avenue South, New York, New York 10010-1710. Tel.: (+1) 212-633-3812; Fax: (+1) 212-462-1935; E-mail: reprints@elsevier.com.

Radiologic Clinics of North America also published in Greek Paschalidis Medical Publications, Athens, Greece.

Radiologic Clinics of North America is covered in *MEDLINE/PubMed (Index Medicus), EMBASE/Excerpta Medica, Current Contents/Life Sciences, Current Contents/Clinical Medicine, RSNA Index to Imaging Literature, BIOSIS, Science Citation Index,* and *ISI/BIOMED.*

Printed in the United States of America.

Contributors

CONSULTING EDITOR

FRANK H. MILLER, MD
Professor of Radiology; Chief, Body Imaging
Section and Fellowship Program and GI
Radiology; and Medical Director MRI,
Department of Radiology, Northwestern
University Feinberg School of Medicine,
Chicago, Illinois

GUEST EDITOR

GIUSEPPE GUGLIELMI, MD
Professor, Department of Radiology,
University of Foggia, Foggia; Scientific Institute
'Casa Sollievo della Sofferenza' Hospital,
San Giovanni Rotondo, Italy

AUTHORS

JUDITH E. ADAMS, MBBS, FRCR, FRCP, FBIR
Professor, Consultant Radiologist, Manchester
Royal Infirmary, Central Manchester
Universities Hospitals NHS Foundation Trust;
Honorary Professor of Diagnostic Radiology,
Imaging Science and Biomedical Engineering,
University of Manchester, Manchester,
United Kingdom

GOPINATHAN ANIL, MD, FRCR
Registrar, Department of Radiology, Changi
General Hospital, Singapore

G.C. ANSELMETTI, MD
Department of Interventional Radiology,
Candiolo Hospital Turin, Italy

ANDREW J. BURGHARDT, BS
Musculoskeletal and Quantitative Imaging
Research, Department of Radiology and
Biomedical Imaging, University of California,
San Francisco, California

**JULIET COMPSTON, MD, FRCPath,
FRCP, FMedSci**
Professor of Bone Medicine, Department of
Medicine, Addenbrooke's Hospital, Cambridge
University Hospitals NHS Foundation Trust,
Cambridge, United Kingdom

BART L. CLARKE, MD
Associate Professor of Medicine, Mayo Clinic
College of Medicine; Consultant, Division of
Endocrinology, Diabetes, Metabolism, and
Nutrition, Mayo Clinic, Rochester, Minnesota

JOHN DAMILAKIS, PhD
Associate Professor, Department of Medical
Physics, Faculty of Medicine, University of Crete,
Iraklion; Department of Medical Physics,
University Hospital of Iraklion, Crete, Greece

LANCE G. DASHER, MD
Department of Radiology, Medical Center
Boulevard, Wake Forest University Baptist
Medical Center, Winston-Salem, North Carolina

FRANCESCA DE TERLIZZI, MSc
MSc Medical Office, IGEA srl, Via Parmenide
Carpi (MO), Italy

DANIELE DIACINTI, MD
Research, Assistant Professor of Radiology,
Department of Radiology, Policlinico Umberto I,
"Sapienza", Rome, Italy

HARRY K. GENANT, MD
University of California San Francisco,
San Francisco, California

JAMES F. GRIFFITH, MB BCh BAO, MRCP, FRCR
Professor, Department of Diagnostic Radiology
and Organ Imaging, Chinese University of Hong
Kong, Prince of Wales Hospital, Shatin, New
Territories, Hong Kong

GIUSEPPE GUGLIELMI, MD
Professor, Department of Radiology, University
of Foggia, Foggia; Scientific Institute
'Casa Sollievo della Sofferenza' Hospital,
San Giovanni Rotondo, Italy

SUNDEEP KHOSLA, MD
Professor of Medicine, Mayo Clinic College
of Medicine; Consultant, Endocrine Research Unit,
Division of Endocrinology, Diabetes, Metabolism,
and Nutrition, Mayo Clinic, Rochester, Minnesota

ROLAND KRUG, PhD
Musculoskeletal and Quantitative Imaging
Research, Department of Radiology and
Biomedical Imaging, University of California San
Francisco, China Basin Landing, San Francisco,
California

THOMAS F. LANG, PhD
Professor in Residence, Joint Bioengineering
Graduate Group, Department of Radiology and
Biomedical Imaging, University of California San
Francisco, San Francisco, California

LEON LENCHIK, MD
Associate Professor, Department of Radiology,
Medical Center Boulevard, Wake Forest University
Baptist Medical Center, Winston-Salem,
North Carolina

THOMAS M. LINK, MD
Musculoskeletal and Quantitative Imaging
Research, Department of Radiology and
Biomedical Imaging, University of California,
San Francisco, California

SHARMILA MAJUMDAR, PhD
Musculoskeletal and Quantitative Imaging
Research, Department of Radiology and
Biomedical Imaging, University of California,
San Francisco; University of California San
Francisco-University of California Berkeley
Joint Graduate Group in Bioengineering,
California

S. MASALA, MD
Department of Interventional Radiology,
University of Rome Tor Vergata; Policlinico
Universitario di Tor Vergata Roma,
Viale Oxford, Roma, Italy

M. MUTO, MD
Neuroradiology, Cardarelli Hospital, Naples, Italy

CHRISTOPHER D. NEWTON, MD
Department of Radiology, Medical Center
Boulevard, Wake Forest University Baptist
Medical Center, Winston-Salem, North Carolina

WILFRED C.G. PEH, MD, FRCPG, FRCPE, FRCR
Clinical Professor of Radiology, Yong Loo Lin
School of Medicine, National University of
Singapore; Senior Consultant and Head,
Department of Diagnostic Radiology, Alexandra
Hospital, Singapore

GIACOMO SCALZO, MD
Department of Radiology, Scientific Institute
Hospital San Giovanni Rotondo, Italy

GIOVANNI SIMONETTI, MD
Department of Radiology, Molecular Imaging,
Interventional Radiology and Radiation Therapy,
"Tor Vergata" University Hospital, Rome, Italy

CORNELIS VAN KUIJK, MD, PhD
Professor and Chair, Department of Radiology,
VU University Medical Center, Amsterdam,
The Netherlands

Contents

> The epidemiology of osteoporosis is reviewed, with a discussion of secular changes in incidence, geographical variation, and economic costs. The morbidity and mortality associated with hip, vertebral, and forearm fractures are outlined. The main pathogenetic factors contributing to age-related bone loss and osteoporosis are reviewed. Finally, there is a discussion of the recent advances in fracture risk prediction and the use of independent clinical risk factors to improve bone mineral density-based prediction.

> The physiology of bone loss in aging women and men is largely explained by the effects of gonadal sex steroid deficiency on the skeleton. In women, estrogen deficiency is the main cause of early rapid postmenopausal bone loss, whereas hyperparathyroidism and vitamin D deficiency are thought to explain age-related bone loss later in life. Surprisingly, estrogen deficiency also plays a dominant role in the physiology of bone loss in aging men. Many other factors contribute to bone loss in aging women and men, including defective bone formation by aging osteoblasts, impairment of the growth hormone/insulin-like growth factor axis, reduced peak bone mass, age-associated sarcopenia, leptin secreted by adipocytes, serotonin secreted by the intestine, and a long list of sporadic secondary causes. Further elucidation of the relative importance of each of these factors will lead to improved preventive and therapeutic approaches for osteoporosis.

> Bone densitometric studies have shown that osteoporosis is a result of prolonged, slow bone loss and that the pattern of loss is different for trabecular and cortical bone. Structurally-insufficient osteoporotic bone is predisposed to fractures. Among the clinically manifest osteoporotic fractures, distal radius leads the list, followed by hip, spine, and proximal humerus. This article examines the use of conventional radiography as well as other imaging-based modalities for the evaluation of osteoporosis and associated fractures in the axial and appendicular skeleton.

Vertebral fractures are usually the first to occur in osteoporosis, provide indisputable evidence of reduced bone strength, and are frequently a harbinger of further vertebral and nonvertebral fracture. Radiologists are best placed to draw attention to the presence of vertebral fractures, most of which are clinically silent. Magnetic resonance imaging supplemented if necessary by computed tomography is usually sufficient to enable distinction between osteoporotic and nonosteoporotic vertebral fracture, without a need for percutaneous biopsy.

Metacarpal morphometry and radiogrammetry are the oldest methods for quantitative assessment of the skeleton. The historical aspects of these measurements are reviewed. Although they were inexpensive and widely available and provided useful research and epidemiologic information, they were labor intensive and imprecise. They were replaced with the current established methods of bone mineral densitometry. With the application of modern computer vision techniques, metacarpal morphometric analysis has been rejuvenated, with improvement in precision and evidence that the method can be applied to studies in adults and children. Evidence for limited normal reference data and the ability to predict future fractures in osteoporosis and reflect activity and predict outcomes in rheumatoid arthritis are presented.

Central DXA is rapid, reliable, and the most commonly used method of measuring bone mineral density in clinical practice. Although interpretation of clinical DXA scans is generally straightforward, it is important for the interpreting physician to be aware of common pitfalls and to maintain rigorous quality assurance. A firm understanding of the clinical utility of DXA allows the interpreting physician to provide valuable recommendations to treating clinicians, thereby improving the care of patients with osteoporosis. This article describes the current approach to and recent advances in the clinical use of central DXA.

Visual semiquantitative (SQ) assessment of the radiographs by a trained and experienced observer is the "gold standard" method to detect vertebral fractures. Vertebral morphometry is a quantitative method to identify osteoporotic vertebral fractures based on the measurement of vertebral heights. Vertebral morphometry may be performed on conventional spinal radiographs (MRX: morphometric x-ray radiography) or on images obtained from dual x-ray absorptiometry (DXA) scans (MXA: morphometric x-ray absorptiometry). Vertebral fracture assessment (VFA) indicates the method for identification of the vertebral fractures using lateral spine views acquired by DXA, with low-dose exposition. For epidemiologic studies and clinical drug trials in osteoporosis research but also in clinical practice, the preferred method is radiographic SQ assessment., because an expert eye can better distinguish between true fractures and vertebral anomalies than can quantitative morphometry. However, vertebral morphometry, calculating the deformity of overall thoracic and lumbar spine, may supply useful data about the vertebral fracture risk. VFA performed during routine densitometry allows identification, by visual or morphometric methods, of most osteoporotic vertebral fractures, even those that are asymptomatic.

Quantitative ultrasound (QUS) has been introduced in the medical field for the study of bone tissue to identify changes in the tissue that could suggest the presence of osteoporosis and bone fragility. The ultrasound technique is simple, versatile, and its low cost and lack of ionizing radiation have led to the diffusion of this method worldwide. The present article is an overview of the most relevant developments in the field of quantitative ultrasound, in clinical and experimental settings. The advantages and limitations of the present technique and suggestions for its use in the clinical practice are reported.

Unlike dual x-ray absorptiometry and high-resolution CT scan and MR imaging techniques, which are largely restricted to the peripheral skeleton owing to radiation dose and signal-to-noise considerations, volumetric quantitative measures provide measures of cortical and trabecular volumetric bone mineral density, cross-sectional geometry, and estimates of whole-bone strength based on patient specific finite element modeling. This article focuses on the application of volumetric quantitative measures to studies of aging, disuse, and drug treatment as related to osteoporosis.

The importance of assessing the bone's microarchitectural make-up in addition to its mineral density in the context of osteoporosis has been emphasized in several publications. The high spatial resolution required to resolve the bone's microstructure in a clinically feasible scan time is challenging. At present, the best suited modalities meeting these requirements in vivo are high-resolution peripheral quantitative imaging (HR-pQCT) and magnetic resonance imaging (MRI). Whereas HR-pQCT is limited to peripheral skeleton regions like the wrist and ankle, MRI can also image other sites like the proximal femur but usually with lower spatial resolution. In addition, multidetector computed tomography has been used for high-resolution imaging of trabecular bone structure; however, the radiation dose is a limiting factor. This article provides an overview of the different modalities, technical requirements, and recent developments in this emerging field. Details regarding imaging protocols as well as image postprocessing methods for bone structure quantification are discussed.

Bone densitometry is an established diagnostic tool in adults to assess bone quantity and to stratify patients and healthy individuals for the prevention of bone fracture. It has become a powerful tool in monitoring diseases and treatments that have an impact on bone metabolism, such as primary osteoporosis or drug-induced secondary osteoporosis. Although there are several techniques to assess bone density (eg, radiogrammetry, dual x-ray absorptiometry [DXA], quantitative CT, and quantitative ultrasound), the most widely used technique is DXA.

GOAL STATEMENT

The goal of the *Radiologic Clinics of North America* is to keep practicing radiologists and radiology residents up to date with current clinical practice in radiology by providing timely articles reviewing the state of the art in patient care.

ACCREDITATION

The *Radiologic Clinics of North America* is planned and implemented in accordance with the Essential Areas and Policies of the Accreditation Council for Continuing Medical Education (ACCME) through the joint sponsorship of the University of Virginia School of Medicine and Elsevier. The University of Virginia School of Medicine is accredited by the ACCME to provide continuing medical education for physicians.

The University of Virginia School of Medicine designates this educational activity for a maximum of 15 *AMA PRA Category 1 Credits*™ for each issue, 90 credits per year. Physicians should only claim credit commensurate with the extent of their participation in the activity.

The American Medical Association has determined that physicians not licensed in the US who participate in this CME activity are eligible for a maximum of *15 AMA PRA Category 1 Credits*™ for each issue, 90 credits per year.

Credit can be earned by reading the text material, taking the CME examination online at http://www.theclinics.com/home/cme, and completing the evaluation. After taking the test, you will be required to review any and all incorrect answers. Following completion of the test and evaluation, your credit will be awarded and you may print your certificate.

FACULTY DISCLOSURE/CONFLICT OF INTEREST

The University of Virginia School of Medicine, as an ACCME accredited provider, endorses and strives to comply with the Accreditation Council for Continuing Medical Education (ACCME) Standards of Commercial Support, Commonwealth of Virginia statutes, University of Virginia policies and procedures, and associated federal and private regulations and guidelines on the need for disclosure and monitoring of proprietary and financial interests that may affect the scientific integrity and balance of content delivered in continuing medical education activities under our auspices.

The University of Virginia School of Medicine requires that all CME activities accredited through this institution be developed independently and be scientifically rigorous, balanced and objective in the presentation/discussion of its content, theories and practices.

All authors/editors participating in an accredited CME activity are expected to disclose to the readers relevant financial relationships with commercial entities occurring within the past 12 months (such as grants or research support, employee, consultant, stock holder, member of speakers bureau, etc.). The University of Virginia School of Medicine will employ appropriate mechanisms to resolve potential conflicts of interest to maintain the standards of fair and balanced education to the reader. Questions about specific strategies can be directed to the Office of Continuing Medical Education, University of Virginia School of Medicine, Charlottesville, Virginia.

The faculty and staff of the University of Virginia Office of Continuing Medical Education have no financial affiliations to disclose.

The authors/editors listed below have identified no financial or professional relationships for themselves or their spouse/partner:
Judith E. Adams, MBBS, FRCR, FRCP, FBIR; Gopinathan Anil, MD, FRCR; G.C. Anselmetti, MD; Andrew J. Burghardt, BS; John Damilakis, PhD; Lance G. Dasher, MD; Daniele Diacinti, MD; Barton Dudlick (Acquisitions Editor); James F. Griffith, MB BCh BAO, MRCP, FRCR; Giuseppe Guglielmi, MD (Guest Editor); Theodore E. Keats, MD (Test Author); Sundeep Khosla, MD; Roland Krug, PhD; Leon Lenchik, MD; Thomas M. Link, MD; Salvatore Masala, MD, PhD; Frank H. Miller, MD (Consulting Editor); Mario Muto, MD; Christopher D. Newton, MD; Wilfred C. G. Peh, MD, FRCPG, FRCPE, FRCR; Giacomo Scalzo, MD; Giovanni Simonetti, MD; and Cornelis van Kuijk, MD, PhD.

The authors/editors listed below have identified the following financial or professional relationships for themselves or their spouse/partner:
Bart L. Clarke, MD is an industry funded research/investigator for NPS Pharmaceuticals.
Juliet Compston, MD, FRCPath, FRCP, FMedSci is a consultant for Servier, Shire, Nycomed, Novartis, Amgen, Procter & Gamble, Wyeth, Alliance for Better Bone Health, Roche, GSK, and Sanofi Aventis; is paid speaking engagements, reimbursement of travel, and accommodations for Servier, Merck, Procter & Gamble, Eli Lilly, Amgen, Nycomed, and Gilead; and has research grants from Servier R & D and Procter & Gamble.
Francesca de Terlizzi, MSc is employed by IGEA S.p.A.
Harry K. Genant, MD is an industry funded research/investigator, a consultant, and an advisory committee/board member for Merck, Lilly, Amgen, Roche, Servier, Pfizer, Genentech, Hologic, and GE/Lunar; and, is a consultant and stockholder for Synarc.
Thomas F. Lang, PhD is an industry funded research/investigator for Merck.
Sharmila Majumdar, PhD is a consultant for Merck and is an industry funded research/investigator for Merck and GlaxoSmithKline.

Disclosure of Discussion of Non-FDA Approved Uses for Pharmaceutical Products and/or Medical Devices.
The University of Virginia School of Medicine, as an ACCME provider, requires that all faculty presenters identify and disclose any off-label uses for pharmaceutical and medical device products. The University of Virginia School of Medicine recommends that each physician fully review all the available data on new products or procedures prior to clinical use.

TO ENROLL

To enroll in the Radiologic Clinics of North America Continuing Medical Education program, call customer service at 1-800-654-2452 or sign up online at http://www.theclinics.com/home/cme. The CME program is available to subscribers for an additional annual fee USD 245.

Radiologic Clinics of North America

THE CLINICS ARE NOW AVAILABLE ONLINE!

Access your subscription at:
www.theclinics.com

Foreword

Osteoporosis is one of the most important diseases involving the elderly. Due to the global aging population, osteoporosis has become a major problem, which is of interest to several medical disciplines implicated in the management of this widespread condition.

Because bone mass declines after menopause in women, with aging in both genders, and as a result of different medical conditions, if it falls below a threshold, in more and more people non-traumatic fractures are occurring during everyday activities. Decreased bone density and the occurrence of nontraumatic fractures define the syndrome of osteoporosis. The most characteristic osteoporotic fractures occur in the vertebrae, the hip, and the distal radius, although a large number of other fractures also are related to osteoporosis. Despite the widely held belief that vertebral fractures receive medical attention because of acute pain, lesser grades of vertebral deformities may be asymptomatic or result in only mild pain. Nonetheless, these can lead to loss of height, postural changes, kyphoscoliosis, restricted activity, and loss of self-esteem.

It is important that radiologists be fully aware of the range of diagnostic techniques that are now available for the diagnosis and follow-up of osteoporosis and know how to apply these sophisticated methods in daily clinical practice.

Dr Giuseppe Guglielmi is a renowned radiologist with a longstanding interest in osteoporosis, and his previous publications on this condition are internationally recognized. He has been successful in engaging several highly qualified experts to contribute to the individual articles in this superb issue.

Although much has been written about osteoporosis, what has been lacking is a definitive comprehensive overview of current knowledge of osteoporosis, focusing on various aspects of imaging in osteoporosis, and this issue of *Radiologic Clinics of North America* fulfills this need. Here, contained in a single volume, is much of what is needed to know about osteoporosis imaging.

I extend my warm congratulations to Dr Guglielmi and colleagues for their excellent achievement in producing this timely and valuable contribution.

Harry K. Genant, MD
University of California San Francisco (UCSF)
505 Parnassus Avenue
San Francisco
CA 94143, USA

E-mail address:
harry.genant@ucsf.edu

Radiol Clin N Am 48 (2010) xi
doi:10.1016/j.rcl.2010.03.003
0033-8389/10/$ – see front matter
© 2010 Elsevier Inc. All rights reserved.

Foreword

The dramatic increase in the incidence of osteoporosis requires up-to-date knowledge of the newest perspectives and the most recent developments in diagnosis and treatment of osteoporotic patients. Bone mineral density is closely related to bone fragility, and the advent of techniques to quantitatively assess bone density has been welcomed, reducing the subjectivity inherent in conventional radiologic assessment of osteoporosis. The ongoing technical process has made various techniques of assessing bone density widely available. These measurement techniques, however, have also incurred some criticism because bone densitometry has sometimes been applied without specific indications and without appropriate clinical ramifications.

Osteoporosis is a disease characterized by reduced bone mass, quality, and strength; changes in skeletal microarchitecture; and increased fracture risk. Osteoporosis, which literally means *porous bone*, is often referred to as the silent disease because symptoms are not noticed until a fracture occurs. A tremendous comprehensive effort has been made in the past 2 decades to improve diagnostic methods, increase awareness, and identify treatments for osteoporosis.

Recently, thanks to my role as expert and technical consultant to the Italian Department of Health, I began considering osteoporosis a fundamental matter to be faced in terms of primary, secondary, and tertiary prevention by conducting an information campaign in schools and, among many other interventions, the creation, for the first time in history, of a registry of fragility fractures of all skeletal segments.

One of the great merits of this issue is that it deals with all aspects of osteoporosis, including morphology and function, providing a perspective on the current status of bone densitometry and its relevance to osteoporosis diagnosis and management. Aside from standard bone densitometry, newer technologies, such as quantitative ultrasound techniques, MR imaging, multidetector CT, and bone structure analysis, are discussed in the context of diagnosing osteoporosis.

I am especially grateful to the authors, who are among the most prominent and knowledgeable in this particular scientific field, for their effort and dedication. The outstanding qualifications and high level of expertise of the editor, Professor Giuseppe Guglielmi, and of the contributing authors are a guarantee for the up-to-date and comprehensive contents of this issue of *Radiologic Clinics of North America*.

I am confident that this issue will guide radiologists and all other clinicians through this minefield of scientific knowledge, and it is my sincere hope that it will assist in daily practice, offering technical suggestions to optimize imaging and treatment in osteoporotic patients.

Giovanni Simonetti, MD
Department of Radiology
Molecular Imaging
Interventional Radiology and Radiation Therapy
"Tor Vergata" University Hospital
Viale Oxford 81
00133 Rome, Italy

E-mail address:
giovanni.simonetti@uniroma2.it

Radiol Clin N Am 48 (2010) xiii
doi:10.1016/j.rcl.2010.03.004
0033-8389/10/$ – see front matter © 2010 Elsevier Inc. All rights reserved.

Preface

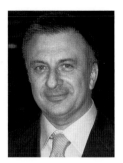

Giuseppe Guglielmi, MD
Guest Editor

It is a great pleasure to introduce this interesting issue of *Radiologic Clinic of North America* on imaging of osteoporosis. The diagnosis of osteoporosis and the determination of fracture risk have always been challenging for radiologists, epidemiologists, and clinicians as well as other researchers and health care professionals working in the field. The need for this issue indicates the great interest among radiologists, and those in several other medical disciplines, in the diagnosis and management of this common condition and its possible complications.

Osteoporosis is one of the leading causes of morbidity and mortality among the elderly. With the prediction that the number of people who are 60 years old or more will increase from approximately 300 million to greater than 700 million in the next 25 years, it can be appreciated that osteoporosis will rapidly reach epidemic proportions with a high socioeconomic impact. Orthopedic procedures in elderly patients are costly, and with the increasing age of the population, these costs will continue to escalate. Thus, although it is primarily radiologists involved in osteoporosis imaging in everyday clinical practice, this book is directed toward endocrinologists, internists, gynecologists, orthopedic surgeons, general practitioners, and every physician who cares for osteoporotic patients. It should be of value to all who work in clinical or scientific studies.

Today's highly sophisticated diagnostic techniques involve conventional radiography as well as quantitative methods: dual energy x-ray absorptiometry, quantitative CT and peripheral quantative CT, vertebral morphometry, and quantitative ultrasound. This issue concludes with the promising techniques of MR imaging and different high-resolution methods, considering also pediatric patients and the interventional modalities available for the treatment of severe osteoporosis conditions.

I would like to thank the authors for their expert contributions to attempt to cover all the important issues encountered in a small and highly specialized field, such osteoporosis imaging.

Finally, my special gratitude goes to Mr Barton Dudlick from Elsevier for inviting me to participate in this project.

Giuseppe Guglielmi, MD
Department of Radiology
University of Foggia
Viale Luigi Pinto, 1
71100 Foggia, Italy

Scientific Institute
'Casa Sollievo della Sofferenza' Hospital
San Giovanni
Rotondo 71013, Italy
E-mail address:
g.guglielmi@unifg.it

Radiol Clin N Am 48 (2010) xv
doi:10.1016/j.rcl.2010.03.002
0033-8389/10/$ – see front matter © 2010 Elsevier Inc. All rights reserved.

Osteoporosis: Social and Economic Impact

Juliet Compston, MD, FRCPath, FRCP, FMedSci

KEYWORDS

- osteoporosis • Fracture • Bone mineral density
- Economic cost • Fracture risk assessment

Osteoporosis is characterized by reduced bone mass and disruption of bone architecture, resulting in increased bone fragility and increased fracture risk.[1] These fractures are a major health problem in the elderly population, leading to significant morbidity, mortality, and cost to health care services. One in two women and one in five men over the age of 50 years will suffer a fracture due to osteoporosis during their remaining lifetime.[2] Demographic changes over the next few decades will result in at least a doubling in the number of these fractures. Worldwide, it is estimated that there are around 9 million osteoporotic fractures each year and that over half of these occur in Europe and the Americas.

A classification of osteoporosis based on bone mineral density (BMD) and fracture was proposed by the World Health Organization in 1994.[3] According to this definition, osteoporosis is defined a BMD T-score less than or equal to -2.5 (ie, 2.5 or more standard deviations [SD] below the mean value in healthy young adults), osteopenia as a T-score between -1 and -2.5 and normal BMD as a T-score higher than -1. Established osteoporosis is defined as a T-score less than or equal to -2.5 and the presence of a fragility fracture. Based on these criteria, osteoporosis is present in 30% of all postmenopausal Caucasian women and 70% of those aged 80 years.[4]

EPIDEMIOLOGY

The incidence of osteoporotic fractures increases markedly with age; in women, the median age for Colles fractures is around 65 years and for hip fracture, 80 years. The age at which vertebral fracture incidence reaches a peak is less well defined but in women is thought to be between 65 and 80 years. In men, no age-related increase in forearm fractures is seen, but hip fracture incidence rises exponentially after the age of 75 years. The prevalence of vertebral fractures rises with age in men, although less steeply than in women.[5]

During the latter part of the 20th century, increases in the age-adjusted incidence of osteoporotic fractures, mainly hip fracture, were reported in Europe and the United States.[6,7] This change was attributed to factors such as reduced physical activity, increased risk of falling, and possibly also changes in hip geometry such as longer hip axis length. Over the past decade, however, stabilization or a decrease in the age-adjusted incidence of osteoporotic fractures has been reported in some countries in the western world (for example Switzerland, Denmark and the United States),[8–10] although others have reported an increase (for example Germany and Japan).[11,12] These data mainly relate to hip fractures, since the incidence of other fracture types is not documented accurately in most countries. Notwithstanding secular changes in fracture incidence, the number of fractures will continue to rise as the population ages, and in Asia and Latin America, a five-fold increase in fractures is predicted during the next 40 to 50 years. Worldwide, it is estimated that the number of hip fractures will rise from 1.66 million in 1990 to 6.26 million in 2050.[13]

Geographical variations in the incidence of hip fractures have been reported in Caucasian women, with higher incidence rates in Scandinavia than in other parts of Europe or the United States.[14] Within Europe alone, there is a more than tenfold variation in incidence rates for

Department of Medicine, Addenbrooke's Hospital, Cambridge University Hospitals NHS Foundation Trust, Box 157, Cambridge CB2 0QQ, UK
E-mail address: jec1001@cam.ac.uk

Radiol Clin N Am 48 (2010) 477–482
doi:10.1016/j.rcl.2010.02.010
0033-8389/10/$ – see front matter © 2010 Elsevier Inc. All rights reserved.

reasons that have yet to be clarified.[15] Smaller differences in vertebral fractures incidence were noted within Europe in the European Vertebral Osteoporosis Study (EVOS).[16] Overall, fracture incidence is higher in white than in black men and women, possibly because of lower BMD, smaller bone size, and greater rates of bone loss in the former.

Fracture is a major risk factor for further fractures, an effect that is partially independent of BMD.[17] Thus the presence of a prevalent vertebral fracture is associated with a seven- to tenfold increase in the risk of subsequent vertebral fracture,[18] and the risk of a new vertebral fracture approaches 20% in the first 12 months after an incident vertebral fracture.[19] A fragility fracture at any site is a risk factor for subsequent fracture at the same or other sites; for example, the risk of a hip fracture is increased 1.4-and 2.7-fold in women and men respectively following a distal forearm fracture,[20] and the risk of hip fracture increases four- to fivefold in women with a vertebral fracture.[21] These observations emphasize the importance of prompt intervention in patients presenting with a fracture to prevent further fractures.

ECONOMIC COSTS

The economic costs of osteoporotic fractures include direct costs of hospitalization and aftercare and indirect costs attributable to the impact of fracture on daily life activities including working days. Together, these costs impose a huge financial burden on health care and social services. In the United States, the direct costs of osteoporotic fractures are estimated at around $18 billion annually,[22] while in Europe the corresponding figure is around €36 billion.[23] In the absence of a significant treatment impact on the global burden of fractures, these costs are set to increase twofold or more by 2050.

HIP FRACTURE

The incidence of hip fractures increases exponentially with age in both women and men,[24,25] with a female/male ratio of 2:1 to 3:1. Of all osteoporotic fractures, hip fractures have the greatest morbidity and mortality.[26,27] They almost always follow a fall, usually backwards or to the side, and require surgical treatment. Because hip fractures characteristically affect frail elderly people, postoperative morbidity and mortality are high. At 6 months after fracture, mortality rates of 12% to 20% have been reported, and only a minority of surviving patients with hip fracture regain their former level of independence, with up to one-third requiring institutionalized care.[28] Mortality after hip fracture is higher in men than in women and increases with increasing age.[29,30] The risk of death is highest immediately after the fracture has occurred and decreases gradually thereafter. Most deaths are related to existing comorbidities rather than a direct result of the fracture, reflecting the frailty of this population.

VERTEBRAL FRACTURE

Vertebral fractures are the most common of all osteoporotic fractures. The diagnosis of vertebral fracture is based on changes in vertebral shape on standard radiographs or images obtained by dual energy X-ray absorptiometry (DXA). There are several different approaches to the definition of vertebral fracture (see the article by Guglielmi and colleagues elsewhere in this issue for further exploration of this topic), but at present there is no universally adopted gold standard for their diagnosis. Estimates of prevalence and incidence are complicated further by the low proportion of vertebral fractures that come to medical attention (20% to 30%).[31]

Data from EVOS have demonstrated that the age standardized prevalence in the European population is 12.0% for women and 12.2% for men aged 50 to 79 years.[16] The similar prevalence in men and women likely reflects the higher risk of traumatic fractures in younger men; the gradient of increased prevalence with age is steeper in women than in men, with rates of 24% and 18% at age 75 to 79 years, respectively. Prospective data in a US population have shown an overall age-standardized incidence of 10.7 per 1000 person–years in women and 5.7 per person–years in men.[32]

Vertebral fractures may occur spontaneously or as a result of normal activities such as lifting, bending, and coughing. A minority of vertebral fractures (possibly around one third) present with acute and severe pain at the site of the fracture, often radiating around the thorax or abdomen. The natural history of this pain is variable; in general, there is a tendency for improvement with time, but resolution is often incomplete. Multiple vertebral fractures result in spinal deformity (kyphosis), height loss, and corresponding alterations in body shape with protuberance of the abdomen and loss of normal body contours. These changes commonly are associated with loss of self-confidence and self-esteem, difficulty with daily activities, and increased social isolation.[33–36] The clinical impact of vertebral fractures is thus substantial, although often underestimated.

Like hip fracture, vertebral fractures are associated with excess mortality mainly as a result of comorbidities. In contrast to hip fracture, however, mortality after vertebral fracture increases with increasing time from fracture. In a study of data from the UK General Practice Research Database, survival in women 12 months after vertebral fracture was 86.5% versus the expected 93.6%, with corresponding figures of 56.5% and 69.9% at 5 years.[37]

WRIST FRACTURE

Fractures of the distal forearm are four times more common in women than in men and show distinct differences in age-related changes in incidence in the two sexes, increasing linearly from age 40 to 65 years and then stabilizing in women and remaining constant in men between ages 20 and 80 years.[38]

Wrist fractures typically occur after a fall forwards onto the outstretched hand. They cause considerable inconvenience, usually requiring 4 to 6 weeks in plaster, and long-term adverse sequelae occur in up to one third of patients. These include pain, sympathetic algodystrophy, deformity, and functional impairment. Only a minority requires hospitalization.

OTHER NONVERTEBRAL FRACTURES

Fractures other than those at the spine, hip, and wrist make an important contribution to the overall morbidity associated with osteoporosis. These include fractures of the humerus, pelvis, ribs, clavicle, and lower leg.

PATHOGENESIS

Bone mass increases through childhood and adolescence, due mainly to increases in bone size. Peak bone mass is attained in the third decade of life, and age-related bone loss is believed to start in both men and women around the beginning of the fifth decade; thereafter bone loss continues throughout life.[39,40] In women, there is an acceleration of the rate of bone loss around the time of the menopause, the duration of which is poorly characterized but may be 5 to 10 years. Because women have a lower peak bone mass than men, lose bone more rapidly during the menopause, and live longer, they are at higher risk of fractures than men.

Bone mass in later life thus depends both on the peak bone mass achieved in early adulthood and on the rate of age-related bone loss. Genetic factors strongly influence peak bone mass, accounting for up to 70% to 80% of its variance.[41] Several genes are likely to be involved; these include the collagen type IA1 gene, a polymorphism of which is associated both with low BMD and fracture risk. Other genes that have been associated with increased risk of osteoporosis and fracture include the osteoprotegerin (OPG) and low-density lipoprotein receptor 5-related (LRP-5) genes.[42] Sex hormone status, nutrition, and physical activity also influence peak bone mass.

In postmenopausal women, estrogen deficiency is the main cause of menopausal bone loss. In older men, estrogen status also is significantly related to BMD levels, whereas the relationship between age-related bone loss and declining testosterone levels is less prominent.[43–45] In elderly patients, vitamin D insufficiency and secondary hyperparathyroidism are common and contribute to age-related bone loss, particularly in cortical bone.[46] Other potential pathogenetic factors include declining levels of physical activity and reduced serum levels of insulin-like growth factor.

ASSESSMENT OF FRACTURE RISK

The use of BMD measurements to predict future fracture risk has a high specificity but a low sensitivity, and most postmenopausal women presenting with a fragility fracture have a BMD T-score higher than -2.5.[47–51] Recently, the importance of clinical risk factors that affect fracture risk independently of BMD has been recognized. These are shown in **Table 1** and are used in the World Health Organization (WHO)-supported FRAX risk algorithm, with or without femoral neck BMD.[52,53] FRAX expresses fracture risk as the 10-year probability of hip fracture and of major osteoporotic fracture (hip, wrist, spine, or humerus), from which intervention thresholds can be derived. Country-specific versions of FRAX are available for several countries.

It should be noted that FRAX is designed only for postmenopausal women and men over the age of 40 who have not previously received bone-protective therapy. It uses only "yes" or "no" responses, and so does not take account of dose–responses for several risk factors including previous fracture, glucocorticoid therapy, and smoking. The weighting given to any previous fragility fracture is the same, and prior clinical vertebral fractures, which carry a higher risk than other previous fractures, are not considered separately.

Falls are not included in the algorithm. For all these reasons, it is important to exercise clinical judgment when using FRAX to assess fracture risk in clinical practice.

Other risk factors for fracture are mediated predominantly through reduction of BMD. These include untreated hypogonadism in men and in women (including aromatase inhibitor and androgen deprivation therapy),[54,55] gastrointestinal disease, chronic liver disease, hyperthyroidism,

Table 1 Risk factors for osteoporosis	
BMD-independent	**BMD-dependent**
Age	Untreated hypogonadism
Previous fragility fracture	Gastrointestinal disease
Maternal history of hip fracture	Endocrine disease
Oral glucocorticoid therapy	Chronic renal disease
Current smoking	Chronic liver disease
Alcohol intake ≥ 3 units/day	Chronic obstructive pulmonary disease
Rheumatoid arthritis	Immobility
BMI ≤ 19 kg/m^2	Drugs (eg, aromatase inhibitors, androgen deprivation therapy, proton pump inhibitors, selective serotonin reuptake inhibitors, thiazolidenediones)
Falls	

Abbreviations: BMD, bone mineral density; BMI, body mass index.

hyperparathyroidism, immobilization, chronic pulmonary disease, and chronic renal disease. Increased fracture risk also has been reported in association with several medications, including proton pump inhibitors, selective serotonin reuptake inhibitors, and thiazolidenediones.[56–60]

SUMMARY

Osteoporotic fractures are a major cause of morbidity and mortality in older people and impose a huge economic burden on health services. Age-related bone loss is a universal phenomenon and is related closely to estrogen deficiency, both in men and women; other pathogenetic factors include vitamin D insufficiency and reduced physical activity. Prediction of fracture risk using BMD measurements has high specificity but low sensitivity. Clinical risk factors for fracture that are to some extent independent of BMD enhance fracture risk prediction and are used with or without BMD in the WHO-supported fracture risk algorithm, FRAX, to generate 10-year probabilities of major osteoporotic and hip fractures.

REFERENCES

1. Consensus Development Conference: diagnosis, prophylaxis and treatment of osteoporosis. Am J Med 1993;941:645–50.
2. World Health Organization. Assessment of fracture risk and its application to screening for postmenopausal osteoporosis. Geneva (Switzerland): World Health Organization; 1994. Technical Report Series: 843.
3. Department of Health and Human Services. Bone health and osteoporosis: a report of the Surgeon General. Rockville (MD): Department of Health and Human Services; 2004.
4. Melton LJ 3rd. How many women have osteoporosis now? J Bone Miner Res 1995;10:175–7.
5. Cooper C, Melton LJ. Epidemiology of osteoporosis. Trends Endocrinol Metab 1992;314:224–9.
6. Kannus P, Palvanen M, Niemi S, et al. Increasing number and incidence of osteoporotic fractures of the proximal humerus in elderly people. BMJ 1996; 313:1051–2.
7. Kannus P, Niemi S, Parkkari J, et al. Hip fractures in Finland between 1970 and 1997 and predictions for the future. Lancet 1999;353:802–5.
8. Abrahamsen B, Vestergaard P. Declining incidence of hip fractures and the extent of use of antiosteoporotic therapy in Denmark 1997–2006. Osteoporos Int 2010;21:373–80.
9. Chevalley T, Guilley E, Herrmann FR, et al. Incidence of hip fracture over a 10-year period (1991–2000): reversal of a secular trend. Bone 2007;40:1284–9.
10. Melton 3rd LJ, Kearns AE, Atkinson EJ, et al. Secular trends in hip fracture incidence and recurrence. Osteoporos Int 2009;20:687–94.
11. Icks A, Haastert B, Wildner M, et al. Trend of hip fracture incidence in Germany 1995–2004: a population-based study. Osteoporos Int 2008;19: 1139–45.
12. Hagino H, Furukawa K, Fujiwara S, et al. Recent trends in the incidence and lifetime risk of hip fracture in Tottori, Japan. Osteoporos Int 2009;20:543–8.
13. Cooper C, Campion G, Melton LJ. Hip fractures in the elderly: a worldwide projection. Osteoporos Int 1992;2:285–9.
14. Johnell O, Gullberg B, Allander E, et al. The apparent incidence of hip fracture in Europe: a study of national register sources. MEDOS Study Group. Osteoporos Int 1992;2:298–302.

15. Elfors I, Allander E, Kanis JA, et al. The variable incidence of hip fracture in southern Europe: the MEDOS study. Osteoporos Int 1994;4:253–63.

16. O'Neill TW, Felsenberg D, Varlow J, et al. The prevalence of vertebral deformity in European men and women: the European Vertebral Osteoporosis Study. J Bone Miner Res 1996;11:1010–8.

17. Kanis JA, Johnell O, De Laet C, et al. A meta-analysis of previous fracture and subsequent fracture risk. Bone 2004;35:375–82.

18. Ross PD, Davis JW, Epstein RS, et al. Pre-existing fractures and bone mass predict vertebral fracture incidence in women. Ann Intern Med 1991;114:919–23.

19. Lindsay R, Silverman S, Cooper C, et al. Risk of new vertebral fracture in the year following a fracture. JAMA 2001;285:320–3.

20. Cuddihy MT, Gabriel SE, Crowson CS, et al. Forearm fractures as predictors of subsequent osteoporotic fractures. Osteoporos Int 1999;9:469–75.

21. Ismail AA, Cockerill W, Cooper C, et al. Prevalent vertebral deformity predicts incident hip though not distal forearm fracture: results from the European Prospective Osteoporosis Study (EPOS). Osteoporos Int 2001;12:85–90.

22. Burge R, Dawson-Hughes B, Solomon DH, et al. Incidence and economic burden of osteoporosis-related fractures in the United States, 2005–2025. J Bone Miner Res 2007;22:465–75.

23. Kanis JA, Johnell O. Requirements for DXA for the management of osteoporosis in Europe. Osteoporos Int 2005;16:229–38.

24. Jones G, Nguyen T, Sambrook PN, et al. Symptomatic fracture incidence in elderly men and women: the Dubbo Osteoporosis Epidemiology Study (DOES). Osteoporos Int 1994;4:277–82.

25. Baron JA, Karagas M, Barrett J, et al. Basic epidemiology of fractures of the upper and lower limb among Americans over 65 years of age. Epidemiology 1996;7:612–8.

26. Cauley JA, Thompson DE, Ensrud KC, et al. Risk of mortality following clinical fractures. Osteoporos Int 2000;11:556–61.

27. Center JR, Nguyen TV, Schneider D, et al. Mortality after all major types of osteoporotic fracture in men and women: an observational study. Lancet 1999;353:878–82.

28. Cooper C, Atkinson EJ, Jacobsen SJ, et al. Population-based study of survival after osteoporotic fractures. Am J Epidemiol 1993;137:1001–5.

29. Wehren LE, Hawkes WG, Orwig DL, et al. Gender differences in mortality after hip fracture: the role of infection. J Bone Miner Res 2003;18:2231–7.

30. Bliuc D, Nguyen ND, Milch VE, et al. Mortality risk associated with low-trauma osteoporotic fracture and subsequent fracture in men and women. JAMA 2009;301:513–21.

31. Melton LJ, Lane AW, Cooper C, et al. Prevalence and incidence of vertebral deformities. Osteoporos Int 1993;3:113–9.

32. Cooper C, Atkinson EJ, O'Fallon WM, et al. Incidence of clinically diagnosed vertebral fractures: a population-based study in Rochester, Minnesota, 1985–1989. J Bone Miner Res 1992;7:221–7.

33. Kanis JA, Johnell O, Oden A, et al. The risk and burden of vertebral fractures in Sweden. Osteoporos Int 2004;15:20–6.

34. Burger H, Van Daele PL, Grashuis K, et al. Vertebral deformities and functional impairment in men and women. J Bone Miner Res 1997;12:152–7.

35. Huang C, Ross PD, Wasnich RD. Vertebral fracture and other predictors of physical impairment and health care utilization. Arch Intern Med 1996;156:2469–75.

36. Nevitt MC, Ettinger B, Black DM, et al. The association of radiographically detected vertebral fractures with back pain and function: a prospective study. Ann Intern Med 1998;128:793–800.

37. Van Staa TP, Dennison EM, Leufkens HG, et al. Epidemiology of fractures in England and Wales. Bone 2001;29:517–22.

38. Owen RA, Melton LJ, Johnson KA, et al. Incidence of Colles' fracture in a North American community. Am J Public Health 1982;72:605–7.

39. Compston J. Sex steroids and bone. Physiol Rev 2001;81:419–47.

40. Parsons TJ, Prentice A, Smith EA, et al. Bone mineral mass consolidation in young British adults. J Bone Miner Res 1996;11:264–74.

41. Ralston SH. Genetics of osteoporosis. Proc Nutr Soc 2007;66:158–65.

42. Richards JB, Rivadeneira F, Inouye M, et al. Bone mineral density, osteoporosis, and osteoporotic fractures: a genome-wide association study. Lancet 2008;371:1505–12.

43. Khosla S, Amin S, Orwoll E. Osteoporosis in men. Endocr Rev 2008;29:441–64.

44. Amin S, Zhang Y, Felson DT, et al. Estradiol, testosterone, and the risk for hip fractures in elderly men from the Framingham Study. Am J Med 2006;119:426–33.

45. Szulc P, Munoz F, Claustrat B, et al. Bioavailable estradiol may be an important determinant of osteoporosis in men: the MINOS study. J Clin Endocrinol Metab 2001;86:192–9.

46. Parfitt AM, Gallagher JC, Heaney RP, et al. Vitamin D and bone health in the elderly. Am J Clin Nutr 1982;36(Suppl 5):1014–31.

47. Siris ES, Miller PD, Barrett-Connor E, et al. Identification and fracture outcomes of undiagnosed low bone mineral density in postmenopausal women. Results from the National Osteoporosis Risk Assessment. JAMA 2001;286:2815–22.

48. Schuit SC, van der Klift M, Weel AE, et al. Fracture incidence and association with bone mineral density

in elderly men and women: the Rotterdam Study. Bone 2004;34:195–202.

49. Wainwright SA, Marshall LM, Ensrud KE, et al. Hip fracture in women without osteoporosis. J Clin Endocrinol Metab 2005;90:2787–93.

50. Sornay-Rendu E, Munoz F, Garnero P, et al. Identification of osteopenic women at high risk of fracture: The OFELY Study. J Bone Miner Res 2005;20:1813–9.

51. Pascoe JA, Seeman E, Henry MJ, et al. The population burden of fractures originates in women with osteopenia, not osteoporosis. Osteoporos Int 2006;17:1404–9.

52. Kanis JA, Oden A, Johnell O, et al. The use of clinical risk factors enhances the performance of BMD in the prediction of hip and osteoporotic fractures in men and women. Osteoporos Int 2007;18:1033–46.

53. Kanis JA, World Health Organization Scientific Group. Assessment of osteoporosis at the primary health care level. Technical Report. Sheffield (UK): WHO Collaborating Centre. UK: University of Sheffield; 2008.

54. McCloskey E. Effects of third-generation aromatase inhibitors on bone. Eur J Cancer 2006;42:1044–51.

55. Smith MR, Boyce SP, Moyneur E, et al. Risk of clinical fractures after gonadotrophin-releasing hormone agonist therapy for prostate cancer. J Urol 2006;175:136–9.

56. Yu EW, Shinoff C, Blackwell T, et al. Use of acid-suppressive medications and risk of bone loss and fracture in postmenopausal women. J Bone Miner Res 2006;21(Suppl 1):S281.

57. Yang Y-X, Lewis JD, Epstein S, et al. Long-term proton pump inhibitor therapy and risk of hip fracture. JAMA 2006;296:2947–53.

58. Haney EM, Chan BK, Diem SJ, et al. Association of low bone mineral density with selective serotonin reuptake inhibitors in older men. Arch Intern Med 2007;167:1246–51.

59. Schwartz AV, Sellmeyer DE, Vittinghoff E, et al. Thiazolidinedione use and bone loss in older diabetic adults. J Clin Endocrinol Metab 2006;91:3276–8.

60. Grey A, Bolland M, Gamble G, et al. The peroxisome proliferator-activated receptor gamma agonist rosiglitazone decreases bone formation and bone mineral density in healthy postmenopausal women: a randomised controlled trial. J Clin Endocrinol Metab 2007;92:1305–10.

Physiology of Bone Loss

Bart L. Clarke, MD[a,*], Sundeep Khosla, MD[b]

KEYWORDS

- Osteoporosis • Osteopenia • Bone loss
- Bone density • Aging • Fractures

Significant bone loss occurs with normal aging in both women and men.[1] Development of osteoporosis, usually in old age, is the natural consequence of age-related bone loss if left untreated. Multiple population-based cross-sectional and longitudinal studies over the last 25 years using areal bone mineral density (aBMD) assessed by dual energy x-ray absorptiometry (DXA) have helped define the general pattern of bone loss with normal aging (Fig. 1). Both sexes lose aBMD at relatively slow rates starting at around age 40, with women losing aBMD more rapidly than men with onset of menopause in their late 40s or early 50s. Postmenopausal women lose trabecular BMD rapidly in their vertebrae, pelvis, and ultradistal wrist. There is less rapid cortical bone loss in the long bones and vertebrae after the menopause. About 8 to 10 years after menopause, slower age-related bone loss becomes prominent, and continues for the rest of life. Men, who do not experience sudden loss of gonadal sex steroid secretion, do not experience accelerated bone loss in their early 50s, as seen in women, but have slower age-related bone loss throughout their adult life past about age 40.

However, because DXA BMD is not able to differentiate changes occurring in trabecular and cortical bone with age, and because DXA BMD cannot assess age-related changes in bone geometry and/or size, more recent studies have used quantitative computed tomography (QCT) scanning[2] to assess bone loss in greater detail. Both peripheral and central QCT, with new image analysis software,[3] have been used to better define the age-related changes in bone volumetric density, geometry, and structure at multiple skeletal sites.

Riggs and colleagues[2] reported large decreases in lumbar spine volumetric BMD (vBMD) with normal aging in a cross-sectional study of men and women aged 20 to 97 years in Rochester, Minnesota, predominantly due to vertebral trabecular bone loss beginning in the third decade. The decrease in lumbar spine vBMD was larger in women than men (55% vs 45%, $P<.001$). The rate of bone loss appeared to increase in middle age in women, accounting for the greater decrease in vBMD seen with aging in women compared with men (Fig. 2). Assessment of changes in radial cortical vBMD at the wrist showed that cortical bone loss did not begin until middle age in either women or men. After middle age, there were linear decreases in cortical vBMD in both women and men, but the decreases were greater in women than men (28% vs 18%, $P<.001$). Normal aging was associated with increases in cross-sectional area at the femoral neck and radius because of continued periosteal apposition with normal aging. The bone marrow space increased more rapidly than cross-sectional area due to continued endosteal bone resorption. Because the rate of periosteal apposition was slower than the rate of endosteal resorption, cortical area and thickness decreased with aging. However, because periosteal apposition increased bone diameter, the ability of bone to resist biomechanical forces increased, partially

This work was supported by Grants AG004875 and AR027065 from the National Institutes of Health.
[a] Division of Endocrinology, Diabetes, Metabolism, and Nutrition, Mayo Clinic College of Medicine, Mayo Clinic, W18-A, 200 1st Street Southwest, Rochester, MN 55905, USA
[b] Endocrine Research Unit, Division of Endocrinology, Diabetes, Metabolism, and Nutrition, Mayo Clinic College of Medicine, Mayo Clinic, Guggenheim 7, 200 1st Street Southwest, Rochester, MN 55905, USA
* Corresponding author.
E-mail address: Clarke.Bart@Mayo.edu

Radiol Clin N Am 48 (2010) 483–495
doi:10.1016/j.rcl.2010.02.014
0033-8389/10/$ – see front matter © 2010 Elsevier Inc. All rights reserved.

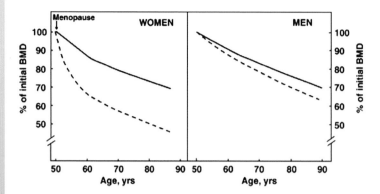

Fig. 1. Patterns of age-related bone loss in women and men. Dashed lines represent trabecular bone and solid lines, cortical bone. The figure is based on multiple cross-sectional and longitudinal studies using DXA. (*From* Khosla S, Riggs BL. Pathophysiology of age-related bone loss and osteoporosis. Endocrinol Metab Clin N Am 2005;34(4):1017; with permission.)

offsetting the decrease in bone strength resulting from decreased cortical area.

Khosla and colleagues[4] subsequently showed that the structural basis for bone loss in the ultra-distal radius with aging is different between men and women. Men have thicker trabeculae in young adulthood, and sustain primarily trabecular thinning without a net change in trabecular number or spacing, whereas women lose trabecular number and have increased trabecular spacing. These changes result in less microstructural damage with aging in men than women, which likely explains the lack of increase in wrist fractures seen in men. Khosla and colleagues[5] then demonstrated that in young men, the apparent conversion of thick trabeculae into more numerous, thinner trabeculae is most closely associated with declining insulin-like growth factor (IGF)-1 levels. By contrast, sex steroids were the major hormonal determinants of trabecular microstructure in elderly men and women. In a subsequent study, Riggs and colleagues[6] showed that the

late onset of cortical bone loss is temporally associated with sex steroid deficiency. However, the early-onset, substantial trabecular bone loss in both sexes during sex steroid sufficiency is unexplained, and indicates that current paradigms on the pathogenesis of osteoporosis are incomplete.

These studies showed that these age-related changes in bone density and structure correlated with the observed increased fracture risk seen in this population in both women and men. Previous studies had shown that distal forearm (Colles') fractures increase rapidly in women after menopause, and then remain constant from about 10 to 15 years after menopause until the end of life (Fig. 3). In contrast, vertebral fractures increase more slowly after menopause, but continue to increase exponentially during later life. Hip fractures in women increase more slowly than vertebral fractures after menopause, but continue to increase throughout life, and increase rapidly in later life. In men, however, distal forearm fractures do not appear to increase with normal aging,

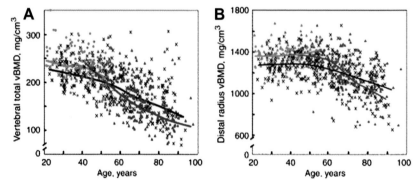

Fig. 2. (A) Values for vBMD (mg/cm³) of the total vertebral body in a population sample of Rochester, Minnesota, women and men between the ages of 20 and 97 years. Individual values and smoother lines are given for premenopausal women in red, for postmenopausal women in blue, and for men in black. (B) Values for cortical vBMD at the distal radius in the same cohort, with color code as in (A). All changes with age were significant (P<.05). (*From* Riggs BL, Melton LJ 3rd, Robb RA, et al. A population-based study of age and sex differences in bone volumetric density, size, geometry, and structure at different skeletal sites. J Bone Miner Res 2004;19(12):1950; with permission.)

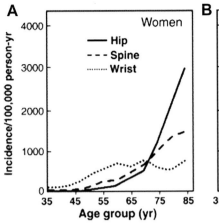

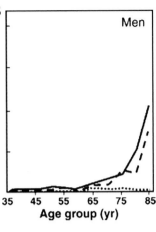

Fig. 3. Age-specific incidence rates for proximal femur (hip), vertebral (spine), and distal forearm (wrist) fractures in Rochester, Minnesota, women (*A*) and men (*B*). (*Adapted from* Cooper C, Melton LJ. Epidemiology of osteoporosis. Trends Endocrinol Metab 1992;3(6):225; with permission.)

probably due to their larger bone size. Vertebral and hip fractures increase gradually with aging in men, beginning about a decade later compared with women, likely due to their lack of significant gonadal steroid deficiency later in life.

Based on these and other studies, it is estimated that 40% of Caucasian women aged 50 years or older will develop a vertebral, hip, or wrist fracture sometime during the remainder of their lives, and that this risk increases to about 50% if nonclinical vertebral fractures detected by radiological imaging are included in the estimate.[7] It is estimated that about 13% of Caucasian men will sustain similar fractures. The risk of these fractures is somewhat lower in non-Caucasian women and men. It is estimated that osteoporotic fractures cost the United States between $12.2 and $17.9 billion each year, as measured in 2002 dollars.[8]

PATHOPHYSIOLOGY OF AGE-RELATED BONE LOSS IN WOMEN
Accelerated Postmenopausal Bone Loss Due to Gonadal Sex Steroid Deficiency

Menopause is associated with onset of rapid bone loss in most women, thought to be caused by decreased ovarian function, leading to decreased estrogen secretion. This rapid bone loss can be prevented by estrogen or hormone replacement.[9,10] During the menopause transition, serum 17β-estradiol levels decrease by 85% to 90% from the mean premenopausal level, and serum estrone levels decrease by 65% to 75% from premenopausal levels.[11] Serum estrone has one-fourth the biologic effect of serum 17β-estradiol. Serum testosterone also decreases following menopause, but to a lesser extent, because testosterone continues to be produced by the adrenal cortex and interstitial cells in the ovary.[12] Khosla and colleagues[13] showed that there may be

a threshold level of serum bioavailable (non-sex hormone binding globulin [SHBG]-bound) estradiol in postmenopausal women below 11 pg/mL, at which trabecular bone loss occurs, whereas a threshold level below 3 pg/mL for bioavailable estradiol leads to cortical bone loss. Some longitudinal clinical studies show that increased bone turnover in perimenopausal women correlates with elevated serum follicle-stimulating hormone (FSH), as well as serum estradiol.[14] The perimenopausal increase in FSH is due to a selective decrease in ovarian inhibin B (InhB). Decreases in inhibin levels across the menopause transition are associated with increasing bone turnover, independent of changes in sex steroids or FSH.[14]

Bone resorption increases by 90% after menopause, as assessed by markers of bone resorption, whereas bone formation also increases, but only by 45% as assessed by markers of bone formation.[15] The difference between bone resorption and formation favors greater bone resorption, which leads to accelerated bone loss during the first 8 to 10 years after menopause. Increased bone resorption leads to an efflux of calcium from the skeleton into the extracellular pool, but compensatory increased renal calcium excretion,[16] decreased intestinal calcium absorption,[17] and partially suppressed parathyroid hormone (PTH) secretion[18] prevent development of hypercalcemia.

The cellular and molecular mechanisms by which estrogen deficiency leads to bone loss are increasingly well understood (**Fig. 4**). Estrogen deficiency increases receptor activator of nuclear factor κB ligand (RANKL),[19] leading to increased osteoclast recruitment and activation and decreased osteoclast apoptosis. RANKL is the final key molecule required for osteoclast development, and is normally expressed by bone marrow stromal/osteoblast precursor cells, T

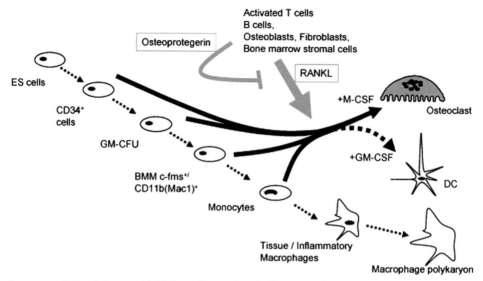

Fig. 4. Summary of stimulatory and inhibitory factors involved in osteoclast development and apoptosis. BMM, bone marrow derived macrophages; ES cells, embryonic stem cells; GM-CFU, granulocyte macrophage colony-forming unit; GM-CSF, granulocyte macrophage colony stimulating factor; M-CSF, macrophage colony stimulating factor; RANKL, receptor activator of nuclear factor κkappa B ligand. (*From* Quinn JMW, Saleh H. Modulation of osteoclast function in bone by the immune system. Mol Cell Endocrinol 2009;310(1–2):42; with permission.)

lymphocytes, and B lymphocytes.[20,21] RANKL binds to its receptor RANK on osteoclast lineage cells,[22] and is neutralized in the bone microenvironment by its soluble decoy receptor osteoprotegerin (OPG), which is produced and secreted by osteoblast lineage cells.[23] Combined in vitro and in vivo studies have shown that estrogen normally suppresses RANKL production by osteoblastic cells and T and B lymphocytes,[20,21] and increases OPG production by osteoblastic cells,[24,25] so that estrogen deficiency leads to an alteration in the RANKL/OPG ratio that favors bone resorption.

Estrogen also modulates production of additional cytokines by bone marrow stromal mononuclear cells and osteoblasts, thereby controlling osteoclast activity by paracrine action.[25] Estrogen is thought to suppress production of bone-resorbing cytokines such as interleukin (IL)-1, IL-6, tumor necrosis factor (TNF)-α, macrophage colony-stimulating factor (M-CSF), and prostaglandins by the appropriate cells.[26] Estrogen-deficient model systems have shown that increased IL-1 and M-CSF levels[27,28] can be reduced by specific antagonists to these molecules.[29–32] The bone-resorptive activity of TNF-α is able to be inhibited by soluble type I TNF receptor.[33] Estrogen deficiency is associated with increased IL-6 levels.[34,35] In vivo, however, it is likely that estrogen suppresses production and activity of multiple cytokines in premenopausal women that would otherwise act cooperatively to cause bone loss. With estrogen deficiency, each cytokine likely accounts for only part of cytokine-mediated age-related bone loss. It is not yet clear that there is a dominant cytokine contributing to estrogen deficiency–associated bone loss.

Estrogen normally also increases the production of transforming growth factor (TGF)-β by osteoblast precursor cells.[36] TGF-β induces apoptosis of osteoclasts.[37] Estrogen also directly stimulates apoptosis of osteoclast precursor cells, and decreases osteoclast precursor differentiation by blocking RANKL/M-CSF-induced activator protein-1–dependent transcription by reducing c-jun activity.[38,39] C-jun activity is reduced by decreasing c-jun transcription and decreasing phosphorylation. Estrogen is also capable of inhibiting the activity of mature osteoclasts by direct, receptor-mediated mechanisms.[40]

Loss of these multiple estrogen-induced restraining actions on osteoclast bone resorption leads to upregulation of rapid bone loss shortly after onset of menopause. The rapid phase of bone loss is sustained for 8 to 10 years before gradually subsiding. Why rapid bone loss gradually subsides after this duration is not yet clear, but it may be that estrogen deficiency alters biomechanical sensing of skeletal mechanical loading by osteocytes within the bone.[41] It is hypothesized that for a given level of skeletal mechanical loading during estrogen deficiency, bone mass is sensed as being excessive by the osteocytes, which then signal the osteoclasts to resorb more bone and/or the osteoblasts to form less bone, leading to net rapid bone loss. Once enough bone is lost, however, it is thought that the proportionately increased skeletal mechanical loading on remaining bone is sufficient to limit further rapid bone loss.

Age-Related Bone Loss Due to Secondary Hyperparathyroidism

While gonadal steroid deficiency may be a major cause for postmenopausal bone loss, other important factors also play a role. During the rapid phase of early postmenopausal bone loss, there is mild suppression of PTH secretion, but during the slower phase of later postmenopausal bone loss there is gradually increasing PTH secretion, with corresponding increasing markers of bone resorption. The increases in serum PTH and markers of bone turnover correlate with each other. Transient suppression of PTH secretion by an intravenous 24-hour calcium infusion in younger premenopausal and elderly postmenopausal women is associated with suppression of markers of bone turnover, strongly suggesting that increased serum PTH was the proximate cause of the increased bone turnover.[42]

The reason for gradually increasing levels of PTH secretion with age is likely multifactorial. Vitamin D deficiency is common in postmenopausal women,[43] and is associated with increased serum PTH levels. Long-standing estrogen deficiency also leads to chronic negative calcium balance because of loss of estrogen effects increasing intestinal calcium absorption[16,44] and renal tubular calcium reabsorption.[45,46] Unless these changes leading to negative calcium balance are compensated for with adequate calcium supplementation, secondary hyperparathyroidism inevitably develops, leading to age-related bone loss.

Bone Loss Due to Decreased Bone Formation

Postmenopausal and age-related bone loss is caused not just by accelerated bone resorption but also by decreased bone formation. Decreased bone formation has generally been attributed to decreased paracrine production of growth factors,[47] and/or decreased growth hormone (GH)[48,49] and IGF-1 levels.[50–52] If estrogen directly stimulates bone formation, estrogen deficiency may also directly result in bone loss. Impaired bone formation is detectable in early menopause.[53] Estrogen increases production of IGF-1,[54] TGF-β,[36] and procollagen synthesis by osteoblast precursor cells in vitro,[54] and increases osteoblast life span by decreasing osteoblast apoptosis.[55,56] Khastgir and colleagues[57]

provided direct evidence that estrogen can stimulate bone formation after cessation of skeletal growth by evaluating iliac crest bone biopsies from 22 elderly women of mean age 65 years before, and 6 years after, percutaneous administration of high doses of estrogen. These investigators found that cancellous bone volume increased by 61%, and trabecular wall thickness by 12%. Tobias and Compston[58] reported similar results. It is not yet clear whether these results are due to the pharmacologic doses of estrogen used, or augmentation of physiologic effects that are normally not of sufficient magnitude to detect. Accumulating data implicate estrogen deficiency as a contributing cause of decreased bone formation with aging, but there is not yet a clear consensus on whether estrogen directly stimulates osteoblast function, and if it does, what the relative magnitude of increased proliferation or decreased apoptosis are.

PATHOPHYSIOLOGY OF AGE-RELATED BONE LOSS IN MEN
Age-Related Bone Loss Due to Gonadal Steroid Deficiency

Although osteoporosis more commonly affects women, men lose about half as much bone with aging as women, and suffer one-third the number of fragility fractures as women.[59,60] Because most men do not develop overt hypogonadism with normal aging, it was thought for many years that gonadal sex steroid deficiency was less significant a cause of bone loss in men than in women. However, multiple studies over the last decade have shown that lack of apparent age-related gonadal sex steroid deficiency in men is due to the doubling of SHBG with aging in men,[61,62] with consequent near-preservation of serum total testosterone and estradiol, but decreased bioavailable and free gonadal sex steroid levels. Serum sex steroids are bound predominantly to circulating albumin or SHBG, but a small fraction circulates in free form. It is estimated that 35% to 55% of circulating testosterone and estradiol is loosely bound to albumin, 42% to 64% circulates bound to SHBG, and that 1% to 3% circulates in free form.[63] Because SHBG binds to testosterone and estradiol with high avidity, this form of gonadal sex steroid is not generally available to diffuse into target tissue cells from the circulation, bind to sex steroid receptors, and exert sex steroid action. The fraction of circulating testosterone and estradiol bound to albumin or circulating free represents bioavailable testosterone and estradiol capable of interacting with sex steroid receptors in target tissues.

A variety of methods have been used to assess serum bioavailable testosterone and estradiol, and multiple groups have reported decreased serum free or bioavailable sex steroids with aging.[64–66] Khosla and colleagues[61] showed in a cross-sectional study of 346 men from age 23 to 90 years in Rochester, Minnesota, that bioavailable testosterone decreased by 64% and bioavailable estrogen by 47%, and that SHBG increased by 124%, luteinizing hormone (LH) by 285%, and FSH by 505% (**Table 1**). Similar data were recently reported from men in the MrOS Study in Sweden.[67] The proximate cause for the increase in SHBG in men, and the failure of the hypothalamic-pituitary-gonadal axis to compensate for decreased circulating bioavailable sex steroids in men are not yet clear, and remain under investigation.[68]

For many years it was assumed that decreased serum testosterone was responsible for age-related bone loss in men, because it has traditionally been viewed as the dominant gonadal steroid in men. However, several cross-sectional observational studies that correlated serum sex steroid levels to BMD at various skeletal sites reported that bone loss in aging men correlated better with serum estradiol than testosterone. The earliest study to report this finding, by Slemenda and colleagues,[65] found correlation coefficients between serum total estradiol and BMD at different skeletal sites ranging from +0.21 to +0.35 ($P = .01$–.05), with inverse correlation coefficients between serum total testosterone and

BMD at various skeletal sites ranging from −0.21 to −0.28 ($P = .03$–.10). Several other cross-sectional studies subsequently confirmed these findings in other male population samples, with positive correlations between serum total or bioavailable estradiol and BMD.[66,67,69–73]

These studies strongly suggested that estrogen deficiency plays the dominant role in age-related bone loss in men as well as women. However, the cross-sectional nature of these studies did not allow discrimination of the effect of estradiol on peak bone density from the effect on preservation or prevention of bone loss with normal aging. Men with low BMD and low estradiol levels may have had low estradiol levels for much or all of their lives, and this would likely have caused low BMD due to decreased acquisition of peak bone density, as well as more rapid bone loss with aging. In addition, correlation studies can never prove causality.

To assess the effect of estrogen deficiency on bone loss in men, Khosla and colleagues[73] evaluated rates of bone loss at different skeletal sites longitudinally over 4 years in young men aged 22 to 39 years, and older men aged 60 to 90 years. Study of these 2 populations allowed separation of the effects of gonadal sex steroids on men reaching peak bone density, from the effects on age-related bone loss. Forearm BMD assessment provided the clearest data, perhaps because of the greater precision of measurement at this site, compared with the lumbar spine and hip sites. In the younger men, forearm BMD increased by 0.42% to 0.43% per year, whereas forearm BMD decreased in the older men by 0.49% to 0.66% each year. The rates of BMD change at the wrist site correlated better with serum bioavailable estradiol levels than serum bioavailable testosterone levels (**Table 2**). Further analysis suggested that there was a serum bioavailable estradiol threshold of 11 pg/mL (40 pmol/L), below which the rate of BMD loss correlated with estradiol. Above this threshold, there was no correlation between rate of bone loss and serum estradiol (**Fig. 5**). The threshold level corresponded to the median serum bioavailable estrogen level in these men, with the corresponding serum total estradiol level of 31 pg/mL, which is near the middle of the normal range for estradiol of 10 to 50 pg/mL in these men. Similar findings were reported by Gennari and colleagues[74] in a cohort of elderly Italian men, with men with serum free estradiol levels below the median for the group losing lumbar spine and femoral neck BMD over 4 years, and men with serum free estradiol levels

Table 1
Changes in serum sex steroids and gonadotropins over life in a random sample of 346 men (Rochester, Minnesota) aged 23 to 90 years

Hormone	Percent Change[a]
Bioavailable estrogen	−47
Bioavailable testosterone	−64
Sex hormone binding globulin	+124
Luteinizing hormone	+285
Follicle-stimulating hormone	+505

[a] $P<.005$.

Data from Khosla S, Melton LJ 3rd, Atkinson EJ, et al. Relationship of serum sex steroid levels and bone turnover markers with bone mineral density in men and women: a key role for bioavailable estrogen. J Clin Endocrinol Metab 1998;83(7):2268; with permission.

Table 2
Spearman correlation coefficients relating rates of change in bone mineral density at the radius and ulna to serum sex steroid levels among a sample of men (Rochester, Minnesota) stratified by age

Spearman Correlation Coefficients	Young		Middle-aged		Elderly	
	Radius	Ulna	Radius	Ulna	Radius	Ulna
T	−0.02	−0.19	−0.18	−0.25[a]	0.13	0.14
E2	0.33[b]	0.22[a]	0.03	0.07	0.21[a]	0.18[a]
E1	0.35[c]	0.34[b]	0.17	0.23[a]	0.16	0.14
Bio T	0.13	−0.04	0.07	0.01	0.23[b]	0.27[b]
Bio E2	0.30[b]	0.20	0.14	0.21[a]	0.29[b]	0.33[c]

Abbreviations: Bio, bioavailable; E1, estrone; E2, estradiol; T, testosterone.
[a] $P<.05$.
[b] $P<.01$.
[c] $P<.001$.
Data from Khosla S, Melton LJ 3rd, Atkinson EJ, et al. Relationship of serum sex steroid levels to longitudinal changes in bone density in young versus elderly men. J Clin Endocrinol Metab 2001;86(8):3558; with permission.

above the median maintaining their BMD at these sites.

Although these cross-sectional studies helped establish that serum estrogen levels are associated with BMD in men, they could not prove that estrogen deficiency was the primary cause of bone loss in aging men. A pivotal experiment giving strong support for estrogen deficiency being more important than testosterone deficiency in causation of bone loss in aging men was performed by Falahati-Nini and colleagues[75] The investigators treated 59 normal elderly men of mean age 68 years with a long-acting gonadotropin-releasing hormone (GnRH) agonist to suppress GnRH, LH, and FSH secretion, and an aromatase inhibitor to block peripheral conversion of testosterone to estrogen, for 3 weeks. Physiologic estrogen and testosterone levels were maintained during suppression of LH and FSH secretion and aromatase blockade by placing the men on estrogen and testosterone patches that mimicked circulating estrogen and testosterone levels for age. After baseline assessment at 3 weeks of the bone resorption markers urinary deoxypyridinoline and NTx-telopeptide, and bone formation markers osteocalcin and P1NP, the

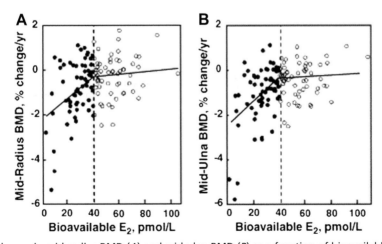

Fig. 5. Rate of change in mid-radius BMD (A) and mid-ulna BMD (B) as a function of bioavailable estradiol levels in elderly men. Model R^2 values were 0.20 and 0.25 for the radius and ulna, respectively, both less than 0.001 for comparison with a one-slope model. Solid circles correspond to subjects with bioavailable estradiol levels less than 40 pmol/L (11 pg/mL) and open circles those with values more than 40 pmol/L. (From Khosla S, Melton LJ 3rd, Atkinson EJ, et al. Relationship of serum sex steroid levels to longitudinal changes in bone density in young versus elderly men. J Clin Endocrinol Metab 2001;86(8);3558; with permission.)

men were randomized to 1 of 4 treatment groups for 3 further weeks. Men in group A (−T, −E) discontinued both their testosterone and estrogen patches; those in Group B (−T, +E) discontinued their testosterone patch but continued their estrogen patch; those in Group C (+T, −E) continued their testosterone patch but discontinued their estrogen patch; and men in Group D (+T, +E) continued both patches. Because GnRH agonist and aromatase inhibitor treatment was maintained during the 3 weeks of patch therapy, the investigators were able to independently assess the effects of testosterone and estrogen on bone metabolism in the men.

The study showed that men in Group A, without either testosterone or estrogen replacement, had significant increases in both markers of bone resorption, whereas these increases were completely blocked in men in Group D, with both testosterone and estrogen replacement (Fig. 6). Men in Group B, who received estrogen but not testosterone, had minimal increases in bone resorption markers, whereas men in Group C, who received testosterone but not estrogen, had significant increases in bone resorption markers. Using a 2-factor analysis of variance (ANOVA) model, the effects of estrogen on urinary deoxypyridinoline and NTx-telopeptide excretion were highly significant (P = .005 and .0002, respectively). Estrogen accounted for more than 70% of the total effect of sex steroids on bone resorption in the men, whereas testosterone accounted for no more than 30% of the effect.

Gonadal steroid-deficient men in Group A had reduced bone formation marker levels, whereas

men in Group D, given combination testosterone and estrogen treatment, maintained normal bone formation markers. Men in Groups B and C, given either testosterone or estrogen treatment, maintained their levels of osteocalcin, which is a marker of function of mature osteoblasts and osteocytes[76] (ANOVA, P = .002 and .013, respectively). Men in Groups B and C maintained their levels of P1NP, representing type I collagen synthesis throughout the various stages of osteoblast differentiation, only with estrogen, but not testosterone (ANOVA, P = .0001).

Leder and colleagues[77] used a slightly different trial design to confirm an independent effect of testosterone on bone resorption, but the cumulative data to date suggest a more prominent role of estrogen in preventing bone resorption in men. Similar findings were reported by Taxel and colleagues[78] in a study of 15 elderly men treated with an aromatase inhibitor for 9 weeks. Suppression of estrogen production caused significant increases in bone resorption markers and suppression of bone formation markers. In another study, Sanyal and colleagues[79] showed that the effects of estrogen on bone in older men were independent of changes in FSH.

The data from these various investigations show that estrogen plays an important and dominant role in bone metabolism in the skeleton of aging men. It therefore appears that decreasing bioavailable estrogen levels in men play a significant role in mediating age-related bone loss in men, similar to women.[80] Declining testosterone levels also play a role, however, because testosterone has antiresorptive effects and is important for maintaining

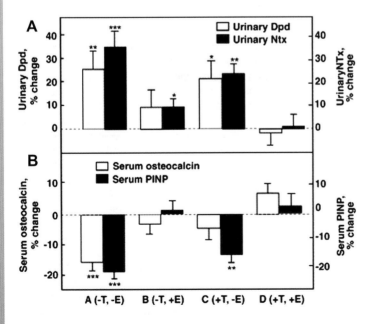

Fig. 6. Percent changes in (A) bone resorption markers (urinary deoxypyridinoline [Dpd] and N-telopeptide of type I collagen [Ntx]) and (B) bone formation markers (serum osteocalcin and N-terminal extension peptide of type I collagen [P1NP]) in a group of elderly men (mean age 68 years) made acutely hypogonadal and treated with an aromatase inhibitor (Group A), treated with estrogen alone (Group B), treated with testosterone alone (Group C), or both (Group D). Significance for change from baseline: *P<.05; **P<.01; ***P<.001. (Adapted from Falahati-Nini A, Riggs BL, Atkinson EJ, et al. Relative contributions of testosterone and estrogen in regulating bone resorption and formation in normal elderly men. J Clin Invest 2000;106(12);1556-7; with permission.)

bone formation. Testosterone also is the substrate for aromatase, which converts testosterone to estrogen. Testosterone has been shown to increase periosteal apposition in bone, at least in rodents.[81] Testosterone also likely contributes to reduced fracture risk in men because of its influence on increasing bone size in men during growth and development.

Age-Related Bone Loss Due to Secondary Hyperparathyroidism

PTH secretion also increases in aging men, similar to what is seen in aging women.[18,59,60] Because higher circulating gonadal sex steroid levels in aging men may help protect against bone resorption promoted by increased PTH levels, it has been more difficult to demonstrate a direct role for PTH in causation of age-related bone loss in men.[82]

FACTORS CONTRIBUTING TO AGE-RELATED BONE LOSS IN BOTH SEXES

Age-related bone loss may be driven primarily by gonadal sex steroid deficiency and physiologic secondary hyperparathyroidism, but multiple other factors also contribute to this process. Vitamin D deficiency, widely prevalent in postmenopausal women with osteoporosis, and common among children and adults without osteoporosis in many countries around the world, worsens age-related physiologic secondary hyperparathyroidism.[43] Age-related decreased bone formation may be due in part to sex steroid deficiency, but other sex steroid–independent factors likely contribute to decreased bone formation. Age-related decreases in production of growth factors necessary for osteoblast differentiation and function most likely contribute to decreased bone formation. The age-related decrease in amplitude and frequency of GH production by the pituitary leads to decreased liver production of IGF-1.[49] IGF-1 levels decrease markedly with age, and IGF-2 levels also decrease, but less rapidly.[50,51] Decreased systemic and local skeletal production of IGF-1 and -2 likely contribute to decreased bone formation with aging. Growth factor binding proteins may also play a role in regulation of age-related bone loss. Amin and colleagues[83] showed that higher serum IGF binding protein (IGFBP)-2 predicts lower BMD, and is associated with increased markers of bone resorption independent of age, body mass, and sex hormones. The association between IGFBP-2 and markers of bone formation may reflect coupling with increased bone resorption, which is not adequate to maintain BMD.

Other changes in endocrine function with aging likely also contribute to the physiology of bone loss. The less potent adrenal androgens dehydroepiandrosterone (DHEA) and DHEA-sulfate both decrease by about 80% with aging, with much of the decrease occurring in young adults,[84] whereas cortisol secretion remains relatively constant throughout life. The decrease in adrenal androgens early in adult life may therefore change the ratio of adrenal catabolic/anabolic hormone activity. This change may contribute to younger adult trabecular bone loss.

Leptin secreted by adipocytes has been demonstrated in mice and humans to regulate bone remodeling through studies of loss-of-function mutations of this hormone or of its receptor. It has been assumed, but not formally demonstrated, that this regulation occurs through neuronal means, possibly via the sympathetic nervous system. It has been difficult to dissociate the influence leptin exerts on appetite and energy expenditure from this function. Shi and colleagues[85] recently showed that deletion of the leptin receptor in mouse neurons results in increased bone formation and bone resorption, resulting in high bone density as seen in leptin-deficient mice. In contrast, osteoblast-specific leptin receptor deletion did not influence bone remodeling. These findings established that leptin regulates bone mass accrual in vivo by acting through neuronal means, and provided a direct demonstration that leptin functions to regulate bone remodeling independently of its regulation of energy metabolism.

Recent studies have demonstrated an important role for circulating serotonin in regulating bone mass in rodents.[86] In addition, patients treated with selective serotonin reuptake inhibitors (SSRIs) have reduced aBMD. The potential physiologic role of serotonin in regulating bone mass in humans remains unclear. Mödder and colleagues[87] measured serum serotonin levels in a population-based sample of 275 women and related these to total body and spine aBMD assessed by DXA, femur neck total and trabecular vBMD, and vertebral trabecular vBMD assessed by QCT, and bone microstructural parameters at the distal radius assessed by high-resolution peripheral QCT. Serotonin levels were inversely associated with body and spine aBMD (age-adjusted $R = -0.17$ and -0.16, $P<.01$, respectively), and with femoral neck total and trabecular vBMD (age-adjusted $R = -0.17$ and -0.25, $P<.01$ and $<.001$, respectively), but not lumbar spine vBMD. Bone volume/tissue volume, trabecular number, and trabecular thickness at the radius were inversely associated with serotonin levels (age-adjusted

$R = -0.16$, -0.16, and -0.14, $P<.05$, respectively). Serotonin levels were also inversely associated with body mass index (BMI [weight in kilograms divided by height in meters squared]; age-adjusted $R = -0.23$, $P<.001$). Multivariable models showed that serotonin levels remained significant negative predictors of femur neck total and trabecular vBMD, as well as trabecular thickness at the radius, after adjusting for age and BMI. Collectively, these data provide support for a physiologic role for circulating serotonin in regulating bone mass in humans.

Lower peak bone density at 25 to 35 years of age also contributes to risk of osteoporosis and fractures later in life. Individuals with lower peak bone density for whatever cause will develop low bone density or osteoporosis sooner than those with higher peak bone density, assuming the rate of bone loss is equivalent as they age.[88]

It has been suggested that bone strength is homeostatically adapted to habitual skeletal loading conditions and that bone loss could, therefore, result simply from age-related reductions in physical activity and muscle mass. In a stratified random sample of women and men 21 to 97 years old in Rochester, Minnesota, Melton and colleagues[89] estimated indices of bone strength, flexural rigidity, and axial rigidity from central QCT measurements at the femoral neck and lumbar spine, and peripheral QCT measurements at the ultradistal radius. Habitual skeletal loading was assessed using lean body mass, total skeletal muscle mass, body weight, and physical activity. This study showed that there was not a close correspondence between changes in habitual load and changes in bone strength, nor any consistent pattern. Moreover, interindividual variation in the strength-to-load ratios was substantial. These data suggest that the hypothesis that reduced skeletal loading is the primary basis for age-related bone loss may be oversimplified.

Numerous sporadic secondary causes of bone loss play a role in age-related bone loss by various mechanisms. It is estimated that about 40% of women and 20% of men have an identifiable sporadic cause of bone loss,[90] such as glucocorticoid therapy, subtle or clinically evident malabsorption, anorexia nervosa, idiopathic hypercalciuria, or behavioral factors such as excess alcohol intake, cigarette smoking, high-caffeine or high-sodium diet, or physical inactivity.

Age-related bone loss and sarcopenia proceed in parallel. It has been suggested that age-related muscle loss is the main factor causing age-related bone loss.[91,92] Although not yet proven, it is likely that age-related muscle loss, causing decreased muscle loading on the skeleton, contributes significantly to age-related bone loss.

SUMMARY

Age-related bone loss in women and men is caused in large part by gonadal sex steroid deficiency and physiologic secondary hyperparathyroidism. Other factors also play key roles, including vitamin D deficiency, intrinsic defects in osteoblast function, impairment of the GH/IGF axis, reduced peak bone mass, age-associated sarcopenia, and various sporadic secondary causes. Further understanding of the relative contributions of each of these factors to age-related bone loss and fracture risk will lead to improved preventive and therapeutic approaches for osteoporosis.

REFERENCES

1. Riggs BL, Khosla S, Melton LJ. Sex steroids and the construction and conservation of the adult skeleton. Endocr Rev 2002;23(3):279–302.
2. Riggs BL, Melton LJ III, Robb RA, et al. A population-based study of age and sex differences in bone volumetric density, size, geometry and structure at different skeletal sites. J Bone Miner Res 2004;19(12):1945–54.
3. Hanson DP, Robb RA, Aharon S, et al. New software toolkits for comprehensive visualization and analysis of three-dimensional multimodal biomedical images. J Digit Imaging 1997;10(3 Suppl 1):229–30.
4. Khosla S, Riggs BL, Atkinson EJ, et al. Effects of sex and age on bone microstructure at the ultradistal radius: a population-based noninvasive in vivo assessment. J Bone Miner Res 2006;21(1):124–31.
5. Khosla S, Melton LJ 3rd, Achenbach SJ, et al. Hormonal and biochemical determinants of trabecular microstructure at the ultradistal radius in women and men. J Clin Endocrinol Metab 2006;91(3):885–91.
6. Riggs BL, Melton LJ, Robb RA, et al. A population-based assessment of rates of bone loss at multiple skeletal sites: evidence for substantial trabecular bone loss in young adult women and men. J Bone Miner Res 2008;23(2):205–14.
7. Cummings SR, Melton LJ. Epidemiology and outcomes of osteoporotic fractures. Lancet 2002; 359(9319):1761–7.
8. Tosteson AN, Hammond CS. Quality of life assessment in osteoporosis: health-status and preference-based measures. Pharmacogenomics 2002; 20(5):289–303.
9. Lindsay R, Aitken JM, Anderson JB, et al. Long-term prevention of postmenopausal osteoporosis by oestrogen: evidence for an increased bone mass after

delayed onset of oestrogen treatment. Lancet 1976; 1(7968):1038–41.

10. Genant HK, Cann CE, Ettinger B, et al. Quantitative computed tomography of vertebral spongiosa: a sensitive method for detecting early bone loss after oophorectomy. Ann Intern Med 1982;97(5):699–705.

11. Khosla SK, Atkinson EJ, Melton LJ III, et al. Effects of age and estrogen status on serum parathyroid hormone levels and biochemical markers of bone turnover in women: a population-based study. J Clin Endocrinol Metab 1997;82(5):1522–7.

12. Horton R, Romanoff E, Walker J. Androstenedione and testosterone in ovarian venous and peripheral plasma during ovariectomy for breast cancer. J Clin Endocrinol Metab 1966;26(11):1267–9.

13. Khosla S, Riggs BL, Robb RA, et al. Relationship of volumetric bone density and structural parameters at different skeletal sites to sex steroid levels in women. J Clin Endocrinol Metab 2005;90(9):5096–103.

14. Perrien DS, Achenbach SJ, Bledsoe SE, et al. Bone turnover across the menopause transition: correlations with inhibins and follicle-stimulating hormone. J Clin Endocrinol Metab 2006;91(5):1848–54.

15. Garnero P, Sornay-Rendu E, Chapuy M, et al. Increased bone turnover in late postmenopausal women is a major determinant of osteoporosis. J Bone Miner Res 1996;11(3):337–49.

16. Young MM, Nordin BE. Calcium metabolism and the menopause. Proc R Soc Med 1967;60(11 Part 1): 1137–8.

17. Gennari C, Agnusdei D, Nardi P, et al. Estrogen preserves a normal intestinal responsiveness to 1,25-dihydroxyvitamin D3 in oophorectomized women. J Clin Endocrinol Metab 1990;71(5):1288–93.

18. Riggs BL, Khosla S, Melton LJ. A unitary model for involutional osteoporosis: estrogen deficiency causes both type I and type II osteoporosis in post-menopausal women and contributes to bone loss in aging men. J Bone Miner Res 1998;13(5):763–73.

19. Lacey DL, Timms E, Tan HL, et al. Osteoprotegerin ligand is a cytokine that regulates osteoclast differentiation and activation. Cell 1998;93(2):165–76.

20. Eghbali-Fatourechi G, Khosla S, Sanyal A, et al. Role of RANK ligand in mediating increased bone resorption in early postmenopausal women. J Clin Invest 2003;111(8):1221–30.

21. Clowes JA, Riggs BL, Khosla S. The role of the immune system in the pathophysiology of osteoporosis. Immunol Rev 2005;208(12):207–27.

22. Hsu H, Lacey DL, Dunstan CR, et al. Tumor necrosis factor receptor family member RANK mediates osteoclast differentiation and activation induced by osteoprotegerin ligand. Proc Natl Acad Sci U S A 1999;96(7):3540–5.

23. Simonet WS, Lacey DL, Dunstan CR, et al. Osteoprotegerin: a novel secreted protein involved in the regulation of bone density. Cell 1997;89(2):309–19.

24. Hofbauer LC, Khosla S, Dunstan CR, et al. Estrogen stimulates gene expression and protein production of osteoprotegerin in human osteoblastic cells. J Clin Endocrinol Metab 1999;140(9):4367–70.

25. Khosla S, Atkinson EJ, Dunstan CR, et al. Effect of estrogen versus testosterone on circulating osteoprotegerin and other cytokine levels in normal elderly men. J Clin Endocrinol Metab 2002;87(4):1550–4.

26. Charatcharoenwitthaya N, Khosla S, Atkinson EJ, et al. Effect of blockade of TNF-alpha and interleukin-1 action on bone resorption in early postmenopausal women. J Bone Miner Res 2007; 22(5):724–9.

27. Manolagas SC, Jilka RL. Bone marrow, cytokines, and bone remodeling: emerging insights into the pathophysiology of osteoporosis. N Engl J Med 1995;332(5):305–11.

28. Pacifici R, Brown C, Puscheck E, et al. Effect of surgical menopause and estrogen replacement on cytokine release from human blood mononuclear cells. Proc Natl Acad Sci U S A 1991; 88(12):5134–88.

29. Tanaka S, Takahashi N, Udagawa N, et al. Macrophage colony-stimulating factor is indispensable for both proliferation and differentiation of osteoclast progenitors. J Clin Invest 1993;91(1):257–63.

30. Kimble RB, Vannice JL, Bloedow DC, et al. Interleukin-1 receptor antagonist decreased bone loss and bone resorption in ovariectomized rats. J Clin Invest 1994;93(5):1959–67.

31. Ammann P, Rizzoli R, Bonjour J, et al. Transgenic mice expressing soluble tumor necrosis factor-receptor are protected against bone loss caused by estrogen deficiency. J Clin Invest 1997;99(7): 1699–703.

32. Kimble RB, Srivastava S, Ross FP, et al. Estrogen deficiency increases the ability of stromal cells to support murine osteoclastogenesis via an interleukin-1- and tumor necrosis factor-mediated stimulation of macrophage colony-stimulating factor production. J Biol Chem 1996;271(46):28890–7.

33. Kitazawa R, Kimble RB, Vannice JL, et al. Interleukin-1 receptor antagonist and tumor necrosis factor binding protein decrease osteoclast formation and bone resorption in ovariectomized mice. J Clin Invest 1994;94(6):2397–406.

34. Girasole G, Jilka RL, Passeri G, et al. 17 beta-estradiol inhibits interleukin-6 production by bone marrow-derived stromal cells and osteoblasts in vitro: a potential mechanism for the antiosteoporotic effect of estrogens. J Clin Invest 1992;89(3):883–91.

35. Jilka RL, Hangoc G, Girasole G, et al. Increased osteoclast development after estrogen loss: mediation by interleukin-6. Science 1992;257(5066):88–91.

36. Oursler MJ, Cortese C, Keeting PE, et al. Modulation of transforming growth factor-beta production in normal human osteoblast-like cells by 17

beta-estradiol and parathyroid hormone. Endocrinology 1991;129(6):3313–20.

37. Hughes DE, Dai A, Tiffee JC, et al. Estrogen promotes apoptosis of murine osteoclasts mediated by TGF-beta. Nat Med 1996;2(10):1132–6.

38. Shevde NK, Bendixon AC, Dienger KM, et al. Estrogens suppress RANK ligand-induced osteoclast differentiation via a stromal cell independent mechanism involving c-Jun repression. Proc Natl Acad Sci U S A 2000;97(14):7829–34.

39. Srivastava S, Toraldo G, Weitzmann MN, et al. Estrogen decreases osteoclast formation by down-regulating receptor activator of NF-κB ligand (RANKL)-induced JNK activation. J Biol Chem 2001;276(12):8836–40.

40. Oursler MJ, Pederson L, Fitzpatrick LA, et al. Human giant cell tumors of the bone (osteoclastomas) are estrogen target cells. Proc Natl Acad Sci U S A 1994;91(12):5227–31.

41. Frost HM. On the estrogen-bone relationship and postmenopausal bone loss: a new model. J Bone Miner Res 1999;14(9):1473–7.

42. Ledger GA, Burritt MF, Kao PC, et al. Role of parathyroid hormone in mediating nocturnal and age-related increases in bone resorption. J Clin Endocrinol Metab 1995;80(11):3304–10.

43. Holick MF. Vitamin D deficiency. N Engl J Med 2007; 357(3):266–81.

44. Gallagher JC, Riggs BL, DeLuca HF. Effect of estrogen on calcium absorption and serum vitamin D metabolites in postmenopausal osteoporosis. J Clin Endocrinol Metab 1980;51(6):1359–64.

45. Nordin BE, Need AG, Morris HA, et al. Evidence for a renal calcium leak in postmenopausal women. J Clin Endocrinol Metab 1991;72(2):401–7.

46. McKane WR, Khosla S, Burritt MF, et al. Mechanism of renal calcium conservation with estrogen replacement therapy in women in early postmenopause—a clinical research center study. J Clin Endocrinol Metab 1995;80(12):3458–64.

47. Marie PJ, Hott M, Launay JM, et al. In vitro production of cytokines by bone surface-derived osteoblastic cells in normal and osteoporotic postmenopausal women: relationship with cell proliferation. J Clin Endocrinol Metab 1993;77(3):824–30.

48. Giustina A, Veldhuis JD. Pathophysiology of the neuroregulation of growth hormone secretion in experimental animals and the human. Endocr Rev 1998; 19(6):717–97.

49. Ho KY, Evans WS, Blizzard WM, et al. Effects of sex and age on the 24-hour profile of growth hormone secretion in man: importance of endogenous estradiol concentrations. J Clin Endocrinol Metab 1987; 64(1):51–8.

50. Bennett AE, Wahner HW, Riggs BL, et al. Insulin-like growth factors I and II, aging and bone density in women. J Clin Endocrinol Metab 1984;59(4):701–4.

51. Boonen S, Mohan S, Dequeker J, et al. Down-regulation of the serum stimulatory components of the insulin-like growth factor (IGF) system (IGF-I, IGF-II, IGF binding protein [BP]-3, and IGFBP-5) in age-related (type II) femoral neck osteoporosis. J Bone Miner Res 1999;14(12):2150–8.

52. Pfeilschifter J, Diel I, Kloppinger T, et al. Concentrations of insulin-like growth factor (IGF)-I, -II, and IGF binding protein-4 and -5 in human bone cell conditioned medium did not change with age. Mech Ageing Dev 2000;117(1–3):109–14.

53. Heaney RP, Recker RR, Saville PD. Menopausal changes in calcium balance performance. J Lab Clin Med 1978;92(6):953–63.

54. Ernst M, Heath JK, Rodan GA. Estradiol effects on proliferation, messenger ribonucleic acid for collagen and insulin-like growth factor-I, and parathyroid hormone-stimulated adenylate cyclase activity in osteoblastic cells from calvariae and long bones. Endocrinology 1989;125(2):825–33.

55. Manolagas SC. Birth and death of bone cells: basic regulatory mechanisms and implications for the pathogenesis and treatment of osteoporosis. Endocr Rev 2000;21(2):115–37.

56. Gohel A, McCarthy MB, Gronowicz G. Estrogen prevents glucocorticoid-induced apoptosis in osteoblasts in vivo and in vitro. Endocrinology 1999; 140(11):5339–47.

57. Khastgir G, Studd J, Holland N, et al. Anabolic effect of estrogen replacement on bone in postmenopausal women with osteoporosis: histomorphometric evidence in a longitudinal study. J Clin Endocrinol Metab 2001;86(1):289–95.

58. Tobias JH, Compston JE. Does estrogen stimulate osteoblast function in postmenopausal women? Bone 1999;24(2):121–4.

59. Khosla S, Amin S, Orwoll E. Osteoporosis in men. Endocr Rev 2008;29(4):441–64.

60. Khosla S. Update in male osteoporosis. J Clin Endocrinol Metab 2010;95(1):3–10.

61. Khosla S, Melton LJ, Atkinson EJ, et al. Relationship of serum sex steroid levels and bone turnover markers with bone mineral density in men and women: a key role for bioavailable estrogen. J Clin Endocrinol Metab 1998;83(7):2266–74.

62. Khosla S. Editorial: sex hormone binding globulin: inhibitor or facilitator (or both) of sex steroid action? J Clin Endocrinol Metab 2006;91(12):4764–6.

63. Clarke BL, Khosla S. Androgens and bone. Steroids 2009;74(3):296–305.

64. Greendale GA, Edelstein S, Barrett-Connor E. Endogenous sex steroids and bone mineral density in older women and men: the Rancho Bernardo study. J Bone Miner Res 1997;12(11): 1833–43.

65. Slemenda CW, Longcope C, Zhou L, et al. Sex steroids and bone mass in older men: positive associations

with serum estrogens and negative associations with androgens. J Clin Invest 1997;100(7):1755–9.

66. Khosla S, Amin S, Singh RJ, et al. Comparison of sex steroid measurements in men by immunoassay versus mass spectroscopy and relationships with cortical and trabecular volumetric bone mineral density. Osteoporos Int 2008;19(10):1465–71.

67. Mellström D, Vandenput L, Mallmin H, et al. Older men with low serum estradiol and high serum SHBG have an increased risk of fractures. J Bone Miner Res 2008;23(10):1552–60.

68. Center JR, Nguyen TV, Sambrook PN, et al. Hormonal and biochemical parameters in the determination of osteoporosis in elderly men. J Clin Endocrinol Metab 1999;84(10):3626–35.

69. Ongphiphadhanakul B, Rajatanavin R, Chanprasertyothin S, et al. Serum oestradiol and oestrogen-receptor gene polymorphism are associated with bone mineral density independently of serum testosterone in normal males. Clin Endocrinol (Oxf) 1998;49(6):803–9.

70. ven den Beld AW, de Jong FH, Grobbee DE, et al. Measures of bioavailable serum testosterone and estradiol and their relationships with muscle strength, bone density, and body composition in elderly men. J Clin Endocrinol Metab 2000;85(9):3276–82.

71. Amin S, Zhang Y, Sawin CT, et al. Association of hypogonadism and estradiol levels with bone mineral density in elderly men in the Framingham study. Ann Intern Med 2000;133(12):951–63.

72. Szulc P, Munoz F, Claustrat B, et al. Bioavailable estradiol may be an important determinant of osteoporosis in men: the MINOS study. J Clin Endocrinol Metab 2001;86(1):192–9.

73. Khosla S, Melton LJ, Atkinson EJ, et al. Relationship of serum sex steroid levels to longitudinal changes in bone density in young versus elderly men. J Clin Endocrinol Metab 2001;86(8):3556–61.

74. Gennari L, Merlotti D, Martini G, et al. Longitudinal association between sex hormone levels, bone loss, and bone turnover in elderly men. J Clin Endocrinol Metab 2003;88(11):5327–33.

75. Falahati-Nini A, Riggs BL, Atkinson EJ, et al. Relative contributions of testosterone and estrogen in regulating bone resorption and formation in normal elderly men. J Clin Invest 2000;106(12):1553–60.

76. Krause C, de Gorter DJJ, Karperian M, et al. Signal transduction cascades controlling osteoblast differentiation. Primer on the metabolic bone diseases and disorders of mineral metabolism. American Society for Bone and Mineral Research: Washington, DC; 2008. p.10–5.

77. Leder BZ, LeBlanc KM, Schoenfeld DA, et al. Differential effects of androgens and estrogens on bone turnover in normal men. J Clin Endocrinol Metab 2003;88(1):204–10.

78. Taxel P, Kennedy DG, Fall PM, et al. The effect of aromatase inhibition on sex steroids, gonadotropins, and markers of bone turnover in older men. J Clin Endocrinol Metab 2001;86(6):2869–74.

79. Sanyal A, Hoey KA, Mödder UI, et al. Regulation of bone turnover by sex steroids in men. J Bone Miner Res 2008;23(5):705–14.

80. Gennari L, Khosla S, Bilezikian JP. Estrogen and fracture risk in men. J Bone Miner Res 2008; 23(10):1548–51.

81. Turner RT, Wakley GK, Hannon KS. Differential effects of androgens on cortical bone histomorphometry in gonadectomized male and female rats. J Orthop Res 1990;8(4):612–7.

82. Kennel KA, Riggs BL, Achenbach SJ, et al. Role of parathyroid hormone in mediating age-related changes in bone resorption in men. Osteoporos Int 2003;14(8):631–6.

83. Amin S, Riggs BL, Melton LJ 3rd, et al. High serum IGFBP-2 is predictive of increased bone turnover in aging men and women. J Bone Miner Res 2007; 22(6):799–807.

84. Labrie F, Belanger A, Cusan L, et al. Marked decline in serum concentrations of adrenal C19 sex steroid precursors and conjugated androgen metabolites during aging. J Clin Endocrinol Metab 1997;82(8): 2396–402.

85. Shi Y, Yadav VK, Suda N, et al. Dissociation of the neuronal regulation of bone mass and energy metabolism by leptin in vivo. Proc Natl Acad Sci U S A 2008;105(51):20529–33.

86. Yadav VK, Oury F, Suda N, et al. A serotonin-dependent mechanism explains the leptin regulation of bone mass, appetite, and energy expenditure. Cell 2009;138(5):976–89.

87. Mödder UI, Achenbach SJ, Amin S, et al. Relation of serum serotonin levels to bone density and structural parameters in women. J Bone Miner Res 2010;25(2):415–22.

88. Seeman E. From density to structure: growing up and growing old on the surfaces of bone. J Bone Miner Res 1997;12(4):509–21.

89. Melton LJ 3rd, Riggs BL, Achenbach SJ, et al. Does reduced skeletal loading account for age-related bone loss? J Bone Miner Res 2006; 21(12):1847–55.

90. Riggs BL, Melton LJ. Medical progress series: involutional osteoporosis. N Engl J Med 1986;314(26): 1676–86.

91. Frost HM. On age-related bone loss: insights from a new paradigm. J Bone Miner Res 1997;12(10): 1539–46.

92. Frost HM. Why the ISMNI and the Utah paradigm? Their role in skeletal and extraskeletal disorders. J Musculoskelet Neuronal Interact 2000;1(1):5–9.

Radiology of Osteoporosis

Gopinathan Anil, MD, FRCR[a], Giuseppe Guglielmi, MD[b,c],
Wilfred C.G. Peh, MD, FRCPG, FRCPE, FRCR[d,e],*

KEYWORDS

- Osteopenia • Osteoporosis • Metabolic bone disorder
- Conventional radiographs

Osteoporosis is a systemic skeletal disease characterized by low bone mass and microarchitectural deterioration of osseous tissue, with consequent increase in bone fragility and susceptibility to fracture.[1] This definition clearly states the systemic nature of the disease, and emphasizes the loss of bone mass and deterioration of its structural integrity as the primary abnormalities. In 1994, the World Health Organization (WHO) provided an objective definition for osteoporosis based on the epidemiologic data from a study on postmenopausal Caucasian women that showed high fracture prevalence when the bone mineral density was lower than 2.5 standard deviations (SD) of normal peak bone mass.[2] This definition used the bone mineral density (BMD) expressed in terms of the T-score, that is, the number of the SDs of the measured BMD from the mean BMD in young adult women. According to the WHO Study Group, the general diagnostic categories are:

- Normal: BMD not more than 1 SD below the young adult mean (T-score above −1)
- Osteopenia (or low bone mass): BMD between 1 and 2.5 SD below young adult mean (T-score between −1 and −2.5)
- Osteoporosis: BMD 2.5 SD or more below the young adult mean (T-score at or below −2.5)
- Severe osteoporosis (or established osteoporosis): BMD 2.5 SD or more below the young adult mean in the presence of one or more fragility fractures.

The same criteria are used for men as well as non-Caucasian women, because no other consensus definition is available. In addition to T-scores, many BMD reports include Z-scores, which represent the number of SDs of the measurement from age-matched mean BMD.

BASIC CONSIDERATIONS

Osteoporosis is the most common metabolic disease of bone.[3,4] Although early references of similar conditions are found in the publications of Sir Astley Cooper,[5] it was Pommer in 1885 who introduced the term "osteoporosis".[6] The term "osteopenia" is more nonspecific and descriptive, merely referring to rarefaction of the skeleton as seen on radiographs (**Table 1**).

The bone mineral and osseous tissue represents a dynamic milieu, with approximately 25% of the serum calcium exchanging with calcium salts in the bone each minute. The annual bone turnover rate is 5% to 10% in normal individuals.[7] Bone densitometric studies have shown that osteoporosis is a result of prolonged, slow bone loss and that the pattern of loss is different for trabecular and cortical bone.[8] In postmenopausal women, the annual remodeling rate is 25% for trabecular bone and 3% for cortical bone.[9] Hence, osteopenia is naturally more obvious in the axial skeleton and ends of long bone where trabecular bone is abundant. The structurally insufficient osteoporotic bone is predisposed to fractures.[3,10] The

[a] Department of Radiology, Changi General Hospital, 2 Simei Street 3, Singapore 529889
[b] Department of Radiology, University of Foggia, Viale L. Pinto, 71100 Foggia, Italy
[c] Scientific Institute 'Casa Sollievo della Sofferenza' Hospital, San Giovanni Rotondo 71013, Italy
[d] Yong Loo Lin School of Medicine, National University of Singapore, Singapore
[e] Department of Diagnostic Radiology, Alexandra Hospital, 378 Alexandra Road, Singapore 159964
* Corresponding author. Department of Diagnostic Radiology, Alexandra Hospital, 378 Alexandra Road, Singapore 159964.
E-mail address: wilfred.peh@gmail.com

Radiol Clin N Am 48 (2010) 497–518
doi:10.1016/j.rcl.2010.02.016
0033-8389/10/$ – see front matter © 2010 Elsevier Inc. All rights reserved.

Table 1
Causes of osteopenia

Restricted	Generalized
Regional	Primary
Migratory osteoporosis	Involutional osteoporosis
Transient osteoporosis	Juvenile osteoporosis
Sudeck dystrophy	Osteogenesis imperfecta
Neuromuscular disorders	
Localized	Secondary
Infection	Chronic disease
Inflammatory arthritis	Endocrine pathologies
Neoplastic conditions	Marrow replacement disorders
	Miscellaneous: alcohol, drugs, etc

cancellous bone fractures the most, with spine being the most frequently affected site.[11] Among the clinically manifest osteoporotic fractures, distal radius leads the list, followed by hip, spine, and proximal humerus.[12,13]

CLASSIFICATION

There is no singular, accepted classification for osteoporosis. Some of the commonly used systems are described here.

I. Osteoporosis may be classified according to the disease distribution into:
   Generalized osteoporosis. The bone density is decreased in the majority of the skeleton, especially the axial components and ends of long bones; this is usually secondary to old age or postmenopausal loss of hormonal support. This group of patients generally belongs to the WHO definition of osteoporosis. Juvenile osteoporosis and congenital diseases such as osteogenesis imperfecta are rarer causes for generalized osteoporosis.
   Regional osteoporosis. The loss of bone density is confined to a region or segment of the body, for example, an entire limb. Disuse atrophy following prolonged immobilization or disuse as well as Sudeck reflex sympathetic dystrophy are classic examples of such regional osteoporosis.

Localized osteoporosis. The loss of bone density is restricted to focal regions of bone, as seen with infections and inflammatory arthritis.

II. According to the cause, osteoporosis may be classified as:
   Primary or secondary osteoporosis. Traditionally osteoporosis with no secondary cause, for example, endocrine disease, chronic illness, drug therapy (eg, heparin, eptoin), are delegated into the broad category of primary osteoporosis. Senile involutional and postmenopausal osteoporosis belongs to this category of primary osteoporosis. This system excludes diseases that need more specific management.
   Idiopathic osteoporosis.[14–16] This rare entity has been described in middle-aged men; it is associated with rapid bone turnover and is often transient with reversal in few years. Different theories like increased secretion of interleukin-1 from monocytes and a disorder of pulsatile parathyroid hormone (PTH) secretion are described, with little conclusive evidence.
   Juvenile osteoporosis.[17] Juvenile idiopathic osteoporosis (JIO) is characterized by prepubertal onset and spontaneous remission with progression of puberty. There is no gender predilection. The bone formation is normal. An increase in osteoclastic activity is presumably responsible for this condition. There is generalized osteopenia with normal bone quality. Vertebral collapse and metaphyseal fractures of long bones are common. The onset is often acute with an aggressive early course. Meticulous investigation to exclude acute leukemia and lymphoma is essential, before making a diagnosis of juvenile osteoporosis.

III. Riggs and colleagues[18,19] classified osteoporosis into 2 subtypes (also popular as Mayo Clinic Classification):
   Type 1 osteoporosis is seen predominantly in postmenopausal women (M:F = 8:1) in the age group of 55 to 65 years; it affects 10% of women during the first 20 years of menopause. The cancellous bone is predominantly affected, and patients usually present with vertebral and wrist fractures. The bone loss in these patients is clearly in excess of that from aging alone.
   Type 2 osteoporosis is seen in old age (often older than 75 years) with decreased bone

turnover and impaired bone formation. Almost half of elderly women and one-fourth of men are victims to this condition. The cortical and trabecular bone is involved proportionately, and usually manifests as hip or vertebral fractures. This form of osteoporosis is associated with a type of secondary hyperparathyroidism whereby the absorption of vitamin D from the gut is decreased. Oral supplementation of calcium and vitamin D can decrease the chances of hip and nonvertebral fractures in this group.[20]

MAGNITUDE OF THE PROBLEM

Osteoporosis affects approximately 75 million people in the United States, Europe, and Japan.[21] Thirty percent of postmenopausal Caucasian women in the United States have osteoporosis at the hip, lumbar spine, or mid-radius, and a further 54% have osteopenia at these sites.[22] Nearly 75% of hip, spine, and distal forearm fractures occur among patients 65 years or older and are presumably of osteoporotic nature.[23] The lifetime risk of osteoporotic fractures is estimated to be around 40%, which is very close to the risk of cardiovascular disease.[24] In white women, the lifetime risk of osteoporotic hip fracture is greater than that of breast carcinoma (1:6 vs 1:9).[25] In Europe, the disability due to osteoporosis is greater than that caused by cancers (with the exception of lung cancer) and is comparable to that from combined effects of a variety of chronic noncommunicable diseases, such as rheumatoid arthritis, asthma, and high blood pressure–related heart disease.[26] In women older than 45 years, osteoporosis accounts for more days spent in hospital than many other diseases, including diabetes, myocardial infarction, and breast cancer.[27] In the Americas and Europe, osteoporotic fractures account for 2.8 million disability-adjusted life years (DALYs) annually, somewhat more than accounted for by hypertension and diabetes mellitus; collectively osteoporosis accounts for 1% of the DALYs attributable to noncommunicable disease.[27,28] The economic impact of this disease is tremendous, as osteoporotic fractures alone cost the United States around $17.9 billion per annum and the United Kingdom around £1.7 billion per annum.[29]

PATHOPHYSIOLOGY

The material composition and structure of the bone is such that it serves 2 contradictory needs, namely, stiffness with flexibility, and lightness with strength.[30] Bone fabric is woven at sub-microscopic and macroscopic levels into an architectural masterpiece of biomechanical engineering—with an optimal mass adapted in size, shape, and architecture for structural strength.[31] The structure undergoes constant modeling and remodeling to maintain the strength and contribute to calcium homeostasis. Bone resorption is a natural process that enables excavation of the marrow cavity and fashions the cortical and trabecular bone during the growth phase, while removing damaged bone in adults. However, for restitution of structure, the volume of bone removed should be replaced by an equal volume of new bone. Osteoporosis is an outcome of disturbances in this balance that is normally regulated by a complex interplay of vitamin D, parathormone, and several other humoral factors. In osteoporosis, the bone tissue per unit volume is less than normal; there are no biochemical changes, but histologically the bone trabeculae and cortex are thinner. The bone mineral makeup is still normal, unlike in osteomalacia or rickets where the bone mineral content is abnormal and hence, the bones are brittle.[3,32]

RISK FACTORS

Age and gender constitute the 2 primary risk factors. The risk of osteoporosis is 10 times greater in a woman in her 80s than one in her 50s, and out of the approximately 10 million osteoporotic persons in the United States, 8 million are women.[9] Total bone mass increases about 50-fold between birth and maturity. The attainment of peak bone mass is typically complete by 35 to 40 years. A lower peak bone density predisposes to osteoporosis.[33] Among postmenopausal women, a low body mass index is an independent risk factor for osteoporosis.[34] A previous fracture is another independent risk factor suggesting that an existing defect in the bony architecture makes a bone more susceptible to fracture again.[35] Twenty percent of the women with an incidental vertebral fracture suffer from a second fracture in the subsequent year.[36] Old age-related muscle wasting and loss of strength, diabetic neuropathy, various joint disorders, and other painful conditions make elderly individuals easy victims for falls and subsequent osteoporotic fractures. The list of risk factors also includes endocrine disease (eg, hypogonadism, hypercorticolism, and hyperthyroidism), alcoholism, cigarette smoking and use of tobacco, physical inactivity and sedentary lifestyle, renal failure, nutritional deficiency, fragility fractures in first-degree relatives, and medications (eg, lithium, heparin, phenobarbitol, immunosuppressants).[37–39] A routine medication such as proton pump inhibitors also can interfere with calcium absorption and predispose to osteoporotic fractures.[40] Similarly, post renal transplant patients have 17 to 34 times greater risk for fragility fractures.[41]

DIAGNOSIS OF OSTEOPOROSIS

Diagnosis of osteoporosis can be made by 3 methods, namely:

1. Bone biopsy. As a diagnostic procedure the use of bone biopsy is restricted to atypical, unclear, and complicated cases for obtaining evidence-based guidelines on diagnosis and treatment. More often, it is done to exclude marrow replacement diseases as the cause of osteoporosis. Histomorphometric analysis of osseous tissue obtained from iliac crest biopsy enables accurate calculation of cellular activity and bone mineral content.[42,43]
2. Biochemical markers, which are mostly markers of bone turnover. Elevated levels of bone turnover markers are associated with future fragility fractures as seen in most prospective studies in postmenopausal women, even when controlled for BMD.[44] The biochemical markers of osteoporosis includes serum β C-telopeptide of type 1 collagen, urinary N-telopeptide of type 1 collagen, N-terminal propeptide of type 1 collagen, bone-specific alkaline phosphatase, circulating osteocalcein, and urine hydroxyproline.[45,46] The concordance between the biochemical markers and bone histomorphometry findings is not very high.[47]
3. Imaging. Of all the 3 diagnostic methods, imaging-based techniques are more practically useful. Various imaging-based techniques, such as conventional radiography, single- and dual-energy x-ray absorptiometry (DXA), morphometry, quantitative computed tomography (QCT), quantitative ultrasound, and high-resolution magnetic resonance imaging (MRI) with virtual biopsy, are available for the evaluation of osteoporosis.

CONVENTIONAL RADIOGRAPHS AND OSTEOPOROSIS

The basic purpose of all the imaging studies is early detection of osteoporosis, to initiate timely therapy and avoid osteoporotic fractures. This approach is essential in the context of osteoporosis because there is a strong sense of denial of personal risk (especially among postmenopausal women), lack of dialog with doctors, restricted access to diagnosis and treatment before the first fracture, and tendency among medical professionals to neglect early evidence of osteoporosis.[48–50] Clinically silent osteoporotic fractures are grossly underdiagnosed during routine radiology reporting, with false-negative interpretation rates as high as about 45% in North America, 46% in Latin America, and 29% in Europe/South Africa/Australia.[48] In such a scenario, the foreboding signs of impending fracture often reflected first on a radiograph are critical to identify and report on. Radiographs are often required in conjunction with other studies like nuclear imaging, DXA, or MRI to confirm complications like fracture or background abnormalities, for example, severe osteoarthritis. Unfortunately, radiographs have low sensitivity to changes of osteoporosis[51] and irrespective of the cause, their appearances are the same. Notwithstanding this limitation, it has to be acknowledged that the abnormalities seen on radiographs closely correlate with pathologic changes in the bone. Radiographs may sometimes hold the key to the cause of generalized bone loss and fragility fractures; for example, association with subperiosteal resorption is typical for hyperparathyroidism, while exuberant callus formation around the fracture is strongly suggestive of Cushing disease.[52] The principal findings of osteoporosis, as seen on a radiograph, are (a) increased radiolucency, (b) cortical thinning, (c) altered trabecular pattern, and (d) fractures and deformities.

Increased Radiolucency

The increase in the radiolucency of the bone is a direct reflection of the "bone poverty" (Fig. 1). The density of the shadow cast by a tissue is in inverse proportion to the amount of x-rays absorbed by it. Absorption rises with the third power of the atomic number and hence, it is a direct function of the amount of calcium in the bone.[53] In osteoporosis, the amount of mineral in the bone is deficient; this decreases the absorption of x-rays and consequently, the final image appears more radiolucent. There must be at least 30% to 50% of bone loss before the change is observable on a radiograph.[51,54]

Cortical Thinning

Osteoporosis affects both the cortical and trabecular bone. Resorption of cortical bone can occur at 3 principal sites, namely, endosteal, periosteal, and intracortical. Any surface of mature bone is a potential site for bone remodeling. In a compact

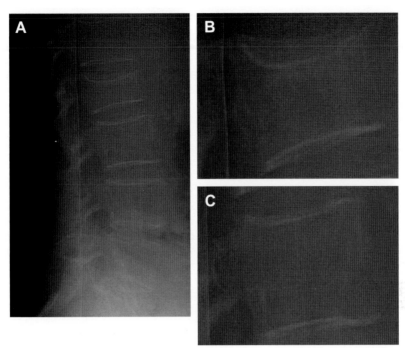

Fig. 1. (*A*) Lateral radiograph of the lumbar spine shows generalized increase in radiolucency, with loss of trabecular impressions and pencil-thin cortices. The generalized loss of bone density mimics the appearance of an "overexposed" radiograph. (*B*) Magnified view of the second lumbar vertebra shows anterior wedging. Note the superior endplate fracture with focal cortical disruption, angular step deformity, and subcortical bandlike increase in density. (*C*) Magnified view of the third lumbar vertebra shows the typical "picture frame" appearance (also known as "ghost vertebra").

bone, most of this activity happens at the highly vascular inner and outer surfaces of the cortex, that is, the periosteal and endosteal surfaces. In involutional osteoporosis, the resorptive process is most active along the endosteal surface. Hence, early subtle changes are difficult to interpret.[55] Moreover, this is a nonspecific pattern of cortical resorption, because most of the other conditions with high bone turnover such as hyperparathyroidism, disuse, osteomalacia, and renal osteodystrophy can show similar changes.[4] Endosteal scalloping may be visible in early osteoporosis, but the usual appearance is of gradual widening of the marrow space with cortical thinning. In severe cases, the cortex becomes thin and frail ("pencil-thin cortex") with a smooth inner surface (see **Fig. 1**). The response of endosteal, periosteal, and intracortical bone resorptive processes differs according to the metabolic stimuli. The pattern of response is determined by the rate of bone turnover initiated by the causative factor. For example, in hyperparathyroidism, where the bone turnover is extremely high, subperiosteal bone resorption is visible, appearing as subtle irregularities along the external surface of the bone; this is especially well seen in metacarpals. Such an unprecedented rate of bone turnover is seldom seen in other conditions and hence, subperiosteal bone resorption with generalized osteopenia is almost pathognomonic for hyperparathyroidism.[56] Intracortical bone loss can be seen at lower rates of bone turnover than is required to cause subperiosteal lucencies or in conditions like hyperthyroidism where the hypermetabolic state results in accelerated catabolism of connective tissue, with cortical bone being affected more than cancellous bone. Intracortical resorption is seen as longitudinal striations or trabeculations, best appreciated in the inner half of the cortex.[57] In involutional osteoporosis, the resorption rate is seldom high enough to produce subperiosteal lucencies or longitudinal cortical tunneling on a radiograph. This knowledge enables one to identify the metabolic cause for loss in bone density and prevents generalized osteopenia with an underlying treatable cause being deemed as senile osteoporosis.

Altered Trabecular Pattern

Cancellous bone offers greater surface area and responds faster to metabolic stimuli, and thus reflects the changes of osteoporosis earlier than cortical bone. In cancellous bone, trabeculae are laid down in intersecting arches corresponding to the compressive and tensile forces acting on it.[58] As the thickness of these trabeculae varies between 50 and 200 μm,[59] theoretically the high resolution of conventional radiographs should permit their characterization. However, due to summation of overlapping shadows on conventional radiographs, the trabecular pattern is accurately depicted only at peripheral sites like the calcaneus, distal radius and, to a lesser extent, the hip[60,61]; whereas in the spine, other factors such as patient habitus and deformities interfere with such assessment. The orderly loss of bone mass in osteoporosis can be studied by observing the trabecular pattern on radiographs. The secondary trabeculae that are not primarily involved in weight bearing disappear first. The primary trabeculae that are parallel to the axis of weight transmission are preserved until late. The weight-bearing trabeculae may sometimes grow thicker, partly due to callus from healing of the microfractures they suffer, and partly as a compensatory mechanism.[62] Thus early on in osteoporosis, the primary trabeculae are accentuated on a radiograph; at a later stage even they disappear, resulting in a "washed-out" appearance (see **Fig. 1**).

Fractures and Deformities

Decreasing BMD increases the likelihood of osteoporotic fracture; nevertheless, the majority of fragility fractures occur in people whose bone mineral densities are not in the osteoporotic range.[63] The common sites for these fragility fractures are the spine, hip, and wrist. The incidence of fractures of the proximal humerus, pelvis, clavicle, scapula, and rib also increase with age in elderly women and to a lesser extent in men. For other fractures—including carpal fractures and fractures of the foot and skull—there appears to be no increase in incidence with aging.[64] Presence of a fragility fracture increases the risk of future fractures. If there is a vertebral fracture, the risk of sustaining a subsequent vertebral fracture is 4 times greater, and this risk increases with increase in the number of preexisting fractures at any given point in time. Similarly, the presence of spine or wrist fracture increases the risk of subsequent hip fracture by 2 times.[65]

TARGET SITES OF INVOLVEMENT
Spine

The radiographic appearance of the spine in involutional osteoporosis may be broadly classified as vertebral fractures and nonfractural changes.

Nonfractural changes
The preservation of vertical trabeculae and involution of the more horizontal ones allows easy delineation of the trabeculae parallel to the line of gravity,[66] which may give the vertebral body

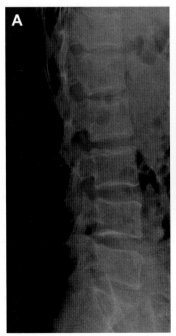
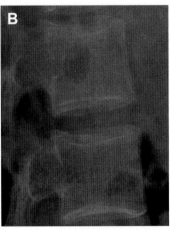

Fig. 2. (A) Lateral radiograph of the spine shows a "coarse striated" appearance of all the vertebral bodies due to resorption of the secondary trabeculae and accentuation of the primary weight-bearing trabeculae. (B) Magnified view depicts the trabecular pattern better.

a coarsely trabeculated/striated appearance (Fig. 2) akin to a hemangioma. Vertebral hemangiomas are also osteopenic (due to replacement of bone with angiomatous tissues) with vertical striations, producing the "corduroy cloth" appearance.[67] However, involvement of multiple consecutive levels and often the entire spine, with no bony expansion or associated soft tissue shadow, aids in differentiating this "pseudo-hemangioma appearance" from a true hemangioma. As the vertebral bodies show progressive decrease in density, it loses its internal features and culminates in the washed-out appearance where the density of the bone approximates with the surrounding soft tissue. Saville[68] classified this progressive loss of features and increase in lucency into 5 grades (Table 2). However, interpretation of such qualitative information involves marked interpersonal variability (probability of correct response = 0.53–0.95).[69] In the spine, cortical thinning is best appreciated on a lateral radiograph at the vertebral endplates, which are otherwise relatively thick. With loss of the trabecular density, the thinned-out linear shadow of the vertebral cortices becomes accentuated, generating the well-known "picture frame" appearance.

Vertebral fractures

Vertebral fractures (VFs) are the hallmark of osteoporosis. Vertebrae generally fail by compression in axial loading. The loss of secondary trabeculae generates the biomechanical environment for fracture of the residual weight-bearing vertical trabeculae. The equation of von Euler states that in a structure with cross ties dividing the length of the vertical columns into 2 halves, the weight required to buckle the structure is inversely proportional to the square of the distance between the cross ties. In short, with loss of the horizontal trabeculae, the vertebra will buckle under one-quarter of the original load required.[62] This process explains the high frequency of osteoporotic vertebral compression fractures.

Osteoporotic VFs are usually identified by characteristic changes in vertebral shape. Biomechanical factors influence the distribution of the fractures. The thoracic kyphosis is most pronounced at the mid-thoracic region, so the loading in flexion is accentuated here. The thoracolumbar junction consists of an articulation between the relatively rigid thoracic spine and the freely mobile lumbar segment, maximizing compressive stresses[70] in this region. Hence, spine fractures are more likely to occur in the mid-thoracic area and at the thoracolumbar junction. Most of the VFs are seen at T8-L1 and L4 vertebral levels.[71] VFs are classified according to the presence or absence of symptoms into "clinical" or "morphometric" VF, respectively. The fractures present at the initial radiograph are termed "prevalent fracture", whereas those appearing on subsequent radiographs are known as "incident fracture". The extent of reduction in vertebral height and morphologic changes that are distinct from other nonfracture deformities are assessed by simple visual analysis of both frontal and lateral radiographs of the entire spine (especially because most of the VFs are multiple). VFs are defined by a reduction in anterior, middle, or posterior vertebral height, although the minimum required reduction (eg, 15% or 20% of vertebral height) varies among definition schemes. Genant and colleagues[72] proposed a semiquantitative scoring system to grade the severity of VFs. These investigators defined a vertebral deformity in T4-L4 vertebrae of more than 20% of loss in height with a reduction in area of more than 10% to 20% as a fracture. Based on this threshold, the Genant scoring system classified VF into 4 grades of severity (Table 3).

Descriptive terminology for VF, depending on the shape (eg, pancake, wedged, fishmouth), severity (mild, moderate, severe), number, and location are popular. Fractures are generally described as wedge-shaped if the anterior height is reduced in relation to posterior height (Fig. 3). In the thoracic vertebrae, the posterior height is greater than anterior height by 1 to 3 mm even in normal individuals; hence a loss of height greater than 4 mm is considered as a true vertebral fracture.[73,74] Some studies have calculated the wedge compression ratio as anterior height/posterior height and have shown the normal lower limit of this ratio to be between 0.8 and 0.92.[75] Traumatic compression fractures of the spine can mimic

Table 2 Saville index	
Grade	**Features Seen on Radiograph**
0	Normal density
1	Minimal loss of density; endplates begin to stand out, giving a stenciled effect
2	Vertical striation is more obvious, endplates are thinner
3	More severe loss of bone density than grade II, endplates becoming less visible
4	Ghostlike vertebral bodies, density is no greater than soft tissue, no trabecular pattern is visible

Grade	Features Seen on Radiograph
0	Normal
1	Approximately 20%–25% reduction in anterior, middle, and/or posterior height
2	Approximately 25%–40% reduction in anterior, middle, and/or posterior height
3	Approximately 40% or greater reduction in anterior, middle, and/or posterior height

Table 3
Genant scoring system

anterior wedging of the vertebral body seen with osteoporosis, but the normal bone density, angular or steplike cortical defects, and normal amount of callus formation may be useful in distinguishing them. In osteoporotic VFs, a demonstrable break in the cortex or significant callus formation is rare.[4] Traumatic fractures are rarely restricted to the endplate alone, which is a frequent feature in osteoporosis. "Vertebra plana" (**Fig. 4**) or "pancake vertebra" is a type of deformity of vertebral body seen with loss of both the anterior and posterior vertebral heights, often in multiple segments. This condition is unusual in osteoporosis and if present, more sinister etiologies like metastasis and myeloma need to be excluded by pertinent laboratory investigation or biopsy correlation (**Fig. 5**). As a direct mechanical sequel of pressure on the weakened bone from the nucleus pulposus, the endplates may show an exaggerated concavity that simulates the vertebral body appearance found in normal fish.[76] In these biconcave deformities, variably described as "codfish", "fishmouth", or "hourglass" vertebrae, the intervertebral disc spaces are usually of normal height. Such deformity may be seen with other conditions with bone softening, such as osteomalacia, Paget disease, or hyperparathyroidism. Isolated endplate deformities due to fracture of the endplate and underlying subcortical bone can also occur in osteoporosis. Endplate deformity may be central or peripheral, and depicted as an altered orientation or step deformity in the endplate with increased density subjacent to the fracture. Central endplate fractures are most frequent at L1 to L4 vertebrae (**Fig. 6**), probably due to the thicker vertebral cortex in the lumbar spine and lumbar lordosis. It is not uncommon to have various types of deformities, and deformities in various stages of temporal evolution within the

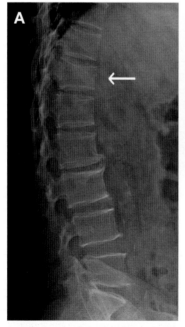
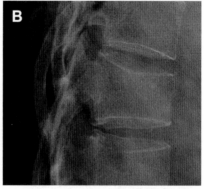

Fig. 3. (*A*) Lateral radiograph of the lumbar spine shows generalized osteopenia with cortical thinning. There is kyphotic deformity at the thoracolumbar junction, secondary to the mild anterior wedging of the T12 body (*arrow*). (*B*) Magnified view of the T12 vertebra better demonstrates the fracture involving the superior endplate and anterior cortex. A careful scrutiny of the endplates is essential to differentiate vertebral fractures of this kind from the physiologic short anterior vertebral height.

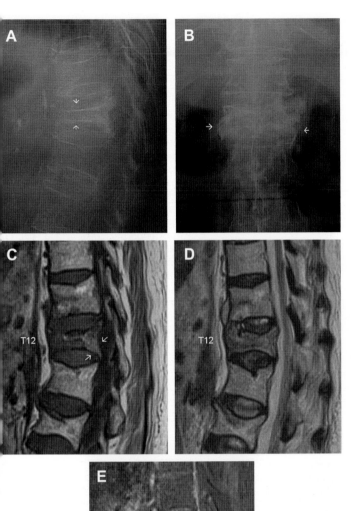

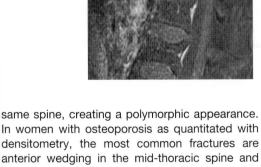

Fig. 4. Example of benign vertebra plana from osteoporotic fracture. (*A*) Lateral and (*B*) frontal radiographs show an osteopenic skeleton with severe compression of T12 vertebral body (*arrows*). T11 and L1 vertebral bodies also show slight decrease in height. Sagittal (*C*) T1-weighted (T1W), (*D*) T2-weighted (T2W), and (*E*) postcontrast fat-suppressed T1W images confirm the benign nature of vertebra plana in this patient. The positive features that favor an osteoporotic fracture seen here are as follows. (1) Preservation of at least some normal T1W marrow signal in an almost completely collapsed T12 vertebral body (*arrows in C*). (2) Fractures involving multiple adjoining vertebrae at the thoracolumbar junction. The superior end plate fracture of L1 is fractured in the center. The horizontal band of low signal seen through the middle of T11 and subjacent to superior endplate of L2 are fracture lines (seen in C and D). (3) Typical enhancement. Note the band-like enhancement with sharp outlines in the collapsed T12 body (*E*), indicating a recent fracture.

same spine, creating a polymorphic appearance. In women with osteoporosis as quantitated with densitometry, the most common fractures are anterior wedging in the mid-thoracic spine and thoracolumbar junction, and central compression fractures from L1 to L4.[77] Isolated fractures above T7 vertebral level should alert the radiologist to a cause other than osteoporosis.[3]

The Genant semiquantitative assessment of standard radiographs is useful in routine clinical practice as well as for research purposes. The alternative, algorithm-based qualitative method (ABQ) is still awaiting further validation for clinical use.[78] As per ABQ method, a vertebra with apparent "reduced" height without evidence of osteoporotic endplate depression is classified as nonosteoporotic short vertebral height (SVH).[79] Adoption of this technique of evaluation may decrease the prevalence of morphometric VF by 30%.

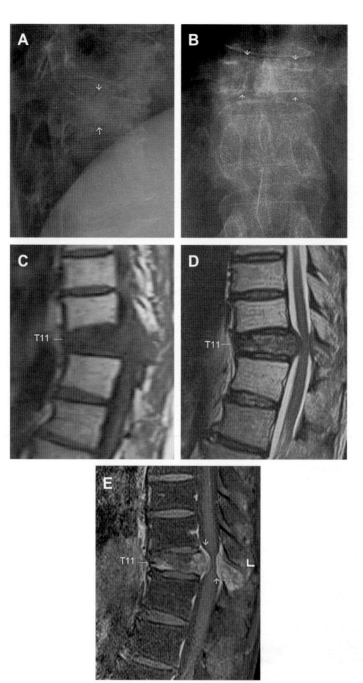

Fig. 5. Example of malignant vertebra plana. (*A*) Frontal and (*B*) lateral radiographs show T11 vertebral body collapse (*arrows*) with background osteopenia. Sagittal (*C*) T1W, (*D*) T2W, and (*E*) postcontrast fat-suppressed T1W images confirm the malignant nature of the vertebra plana in this patient. The positive features that favor an malignant collapse are: (1) there is complete loss of normal marrow signal from the collapsed T11 vertebral body (*C*); (2) convex posterior border of the vertebra compressing the spinal cord (*D*)—compare this with the concave posterior border in osteoporotic collapse (**Fig. 4D**); (3) solid pattern of inhomogeneous enhancement (*E*); (4) involvement of posterior elements (*arrowhead in E*) and epidural soft tissue component (*arrows in E*).

Differential diagnoses for vertebral osteoporosis

Notochordal remnants can cause impressions on the vertebral endplates simulating fish vertebrae. On a frontal radiograph, they produce parasagittal concavity in the endplates that gives rise to a "cupid's bow" appearance.[80] The impressions focally involve the posterior two-thirds of the endplate, and their pits are smooth and lined by cortical bone. On computed tomography (CT), they are seen as posterolaterally located parasagittal depressions with an "owl's eye" appearance. Schmorl node, characterized by displacement of a portion of the intervertebral disc into the vertebral body due to disruption of the endplate, can be seen in osteoporosis, besides other conditions such as hyperparathyroidism, neoplasms, trauma, osteomalacia, and infection.[81]

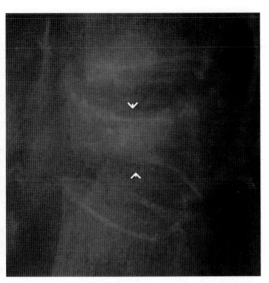

Fig. 6. Lateral radiograph of L1 vertebral body shows osteoporotic central endplate fractures. Both the superior and inferior endplates are involved.

The depression formed by a Schmorl node leads to discontinuity and an irregular contour of the vertebral endplate, and can involve any portion of the vertebral endplate; this distinguishes them from the impression caused by notochordal remnants.[82] Schmorl nodes of osteoporosis are smaller and exhibit more irregular borders than those of the juvenile-onset variety. In Schuermann disease (osteochondritis of secondary ossification centers of vertebrae), there is anterior vertebral wedging with multiple Schmorl nodes and loss of disc height with kyphotic deformity. Schuermann disease affects the mid and lower thoracic spine, and hence overlaps with the preferred site for osteoporosis. Preferential involvement of male gender, early age of onset (13–17 years), lack of universal osteopenia, coexisting degenerative changes disproportionate for age, and other vertebral anomalies such as partial vertebral fusion and limbus vertebrae serve as unique features for recognizing this condition. Metastasis (see **Fig. 5**) and myeloma are the most sinister differential diagnoses that need to be considered. The obvious indicators of malignant vertebral collapse include fractures located in the upper thoracic spine, expansile lesions, bulging posterior border with smooth contours (in osteoporosis it is generally concave, traumatic fractures of osteoporotic bone that may cause posterior bulging but with sharp angular margins or retropulsed fragments), destructive lesions, involvement of the pedicle and neural arch, para-/prevertebral soft tissue component, involvement of multiple discontinuous vertebral segments, and differential loss of bone density within the same bone or adjoining vertebra (in osteoporosis the bone loss is fairly uniform in the entire skeleton). In metastatic disease, there is a haphazard destruction of the trabecular network in a moth-eaten or permeative pattern. Close inspection may show erosion or destruction of endplates. Focal lytic/sclerotic lesions, if present, make the diagnosis more obvious. However, the sensitivity and specificity of these radiographic findings are low. The best problem-solving tool to distinguish a pathologic fracture from fragility

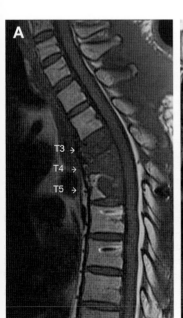
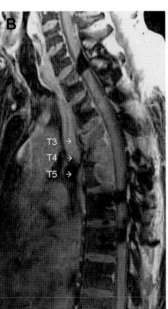

Fig. 7. Sagittal (*A*) pre- and (*B*) post-contrast T1W images of a patient diagnosed with myeloma. The upper thoracic vertebral body collapse (T3 and T4) is highly suggestive of a malignant etiology. In both T3 and T4 vertebral bodies, there is complete loss of normal T1 marrow signal. In T5 vertebral body, there is partial loss of normal signal; however, the area of T1 signal loss has a round configuration (compare with the bandlike configuration in **Fig. 8**).

fracture would be MRI. A smoothly convex posterior border, abnormal signal intensity of the pedicle or posterior elements, an epidural mass, a focal paraspinal mass, and other spinal metastases are features of malignant compression fractures sought for in an MRI (**Figs. 5** and **7**).[83] A low signal intensity band on T1- and T2-weighted images, persistent normal bone marrow signal intensity of the vertebral body, retropulsion of a posterior bone fragment, and multiple compression fractures favor acute osteoporotic compression fractures (**Fig. 8**).[84] T1-weighted images are more reliable in distinguishing metastatic from osteoporotic collapse. Malignant vertebral collapse typically exhibits low signal intensity on T1-weighted images, whereas chronic osteoporotic vertebral collapse exhibits normal signal intensity.[85] In acute osteoporotic fractures, (1) at least one or more areas of normal marrow signal intensity persists, (2) the area of low T1-weighted signal is often restricted to the vicinity of the fracture line, and (3) it is usual to have a sharp demarcation between the areas of low signal and normal marrow signal (see **Fig. 4**). The T1-weighted hypointensities seen in acute compression fractures have a band-like configuration. With metastases, the usual pattern is a complete loss of the normal T1 marrow signal (see **Fig. 5**); even if areas of normal signal persist, they are round in configuration (see **Fig. 7**).[86] In post-gadolinium T1-weighted MRI, the areas corresponding to impacted, fractured bone are seen as dark bands with linear enhancement due to vascular reactive process reparative to the fracture surrounding it. In metastasis, the marrow enhancement is more extensive, patchy, nonlinear, and of solid pattern.[83] The presence of focal, linear, or triangular areas of high signal intensity ("fluid sign") adjacent to vertebral endplate on short-tau inversion recovery (STIR) images is said to be a feature of acute and subacute osteoporotic compression fractures and is rarely seen in metastatic fractures.[86] CT is not as informative as MRI, but it may still be used as a less resource intensive and easily available technique. CT can also show the vacuum sign (analogous to fluid sign on MRI), which is an indicator of benign disease.[87]

Several systemic diseases may present with an osteoporosis-like radiographic picture; however, the presence of certain diagnostic features may aid the differentiation. In osteomalacia, the Looser zones, prominent cortical tunneling,[7] and indistinct outlines of the coarse trabeculae besides other features of bone softening are prominently seen, while subperiosteal bone resorption is almost pathognomonic for hyperparathyroidism. Exuberant callus formation (seen as "marginal condensation" subjacent to vertebral endplates), when seen with radiographic findings of osteoporosis, is characteristic for Cushing disease. Additional findings such as osteonecrosis of the femoral head are frequently seen with exogenous steroid administration.[88] In hemoglobinopathies, the replacement of trabeculae with hemopoietic tissue causes osteoporosis-like radiographic appearance. In sickle cell disease, characteristic H-shaped vertebrae are seen, due to steplike depression of the superior and inferior vertebral margins, which is attributed to disturbance in

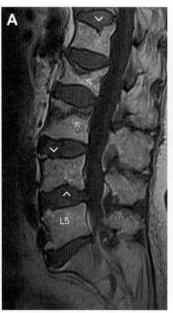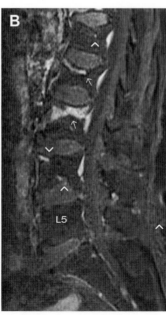

Fig. 8. Sagittal (*A*) pre- and (*B*) post-contrast T1W images in a patient with multiple osteoporotic vertebral fractures. The linear hypointensity (*arrows in A*) that run parallel to the superior endplate in L2 and L3 vertebral bodies represents fracture lines. Postcontrast images show a corresponding bandlike enhancement (*arrows in B*) from reactionary changes along these recent fractures. The arrowheads show the focal endplate fractures. The endplate fractures involving the L4 vertebral body show minimal enhancement, while the one adjacent to the L1 superior endplate does not enhance, suggesting an old fracture.

growth at the chondro-osseous junction resulting from venous occlusion by abnormal red blood cells. This configuration is pathognomonic for sickle cell disease, and may occasionally be seen with Gaucher disease. In renal osteodystrophy, bone changes are a result of combination of different processes including secondary hyperparathyroidism, osteomalacia, osteoporosis, osteosclerosis, and aluminum toxicity. Here the vertebrae have a so-called rugger jersey appearance, consisting of bands of subchondral sclerosis beneath the endplates of the vertebrae and more lucent areas in between. The presence of an intravertebral gas cleft (ie, cleft sign, intravertebral vacuum phenomenon) in vertebral compression fractures (VCFs) is a feature of osteonecrosis, also referred to as Kümmell disease.[89,90] This feature appears as a transverse, linear, or semilunar radiolucent shadow that is located centrally within or adjacent to the endplate of a collapsed vertebral body. Prolonged supine posture can result in accumulation of fluid within these clefts.[91] These areas of corticocancellous disruption are unusual with pathologic fractures, and represent benign collapse.[87,92]

Pelvis and Hip

Radiographic manifestations of osteoporosis in the hip and pelvis are identical to most other sites. The iliac blades in the region of iliac fossa, the pubis, supracetabular region, femoral neck, and greater trochanter are the sites most affected in osteoporosis. The trabecular changes of osteoporosis are most accentuated in the proximal end of the femur, and in the region between the sacroiliac joint and hip joint. The cortical thinning is most distinctive at the iliac crests, pubic rami, ischia, and femoral head and neck.

As early as 1867, Von Meyer stated that the trabeculae in the proximal femur corresponded in position to the trajectories of maximum compression and tensile stress.[58] Fifty years later, Koch provided mathematical evidence for this theory and stated that the transmission of weight from the head of the femur to the shaft determined the arrangement of trabeculae in the upper end of femur.[93] The absence of adult trabecular pattern in the infant femur until onset of weight bearing and lack of organized trabecular pattern in proximal femur of a sloth (an animal that hangs upside down) endorses this fact.[94,95] The trabeculae in the proximal femur can be divided into 5 groups according to their orientation (Fig. 9),[96] namely:

Principal compressive group. These trabeculae are the uppermost, thickest, and most closely packed of all the trabeculae.

They extend from medial metaphyseal cortex to the superior femoral head. They are oriented as slightly curved radial lines. In osteoporosis, they appear accentuated and are the last to undergo resorption.

Secondary compressive group. These trabeculae arise below the principal compressive group, adjacent to the cortex, near the lesser trochanter, and curve upwards and laterally toward the greater trochanter and upper femoral neck; they are thin and sparsely arranged.

Greater trochanteric group. These trabeculae consist of some slender and poorly defined tensile ones that arise from the lateral cortex just below the greater trochanter and sweep upward to end near its superior surface.

Principal tensile group. These trabeculae spring from the lateral cortex immediately below the greater trochanter group. These trabeculae are the thickest among the tensile group. They curve upward and inward across the neck of the femur, to end in the inferior portion of the femoral head.

Secondary tensile group. These trabeculae arise from the lateral cortex below the principal tensile trabeculae. They arch upward and medially across the upper end of femur and end more or less irregularly after crossing the midline.

In the neck of the femur, the principal compressive, the secondary compressive, and the principal tensile trabeculae enclose an area containing some thin and loosely arranged trabeculae, called Ward's triangle (see Fig. 9C). In early osteoporosis, this triangle becomes more radiolucent and is prominently seen as the less visible trabeculae involute and the bordering groups are better demarcated. As the severity of osteoporosis increases, the tensile group regresses from medial to lateral, thereby opening the Ward's triangle laterally. Based on this predictable sequence of involution of trabeculae, Singh and colleagues[96] suggested an index that could serve as a radiographic scale for diagnosis and grading of the severity of osteoporosis (Table 4). As per this index, grade 4 is borderline osteoporosis with definite osteoporosis beginning at grade 3. In grades 5 and 6, the bone is histologically normal. Later, a grade 7 was added to this scale for individuals who have dense bone.[97]

The hip fractures are usually a consequence of direct fall that generates an impact up to 3 times greater than the fractural strength of femoral

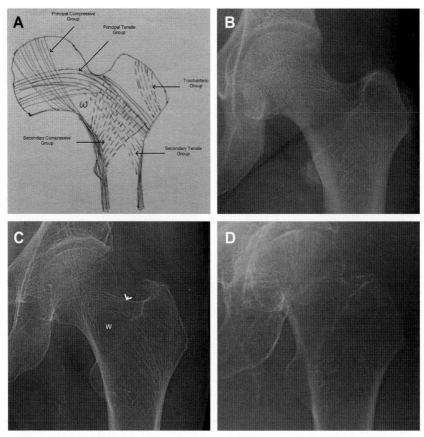

Fig. 9. (*A*) Line diagram shows the normal trabecular pattern in the proximal femur. W, Ward's triangle. (*B*) Radiograph of a normal subject shows all the trabeculae depicted in the previous line diagram. (*C*) Radiograph shows osteoporotic changes (Singh index Grade 3) with increased lucency of Ward's triangle and break in the continuity of the principal tensile trabeculae (*arrowhead*). (*D*) Radiograph shows an undisplaced cervical fracture of the femur with background changes of severe osteoporosis. The fracture line is represented by the subcapital line of sclerosis.

neck and trochanteric region.[98] Fractures of the proximal femur can usually be classified as cervical (femoral neck or intracapsular) fractures or trochanteric (extracapsular) fractures (**Fig. 10**). Trochanteric fractures are seen in more elderly individuals, with a greater degree of generalized osteoporosis. These patients are at greater risk of future fractures and their risk of fracture is more closely related to femoral BMD measurements.[99,100] The intertrochanteric fractures are often comminuted, with separation of the greater and/or lesser trochanter. The risk of cervical fractures is associated with the biomechanical properties that result in part from the pelvic anatomy, and hence structural information or measures of geometric properties may be beneficial for identifying women with cervical fractures.[100] From a therapeutic viewpoint, cervical fractures are at greater risk of avascular necrosis of femoral head as most of the blood vessels supplying the femoral

head traverse the femoral neck. Open reduction and internal fixation is often required in cervical fractures to restore anatomic continuity and vascular integrity to the femoral head. Most of the displaced or impacted hip fractures are seen on radiographs. An undisplaced femoral neck fracture may be represented by a band of sclerosis traversing the femoral neck (see **Fig. 9**D) or subtle disruption of the normal trabecular pattern, with valgus angulation of the primary compressive trabeculae. It is not uncommon for subtle nondisplaced fractures to go undiagnosed initially, only to present at a later date after displacement has occurred. In equivocal cases of undisplaced fractures, MRI is valuable. MRI shows the actual fracture line as linear area of hypointensity, surrounded by bone marrow edema. MRI can demonstrate positive findings within 2 to 6 hours of injury, whereas scintigraphy has a lag time of 24 to 72 hours following the trauma before the

Table 4
Singh index (radiographic findings are progressive from one grade to the next)

Grade	Radiographic Findings
6	Normal
5	Secondary compressive trabeculae are not seen and Ward's triangle is prominent
4	Principal tensile trabeculae start involuting but still traceable in continuity
3	Break in continuity of principal tensile trabeculae opposite the greater trochanter
2	Only principal compressive trabeculae are seen as the rest get resorbed
1	Principal compressive trabeculae are no longer seen

fracture is visualized. When osteoporosis and severe degenerative joint disease coexist, stress fractures occasionally occur through the medial aspect of the femoral neck and pubic rami. However, osteoarthritic hip is associated with diminished risk for osteoporotic VF, while the prevalence of osteoarthritis of hip is low in the presence of osteoporosis.[101]

Subchondral insufficiency fractures of the hip have recently been recognized as a distinct clinical entity, mainly based on radiological studies.[102,103] Subchondral insufficiency typically occurs in osteoporotic elderly women who present with acute hip pain and often have insufficiency fractures elsewhere. This entity is easily overlooked or confused with avascular necrosis and when there is significant joint involvement with osteoarthritis.[98] These fractures are often difficult to diagnose clinically, rapidly progress to destructive hip disease and, if detected early, can be treated conservatively with good outcome. Initial radiographs are often normal. Subsequently, they show a curvilinear subchondral lucency or sclerosis (representing the fracture line) in the superior or superolateral aspects of the femoral head (**Fig. 11**A). Focal depression, contoural abnormality, step deformity and, eventually, collapse of the femoral head follow. Scintigrams show nonspecific increased in activity (**Fig. 11**B), while MRI can accurately diagnose this condition, where it is seen as a T1- and T2-hypointense band parallel to the articular surface in the subchondral region, which represents the fracture and associated repair tissue.[104] There may be extensive marrow edema and focal contour defects of the femoral head. These changes are reversible and resolve on follow-up MRI.[101] Besides osteoporosis, this entity may be encountered in patients on corticosteroid therapy, postradiation injury, and post renal transplantation. The proximal femur is a favored site for metastatic lesions. Hence, it is essential to exclude pathologic fracture in every deemed case of osteoporotic hip fracture. Of particular note are the proximal femoral fractures in the subtrochanteric region or stand-alone fracture involving the lesser trochanter. These fractures have a high probability of being secondary to metastatic disease.[105]

In osteoporosis, stress fracture of sacrum and pubis is common. Stress fractures occur due to chronic repetitive trauma, ultimately resulting in structural failure of bone; they can be subgrouped into "insufficiency" and "fatigue" stress fractures.

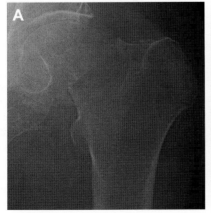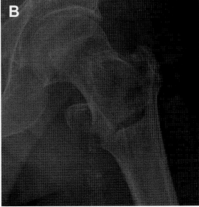

Fig. 10. Radiographs from 2 different patients with osteoporosis show (*A*) transcervical fracture of the femoral neck and (*B*) intertrochanteric fracture.

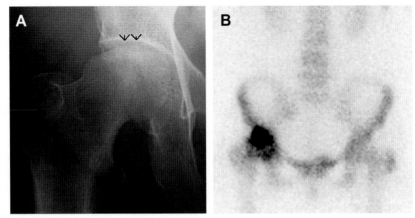

Fig. 11. (A) Radiograph shows an advanced case of subchondral insufficiency fracture with contour deformity seen along the superolateral aspect of the femoral head. The area of linear sclerosis (*arrowheads*) represents the sub-chondral fracture. (B) Tc-99m bone scintigram in the same patient shows a localized increase in the uptake of the radioactive tracer in the region, corresponding to the subchondral insufficiency fracture seen on the radiograph.

If a stress fracture occurs in a healthy bone due to unusual activity, it is termed a fatigue fracture. An insufficiency fracture occurs when normal or phys-iologic muscular activity stresses a bone that is deficient in mineral or elastic resistance.[106] The term pathologic fracture should be restricted to any situation in which preexisting neoplasm or infection has weakened the bone. Fatigue fractures of the sacrum are extremely rare, and most of the stress fractures of the sacrum are of insufficiency type.[107] These fractures are 5 times more common in osteoporotic women than men. When present, a stress fracture site is identified by localized peri-osteal response and transverse opaque zones of callus formation. In elderly patients, the insuffi-ciency fractures of sacrum are frequently identified when they undergo a bone scan to exclude skeletal metastatic disease. Isotope bone scan is the most sensitive method for detecting these fractures.[108] The common patterns identified at bone scinti-grams in sacral insufficiency fractures are H-pattern (Honda sign) from bilateral vertical fractures through sacral ala connected by a transverse frac-ture through sacral body (**Fig. 12**), I-pattern from single vertical fracture passing through the sacral ala, and the arc-pattern from transverse fracture running horizontally across the sacrum. Once de-tected on bone scan, these can be confirmed by CT or MRI. Pubic insufficiency fractures most often involve the body of pubis, are frequently bilateral, and may coexist with fractures elsewhere in the pelvic ring.[109] Sometimes they may progress to pubic osteolysis, which mimics neoplastic destruc-tion. Insufficiency fractures in the pelvis can involve the acetabulum, seen as hazy, sclerotic bands at the lateral supra-acetabular margin, sometimes parallel to acetabular cortex medially and occa-sionally extending into the pelvic inlet.

Nonhip Appendicular Skeleton

The radius, calcaneus, humerus, mandible, and metacarpals are common sites of nonhip appen-dicular skeleton affected by osteoporosis. Most of the fractures involve the distal radius, humeral neck, and ankle malleoli. The distal forearm frac-tures usually follow a fall on the outstretched arm and are of the Colles type, with dorsal displace-ment of the distal radial segment (**Fig. 13**). These fractures are more frequently left-sided, which may in part be related to differences in bone mass between dominant and nondominant (usually left) arms or fall characteristics.[110] Residual deformities often follow osteoporotic forearm fractures. Up to 20% may experience some long-term complication, including reflex sympathetic dystrophy, malunion, neuropathy, and secondary osteoarthritis.[111] Osteoporotic fractures of the proximal humerus most commonly involve the surgical neck (**Fig. 14**). These fractures occur when the individual is unable to break his or her forward or oblique fall and therefore lands directly on the shoulder, a mechanism similar to that seen in osteoporotic hip fractures.[112] An inci-dent humeral fracture is associated with an 83% increase in the risk of a subsequent incident hip fracture.[113]

Radiologic imaging of the hand is a fundamental step in evaluating grade and type of osteoporosis. Barnett and Nordin[114] devised a fairly precise "metacarpal cortical index" for objectively measuring osteoporosis. These investigators

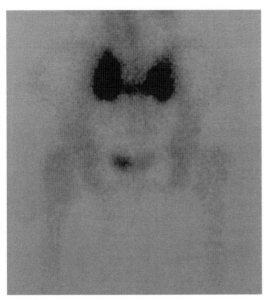

Fig. 12. Tc-99m bone scintigram shows increased uptake in the sacrum with an H-shaped configuration, typical of a sacral insufficiency fracture. This pattern is popularly known as the "Honda sign".

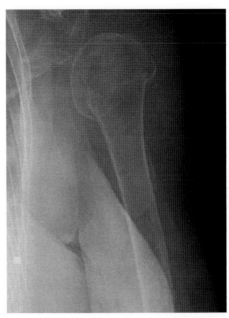

Fig. 14. Radiograph shows a fracture of the humeral neck with impaction. Background changes of generalized decrease of bone density and cortical thinning are those of osteoporosis.

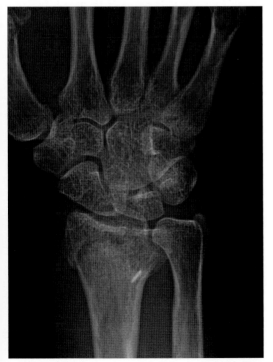

Fig. 13. Radiograph shows a distal radial fracture (Colles type). This is the most commonly manifested osteoporotic fracture.

divided the sum of the thickness of the medial and lateral cortices of the shaft of either second metacarpal bone at the thickest point of the cortex by the total diameter of the shaft at that level. This fraction was multiplied by 100 to obtain the metacarpal cortical index (MCI). In a similar manner, they also calculated a cortical index for the femur and spine. A reasonable relationship was found between these scores and findings at iliac bone biopsy. Digital x-ray radiogrammetry, the modern version of MCI, is an easy to measure and inexpensive test that requires just an analog radiograph and minimal hardware support for computing purposes. Digital x-ray radiogrammetry is useful as a measure of bone size and bone mass, for observing the course of osteoporosis and its treatment, and for epidemiologic studies.[115]

The calcaneus is an optimal site for the morphologic evaluation of trabecular pattern (Fig. 15). The calcaneal trabecular pattern (expressed as the "calcaneal index") closely parallels that in the upper end of the femur (Singh index) and is easier to assess. Both indices have a significant correlation with age.[116] Like the proximal femur, the calcaneus has compression and tensile trabeculae. The compression trabeculae are in 2 sets. One begins at the subtalar articular surface and diverges downward and backward through the waist of calcaneus, thins out gradually, and fans

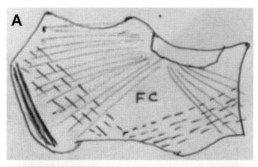

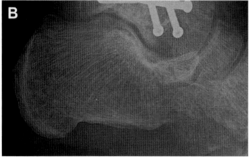

Fig. 15. The calcaneal trabecular pattern. (*A*) Line diagram and (*B*) radiograph show the continuous thin lines that represent compressive trabeculae while the interrupted lines represent tensile trabeculae. Another set of trajectory trabeculae are seen parallel to the calcaneal attachment of the Achilles tendon. FC (foramen calcanei) is an area with few thin vertical trabeculae between the anterior and posterior compressive trabeculae. Interruption or buckling of these trabeculae may be the only evidence of fracture in some cases.

out over the entire posterior surface. The second set of compression trabeculae pass anteriorly from the subtalar articular surface toward the articulation with the cuboid. Tensile trabeculae start in front of the tuberosity of the calcaneus, and sweep both backward and forward between the 2 compression struts. Another set of trajectory trabeculae is seen in the line of pull of the calcaneal tendon; this is a thick compact group of parallel trabeculae along the subcutaneous part of the bone. Depending on the degree of resorption of these trabeculae, Jhamaria and colleagues[116] classified osteoporosis from grade V (normal) to grade I (severe osteoporosis). Unlike at the hip, there is no soft tissue overlap at the calcaneus, and the probability of errors due to limb rotation and neck-shaft angle is absent.

BEYOND CONVENTIONAL RADIOGRAPHS

In the contemporary initiative against osteoporosis, several techniques beyond conventional radiographs have come into the fray. BMD measurement

using DXA is the current gold standard in defining, as well as evaluating, osteoporosis. Vertebral fracture assessment (VFA) done with x-ray absorptiometry that can be performed as a point-of-service convenience for the patient when done at the same visit as for BMD is also gaining popularity.[117] The ease of availability, lower cost and radiation involved, and reliable information available are the attractive features of this technique. VFA compares favorably with standard spine radiographs in detecting VFs using the Genant SQ method.[118,119] QCT is another method of measuring BMD .Unlike DXA, QCT gives estimates of cortical and trabecular bone separately and hence is sensitive to changes from higher turnover of trabecular bone. BMD can be measured by QCT on any computed tomographic system provided it is calibrated with standardized densities of calcium hydroxyapatite.[120] The accuracy of QCT in predicting spine fractures compares well with DXA. In addition, it also provides volumetric information as compared with the 2-dimensional information obtained with DXA. Quantitative ultrasound (QUS) techniques have been widely applied to the investigation of diseases associated with bone loss and increased fracture risk, and are especially useful in peripheral skeletal sites like the calcaneus, tibia, and the phalanges.[121] QUS reflects the quality aspects of bone, such as microstructure and geometry, independent of bone mass. QUS is valuable in predicting osteoporotic fracture risk.[121] Lack of radiation, low cost of equipment, provision for bedside performance, and safety in the pediatric population are some of the attractive features of QUS. QUS operates on the principle of decrease in the attenuation of sound waves with decrease in the number of trabeculae. High-resolution MRI to assess the trabecular bone is based on the modification of the T1 and T2 relaxation time of the bone marrow due to the magnetic field inhomogeneities created from the close proximity of marrow and bony trabeculae. The greater the number of interphases that marrow shares with bone, the greater will be the changes in relaxation time. This technique enables virtual biopsy from multiple sites and is an attractive alternative for assessing trabecular bone structure, with a potential for quantifying bone marrow composition. High-resolution MRI holds promise as a modality for comprehensive characterization of age-related or therapy-related metabolic changes in the skeleton.[122–124]

SUMMARY

Radiology has a central role in several aspects of the diagnosis and treatment of osteoporosis. Radiographs depict a plethora of manifestations of this ubiquitous disease. It is critical for a radiologist to be aware of the myriad appearances of osteoporosis and to distinguish them from the routine differential diagnoses. A conscious effort to overcome the tendency of underdiagnosing osteoporosis is essential and when detected, efforts to identify a cause for the same should be made with a prudent use of CT, MRI, and nuclear imaging as problem-solving tools. Reasonable awareness of the scope of specialized modalities like DXA, QUS, QCT, and MRI-guided virtual bone biopsy among general radiologists is also needed.

REFERENCES

1. Consensus development conference: diagnosis, prophylaxis, and treatment of osteoporosis. Am J Med 1993;94:646–650. Available at: http://www.ncbi.nlm.nih.gov/pubmed/8506892. Accessed February 20, 2010.

2. Assessment of fracture risk and its application to screening for postmenopausal osteoporosis: report of a WHO Study Group. WHO technical report series. Geneva (Switzerland): World Health Organization; 1994. p. 843. Available at: http://www.ncbi.nlm.nih.gov/pubmed/7941614. Accessed February 20, 2010.

3. Quek ST, Peh WCG. Radiology of osteoporosis. Semin Musculoskelet Radiol 2002;6:197–206.

4. Guglielmi G, Muscarella S, Leone A, et al. Imaging of metabolic bone diseases. Radiol Clin North Am 2008;46:703–33.

5. Cooper AP. A treatise on dislocation and fractures of the joints. London: John Churchill; 1842.

6. National Institute of Health, Consensus Panel. Consensus development conference on osteoporosis. JAMA 1984;252:799–802.

7. Wilson JS, Genant HK. In vivo assessment of bone metabolism using the cortical striation index. Invest Radiol 1979;14:131–6.

8. Riggs BL, Wahner HW, Seeman E, et al. Changes in bone mineral density of the proximal femur and spine with aging. J Clin Invest 1982;70:716–23.

9. Lash WL, Nicholson JM, Velez L, et al. Diagnosis and management of osteoporosis. Prim Care Clin Office Pract 2009;36:181–98.

10. Seeman E, Delmas PD. Bone quality—the material and structural basis of bone strength and fragility. N Engl J Med 2006;354:2250–61.

11. McKiernan FE. The broadening spectrum of osteoporotic vertebral fracture. Skeletal Radiol 2009;38: 303–8.

12. Cummings SR, Kelsey JL, Nevitt MC, et al. Epidemiology of osteoporosis and osteoporotic fractures. Epidemiol Rev 1985;7:178–208.

13. Hegeman JH, Oskam J, Van der Palen J, et al. The distal radial fracture in elderly women and the bone mineral density of the lumbar spine and hip. J Hand Surg Br 2004;29:473–6.

14. Bordier PJ, Miravet L, Hioco D. Young adult osteoporosis. Clin Endocrinol Metab 1973;2:277–92.

15. Pacifici R, Rothstein M, Rifas L, et al. Increased monocyte interleukin-1 activity and decreased vertebral bone density in patients with fasting idiopathic hypercalciuria. J Clin Endocrinol Metab 1990;71:138–45.

16. Harms HM, Kaptaina U, Kulpmann WR, et al. Pulse amplitude and frequency modulation of parathyroid hormone in plasma. J Clin Endocrinol Metab 1989;69:843–51.

17. Smith R. Idiopathic osteoporosis in the young. J Bone Joint Surg Br 1980;62:417–27.

18. Riggs BL, Melton LJ III. Involutional osteoporosis. N Engl J Med 1986;314:1676–86.

19. Riggs BL, Melton LJ III. Evidence for two distinct syndromes of involutional osteoporosis. Am J Med 1983;75:889–901.

20. Chapuy MC, Arlot ME, Duboeuf F, et al. Vitamin D3 and calcium to prevent hip fractures in the elderly women. N Engl J Med 1992;327:1637–42.

21. Consensus development statement. Who are candidates for prevention and treatment for osteoporosis? Osteoporos Int 1997;7:1–6. Available at: http://www.springerlink.com/content/q8757186x4765151/. Accessed February 20, 2010.

22. Melton LJ 3rd. Perspectives. How many women have osteoporosis now? J Bone Miner Res 1995;10:175–7.

23. Melton LJ 3rd, Crowson CS, O'Fallon WM. Fracture incidence in Olmsted County, Minnesota: comparison of urban with rural rates and changes in urban rates over time. Osteoporos Int 1999;9:29–37.

24. Kanis JA. Diagnosis of osteoporosis and assessment of fracture risk. Lancet 2002;359(9321):1929.

25. Cummings SR, Melton LJ. Epidemiology and outcomes of osteoporotic fractures. Lancet 2002; 359(9319):1761.

26. Johnell O, Kanis JA. An estimate of the worldwide prevalence and disability associated with osteoporotic fractures. Osteoporos Int 2006;17:1726–33.

27. Kanis JA, Delmas P, Burckhardt P, et al. Guidelines for diagnosis and management of osteoporosis. The European Foundation for Osteoporosis and Bone Disease. Osteoporos Int 1997;7:390–406.

28. Delmas PD. Clinical potential of RANKL inhibition for the management of postmenopausal osteoporosis and other metabolic bone diseases. J Clin Densitom 2008;11:325–38.

29. Cooper C. Epidemiology of osteoporosis. Osteoporos Int 1999;9(Suppl 2):S2–8.

30. Wainwright SA, Biggs WD, Currey JD, et al. Mechanical design in organisms. Princeton (NJ): Princeton University Press; 1982. p. 1–436.

31. Yeni YN, Brown CU, Wang Z, et al. The influence of bone morphology on fracture toughness of the human femur and tibia. Bone 1997;21:453–9.

32. Nicholas JA, Saville PD, Bronner F. Osteoporosis, osteomalacia, and the skeletal system. J Bone Joint Surg Am 1963;45:391–405.

33. Mora S, Gilsanz V. Establishment of peak bone mass. Endocrinol Metab Clin North Am 2003;32: 39–63.

34. Ravn P, Cizza G, Bjarnason NH, et al. Low body mass index is an important risk factor for low bone mass and increased bone loss in early postmenopausal women. Early Postmenopausal Intervention Cohort (EPIC) study group. J Bone Miner Res 1999;14:1622–7.

35. Klotzbuecher CM, Ross PD, Landsman PB, et al. Patients with prior fractures have an increased risk of future fractures: a summary of the literature and statistical synthesis. J Bone Miner Res 2000; 15:721–39.

36. Lindsay R, Silverman SL, Cooper C, et al. Risk of new vertebral fracture in the year following a fracture. JAMA 2001;285:320–3.

37. National Osteoporosis Foundation. Physician's guide to prevention and treatment of osteoporosis. Washington, DC: National Osteoporosis Foundation; 2003. p. 1–7.

38. Freaney R, McBrinn Y, McKenna MJ. Secondary hyperparathyroidism in elderly people: combined effect of renal insufficiency and vitamin D deficiency. Am J Clin Nutr 1993;58:187–91.

39. Cooper C, Atkinson EJ, Jacobsen SJ, et al. Population-based study of survival after osteoporotic fractures. Am J Epidemiol 1993;137:1001–5.

40. Targownik LE, Lix LM, Metge CJ, et al. Use of proton pump inhibitors and risk of osteoporosis-related fractures. CMAJ 2008;179:319–26.

41. Ramsey-Goldman R, Dunn JE, Dunlop DD, et al. Increased risk of fracture in patients receiving solid organ transplants. J Bone Miner Res 1999; 14:456–63.

42. Rehman MT, Hoyland JA, Denton J, et al. Histomorphometric classification of postmenopausal osteoporosis: implications for the management of osteoporosis. J Clin Pathol 1995;48:229–35.

43. Kann PH, Pfützner A, Delling G, et al. Transiliac bone biopsy in osteoporosis: frequency, indications, consequences and complications. An evaluation of 99 consecutive cases over a period of 14 years. Clin Rheumatol 2005;25:30–4.

44. Garnero P. Biomarkers for osteoporosis management: utility in diagnosis, fracture risk prediction and therapy monitoring. Mol Diagn Ther 2008;12: 157–70.

45. Davison KS, Kendler D, Ammann P, et al. Assessing fracture risk and effects of osteoporosis drugs: bone mineral density and beyond. Am J Med 2009; 122:992–7.

46. Weinstein RS, Parfitt AM, Marcus R, et al. Effects of raloxifene, hormone replacement therapy, and placebo on bone turnover in postmenopausal women. Osteoporos Int 2003;14:814–22.

47. Fink HA, Milavetz DL, Palermo L, et al. Fracture Intervention Trial Research Group. What proportion of incident radiographic deformities is clinically diagnosed and vice versa? J Bone Miner Res 2005;20:1216–20.

48. Delmas PD, van de Langerijt L, Watts NB, et al. Under-diagnosis of vertebral fractures is a worldwide problem: the IMPACT study. J Bone Miner Res 2005;20:557–63.

49. Gehlbach SH, Bigelow C, Heimisdottir M, et al. Recognition of vertebral fractures in a clinical setting. Osteoporos Int 2000;11:577–82.

50. How fragile is her future? A report investigating the current understanding and management of osteoporosis world-wide. A survey published by IOF (International Osteoporosis Foundation) in 2000. Available at: http://www.iofbonehealth.org/publications/how-fragile-is-her-future.html. Accessed October 23, 2009.

51. Harris WH, Heaney RP. Skeletal renewal and metabolic bone disease. N Engl J Med 1969; 280:303–11.

52. Vogler JB, Kim JH. Metabolic and endocrine diseases of the skeleton. In: Grainger RG, Allison D, Adam A, et al, editors. Diagnostic radiology. A textbook of medical imaging. 4th edition. London: Churchill Livingstone; 2001. p. 1925–65.

53. Wolbarst AB. Dependence of attenuation on atomic number and photon energy. In: Wolbarst AB, editor. Physics of radiology. Norwalk (CT): Appleton and Lange; 1993. p. 113–21.

54. Ardran GM. Bone destruction not demonstrable by radiography. Br J Radiol 1951;24(278):107–9.

55. Grampp S, Steiner E, Imhof H. Radiological diagnosis of osteoporosis. Eur Radiol 1997;7(Suppl 2): S11–9.

56. Genant HK, Heck LL, Lanzl LH, et al. Primary hyperparathyroidism: a comprehensive study of clinical, biochemical, and radiographic manifestations. Radiology 1973;109:513–24.

57. Meunier PJ, S-Bianchi GG, Edouard CM, et al. Bony manifestations of thyrotoxicosis. Orthop Clin North Am 1972;3:745–52.

58. von Meyer H. Die Architektur der Spongiosa [The architecture of the spongiosa]. Reichert und Dubois-Reymonds Archiv 1867;34:615–28 [in German].

59. Link TM, Majumdar S, Grampp S, et al. Imaging of trabecular bone structure in osteoporosis. Eur Radiol 1999;9:1781–8.

60. Benhamou C, Lespessailles E, Jacquet G, et al. Fractal organization of trabecular bone images on calcaneus radiographs. J Bone Miner Res 1994; 9:1909–18.

61. Geraets W, van der Stelt P, Netelenbos C, et al. A new method for automatic recognition of the

radiographic trabecular pattern. J Bone Miner Res 1990;5:227–32.

62. Vernon-Roberts B, Pirie J. Healing trabecular microfractures in the bodies of lumbar vertebrae. Ann Rheum Dis 1973;32:406–12.

63. Cranney A, Jamal SA, Tsang JF, et al. Low bone mineral density and fracture burden in postmenopausal women. CMAJ 2007;177:575–80.

64. van Staa TP, Dennison EM, Leufkens HGM, et al. Epidemiology of fractures in England and Wales. Bone 2001;29:517–22.

65. Johnell O, Kanis JA, Oden A, et al. Fracture risk following an osteoporotic fracture. Osteoporos Int 2004;15:175–9.

66. Atkinson PJ. Variation in trabecular structure of vertebrae with age. Calcif Tissue Res 1967;1: 24–32.

67. Sherman RS, Wilner D. The Roentgen diagnosis of hemangioma of bone. AJR Am J Roentgenol 1961; 86:1146–57.

68. Saville PD. A quantitative approach to simple radiographic diagnosis of osteoporosis: its application to the osteoporosis of rheumatoid arthritis. Arthritis Rheum 1967;10:416–22.

69. Finsen V, Anda S. Accuracy of visually estimated bone mineralization in routine radiographs of the lower extremity. Skeletal Radiol 1988;17:270–5.

70. Ismail AA, Cooper C, Felsenberg D, et al. Number and type of vertebral deformities: epidemiological characteristics and relation to back pain and height loss. Osteoporos Int 1999;9: 206–13.

71. Patel U, Skingle S, Campbell GA, et al. Clinical profile of acute vertebral compression fractures in osteoporosis. Br J Rheumatol 1991;30:418–21.

72. Genant HK, Wu CY, van Kuijk C, et al. Vertebral fracture assessment using a semiquantitative technique. J Bone Miner Res 1993;8:1137–48.

73. Hurxthal LM. Measurement of anterior vertebral compressions and biconcave vertebrae. Am J Roentgenol Radium Ther Nucl Med 1968;103: 635–44.

74. Lunt M, Ismail AA, Felsenberg D, et al. Defining incident vertebral deformities in population studies: a comparison of morphometric criteria. Osteoporos Int 2002;13:809–15.

75. Launidsen KN, De Carvalho A, Andersen AH. Degree of vertebral wedging of the dorso-lumbar spine. Acta Radiol Diagn 1984;25:29–32.

76. Resnick DL. Fish vertebrae. Arthritis Rheum 1982; 25:1073–7.

77. De Smet AA, Robinson RG, Johnson BE, et al. Spinal compression fractures in osteoporotic women: patterns and relationship to hyperkyphosis. Radiology 1988;166:497–500.

78. Grados F, Fechtenbaum J, Flipon E, et al. Radiographic methods for evaluating osteoporotic vertebral fractures. Joint Bone Spine 2009;76: 241–7.

79. Ferrar L, Jiang G, Armbrecht G, et al. Is short vertebral height always an osteoporotic fracture? The Osteoporosis and Ultrasound Study (OPUS). Bone 2007;41:5–12.

80. Dietz GW, Christensen EE. Normal "Cupid's bow" contour of the lower lumbar vertebrae. Radiology 1976;121:577–9.

81. Yochum TR, Wylie J, Green RL. Schmorl's node phenomenon. JNMS 1994;2:19–22.

82. Chan KK, Sartoris DJ, Haghighi P, et al. Cupid's bow contour of the vertebral body: evaluation of pathogenesis with bone densitometry and imaging-histopathologic correlation. Radiology 1997;202:253–6.

83. Cuenod CA, Laredo JD, Chevret S, et al. Acute vertebral collapse due to osteoporosis or malignancy: appearance on unenhanced and gadolinium-enhanced MR images. Radiology 1996;199:541–9.

84. Jung HS, Jee WH, McCauley TR, et al. Discrimination of metastatic from acute osteoporotic compression spinal fractures with MR imaging. Radiographics 2003;23:179–87.

85. Colman UK, Porter BA, Redmond JI, et al. Early diagnosis of spinal metastases by CT and MR studies. J Comput Assist Tomogr 1988;12:423–6.

86. Baur A, Stabler A, Arbogast S, et al. Acute osteoporotic and neoplastic vertebral compression fractures: fluid sign at MR imaging. Radiology 2002; 225:730–5.

87. Laredo JD, Lakhdari K, Bellaiche L, et al. Acute vertebral collapse: CT findings in benign and malignant nontraumatic cases. Radiology 1995; 194:41–8.

88. Madell SH, Freeman LM. Avascular necrosis of bone in Cushing's Syndrome. Radiology 1964;83: 1068–70.

89. Kümmell H. Die rarefizierende Ostitis der Wirbelkörper [The rarefying osteitis of vertebral body]. Deutsche Med 1895;21:180–1 [in German].

90. Resnick D, Niwayama G, Guerra J Jr, et al. Spinal vacuum phenomena: anatomical study and review. Radiology 1981;139:341–8.

91. Malghem J, Maldague B, Labaisse M. Intravertebral vacuum cleft: changes in content after supine positioning. Radiology 1993;187:483–7.

92. McKiernan FE, Faciszewski T, Jensen R. The dynamic mobility of vertebral compression fractures. J Bone Miner Res 2003;18:24–30.

93. Koch JC. The laws of bone architecture. Am J Anat 1917;21:177–298. Available at: http://www3.inter-science.wiley.com/journal/109887566/abstract. Accessed February 20, 2010.

94. Tobin WJ. The internal architecture of the femur and its clinical significance. The upper end. J Bone Joint Surg Am 1955;37:S7–71.

95. Townsley W. The influence of mechanical factors on the development and structure of bone. Am J Phys Anthropol 1948;6:25–39.

96. Singh M, Nagrath AR, Maini MS. Changes in the trabecular pattern of the upper end of femur as an index of osteoporosis. J Bone Joint Surg Am 1970;52(3):457–67.

97. Singh M, Riggs BL, Beabout JW, et al. Femoral trabecular-pattern index for evaluation of spinal osteoporosis. Ann Intern Med 1972;77:63–7.

98. Cheong HW, Peh WCG, Guglielmi G. Imaging of diseases of the axial and peripheral skeleton. Radiol Clin North Am 2008;46:703–33.

99. Greenspan SL, Myers ER, Maitland LA, et al. Trochanteric bone mineral density is associated with type of hip fracture in the elderly. J Bone Miner Res 1994;9:1889–94.

100. Mautalen CA, Vega EM, Einhorn TA. Are the etiologies of cervical and trochanteric hip fractures different. Bone 1996;18:S133–7.

101. Healey JH, Vigorita VJ, Lane JM. The coexistence and characteristics of osteoarthritis and osteoporosis. J Bone Joint Surg Am 1985;67(4):586–92.

102. Rafii M, Mitnick H, Klug J, et al. Insufficiency fracture of the femoral head: MR imaging in three patients. Am J Roentgenol 1997;168:159–63.

103. Yamamoto T, Schneider R, Bullough PG. Insufficiency subchondral fracture of the femoral head. Am J Surg Pathol 2000;24:464–8.

104. Yamamoto T, Bullough PG. Subchondral insufficiency fracture of the femoral head: a differential diagnosis in acute onset of coxarthrosis in the elderly. Arthritis Rheum 1999;42:2719–23.

105. Dijkstra PD, Oudkerk M, Wiggers T. Prediction of pathological subtrochanteric fractures due to metastatic lesions. Arch Orthop Trauma Surg 1997;116:221–4.

106. Daffner RH, Pavlov H. Stress fractures: current concepts. Am J Roentgenol 1992;159:245–52.

107. Ahovuo JA, Kiuru MJ, Visuri T. Fatigue stress fractures of the sacrum: diagnosis with MR imaging. Eur Radiol 2004;14:500–5.

108. Ries T. Detection of osteoporotic sacral fracture with radionuclides. Radiology 1983;146:783–5.

109. De Smet AA, Neff JR. Pubic and sacral insufficiency fractures: clinical course and radiologic findings. AJR Am J Roentgenol 1985;145:601–6.

110. O'Neill TW, Cooper C, Finn JD, et al. Incidence of distal forearm fracture in British men and women. Osteoporos Int 2001;12:555–8.

111. Cooney WP III, Dobyns JH, Linscheid RL. Complications of Colles' fractures. J Bone Joint Surg Am 1980;62:613–9.

112. Palvanen M, Kannus P, Parkkari J, et al. The injury mechanisms of osteoporotic upper extremity fractures among older adults: a controlled study of 287 consecutive patients and their 108 controls. Osteoporos Int 2000;11:822–31.

113. Clinton J, Franta A, Nayak L, et al. Proximal humeral fracture as a risk factor for subsequent hip fractures. J Bone Joint Surg Am 2009;91:503–11.

114. Barnett E, Nordin BEC. The radiological diagnosis of osteoporosis: a new approach. Clin Radiol 1960;11:166–74.

115. Nielsen SP. The metacarpal index revisited: a brief overview. J Clin Densitom 2001;4:199–207.

116. Jhamaria NL, Lal KB, Udawat M, et al. The trabecular pattern of calcaneum as an index of osteoporosis. J Bone Joint Surg Br 1983;65:195–8.

117. Greenspan SL, von Stetten E, Emond SK, et al. Instant vertebral assessment: a noninvasive dual x-ray absorptiometry technique to avoid misclassification and clinical management of osteoporosis. J Clin Densitom 2001;4:373–80.

118. Vokes TJ, Dixon LB, Favus MJ. Clinical utility of dual-energy vertebral assessment (DVA). Osteoporos Int 2003;14:871–8.

119. Schousboe JT, DeBold CR. Reliability and accuracy of vertebral fracture assessment with densitometry compared to radiography in clinical practice. Osteoporos Int 2006;17:281–9.

120. Link TM, Majumdar S. Osteoporosis imaging. Radiol Clin North Am 2003;41:813–39.

121. Guglielmi G, Adams J, Link TM. Quantitative ultrasound in the assessment of skeletal status. Eur Radiol 2009;19:1837–48.

122. Ballon D, Jakubowski A, Gabrilove J, et al. In vivo measurements of bone marrow cellularity using volume- localized proton NMR spectroscopy. Magn Reson Med 1991;19:85–95.

123. Derby K, Kramer DM, Kaufman L. A technique for assessment of bone marrow composition using magnetic resonance phase interference at low field. Magn Reson Med 1993;29:465–9.

124. Ishizaka H, Tomiyoshi K, Matsumoto M. MR quantification of bone marrow cellularity: use of chemical shift misregistration artifact. AJR Am J Roentgenol 1993;160:572–4.

Vertebral Fracture

James F. Griffith, MB BCh BAO, MRCP, FRCR[a],*,
Giuseppe Guglielmi, MD[b,c]

KEYWORDS

- Vertebral fracture • Osteoporosis • Metastases
- Radiography • Magnetic resonance imaging

SIGNIFICANCE OF VERTEBRAL FRACTURE

Vertebral fractures are uncommon in younger years, although their incidence increases considerably in later years with increasing prevalence of low bone mass as a result of osteoporosis. Because osteopenia is much more common than osteoporosis, almost half of all vertebral fractures tend to occur in subjects with osteopenia rather than with osteoporosis, as assessed by T score.[1,2] Nevertheless, the occurrence of a less-traumatic or nontraumatic vertebral fracture in an otherwise healthy individual is indisputable evidence of reduced bone strength, and, in this respect, osteoporosis, irrespective of T-score measurement.

Vertebral fractures provide a significant warning of subsequent osteoporotic fracture, as they tend to occur more frequently and earlier than other osteoporosis-related fractures of the proximal femur, distal radius, and other sites.[3] The presence, severity, and multiplicity of osteoporotic vertebral fracture are important predictors of further vertebral fracture risk. Over an 8-year period, subjects with prevalent (ie, preexisting) vertebral fractures had a 5-fold increased risk of further vertebral fracture and a 3-fold increased risk of proximal femoral fracture.[4] Similarly, during a 4-year period following an incident (ie, new) vertebral fracture, postmenopausal women are 4 times more likely to develop a further vertebral fracture and twice as likely to develop a proximal femoral fracture than those without an incident vertebral fracture.[4] The overall risk of further vertebral fracture is 20% in the year following incident fracture, with relative risk being 4 times greater in those with severe rather than mild fractures and

3 times greater in those with multiple (>3) rather than single vertebral fractures.[5]

Vertebral fractures are associated with a poorer quality of life because of limitation in physical ability and impaired social function, an effect particularly noticeable in patients with more severe fractures, multiple fractures, and lumbar fractures.[6,7] As well as increased morbidity, increased mortality is also associated with vertebral fracture. For example, subjects with incident fracture have a 3-fold increased mortality risk during the ensuing 4 years compared with nonfractured counterparts, particularly because of pulmonary disease and cancer.[8,9]

A clinical scenario therefore exists of patients sustaining an isolated vertebral fracture and going on to develop several new fractures over the ensuing years. This process, referred to as the vertebral fracture cascade, is likely to be multifactorial in origin, related in part to poor bone quality, disordered spine biomechanics, and neuromuscular dysfunction.[10] A vertebral fracture cascade leads to deteriorating physical and psychosocial function, which progressively declines with each new vertebral fracture. The World Health Organization has recognized the clinical importance of vertebral fracture, although defining "severe osteoporosis" as a T score of 2.5 and the presence of an osteoporotic fracture. Recognition is important because subjects with a vertebral fracture and a T score of less than 2.5 appear to be those most likely to benefit from timely antiosteoporotic drug therapy.

Yet, despite the clear undisputed clinical relevance of vertebral fractures, these remain sorely

[a] Department of Diagnostic Radiology and Organ Imaging, Chinese University of Hong Kong, Prince of Wales Hospital, Ngan Shing Street, Shatin, New Territories, Hong Kong
[b] Department of Radiology, University of Foggia, San Giovanni Rotondo, Viale L. Pinto, 71100 Foggia, Italy
[c] Scientific Institute 'Casa Sollievo della Sofferenza' Hospital, San Giovanni Rotondo 71013, Italy
* Corresponding author.
E-mail address: griffith@cuhk.edu.hk

Radiol Clin N Am 48 (2010) 519–529
doi:10.1016/j.rcl.2010.02.012
0033-8389/10/$ – see front matter © 2010 Elsevier Inc. All rights reserved.

underdiagnosed in everyday practice.[11–13] Two main reasons account for this inadequacy. First, vertebral fractures frequently do not present as a clinically recognizable event. Typical symptoms of vertebral fracture are back pain and limitation of movement. Both of these symptoms are common in elderly subjects, and as such, unlike patients with appendicular skeletal fractures, three-quarters of patients with vertebral fractures do not seek medical attention.[13] Improving patient awareness may not necessarily help given that only about one-third of prevalent vertebral fractures on hindsight correspond with a symptomatic period.[14] Second, many radiologically apparent vertebral fractures go unreported. Of patients older than 60 years presenting at emergency departments, about one-sixth had a moderate-to-severe vertebral fracture that was evident on lateral chest radiographs, of which only about one-half were noted on radiology reports and fewer still received specific medical attention.[15] This study probably represents an underestimation of the true vertebral fracture prevalence because mild fractures were not included and lumbar radiographs were not available for analysis.[15]

PREVALENCE OF VERTEBRAL FRACTURE

In a cross-sectional study of more than 15,500 subjects aged 50 to 79 years across Europe, in which all spine radiographs were read at a single center, the prevalence of vertebral fracture ranged from 6% to 21%.[16] As expected, in younger subjects there was a higher prevalence of fracture in men largely related to trauma, although the trend changed in the case of older subjects whereby vertebral fracture was more prevalent in females. In a 4-year longitudinal study of older subjects, the overall yearly incidence of vertebral fracture was 7 in 1000 for men and 12 in 1000 for women. This prevalence was very much age dependent. For example, the yearly incidence of 6 in 1000 for women aged 55 to 57 years increased to 23 in 1000 for women aged 75 to 79 years.[17] White Caucasian women tend to have a higher vertebral fracture rate than Hispanic, African, and Asian women.[18] Vertebral fracture is also more common in subjects with chronic obstructive airways disease, inflammatory bowel disease, diabetes, and chronic rheumatologic disease.

PATHOPHYSIOLOGY OF VERTEBRAL FRACTURE

The vertebral body, similar to the proximal femur and distal radius, has a relatively larger trabecular rather than cortical bone component and largely depends on this trabecular bone for its strength. Because trabecular bone is thin and has a large surface area, it is more responsive to changes in its microenvironment than cortical bone and is the first to be visibly affected in the osteoporotic process. Osteoporotic fractures, therefore, tend to occur in those bone parts, such as the vertebral body, that rely heavily on trabecular bone for their strength. Trabecular bone and density are not evenly distributed throughout the vertebral body. The weakest parts of the vertebral body are found anteriorly and superiorly where lower density is not compensated for by higher trabecular structural architecture.[19] Central trabeculae tend to be about 15% thicker and have fewer free ends than those near the endplates.[19] Although all trabeculae are prone to thinning and eventual perforation during the osteoporotic process, the effect on horizontally and vertically orientated trabeculae is slightly different. With aging, horizontal and probably vertical trabeculae reduce in number, though only horizontal trabeculae reduce in thickness.[20] Finite element modeling analysis has indicated that this differential response may be a result of different mechanisms stimulating the resorption of horizontal and vertical trabeculae, with horizontal trabeculae being reabsorbed preferentially as a result of strain adaptive resorption and vertical trabeculae being reabsorbed as a result of microdamage.[21]

Progressive bone loss reduces the volumetric bone mineral density of the vertebral body to about 20% of normal, whereas vertebral body strength reduces to only about 10% of normal.[22,23] This makes the vertebral body, and particularly its anterosuperior portion, more prone to fracture during everyday off-axial or even axial loading. Depending on the external force applied and inherent vertebral body strength, initial fracture severity may vary from a small incremental fracture to an almost complete vertebral body fracture. This incremental nature of vertebral fractures has been seen histologically in that osteoporotic vertebral fractures frequently demonstrate overlapping of the various fracture healing stages as a result of repeated microfractures being superimposed on prior healing fractures.[24] As the vertebrae and intervertebral discs function very much as an integrated unit, isolated fracture of 1 vertebral body can affect spinal kinetics and loading of adjacent vertebral bodies sufficiently to result in further vertebral fracture.

Increasing vertebral body cross-sectional area reduces fracture risk. The vertebral body cross-sectional area is about 25% greater in men than in women.[25] However, although men have larger bones, these bones are loaded substantially more than the smaller bones of females. Periosteal bone apposition, especially in men, may potentially offset the increased fragility precipitated by reduced bone mass through increasing vertebral body cross-sectional area. Longitudinal volumetric quantitative computed tomography–based study has shown that women, in addition to possessing smaller vertebral bodies and losing bone more rapidly than men, also increase vertebral cross-sectional area more slowly than men, thus potentially predisposing women to increased vertebral fracture risk.[26]

DIAGNOSIS AND AGING OF VERTEBRAL FRACTURE

Although the radiologic diagnosis of a moderate-to-severe vertebral body fracture is straightforward, radiologic assessment of a mild vertebral fracture remains contentious. This difficulty in defining the presence of a mild vertebral fracture is a reflection of several potential pitfalls that are addressed by G Guglielmi and D Diacinti elsewhere in this issue for further exploration of this topic. First, mild anterior or posterior wedging is a normal feature of thoracic and lumbar vertebral bodies (Fig. 1). Second, short vertebral height is a feature of aging and spinal degeneration in the absence of detectable osteoporosis fracture as well as a feature of other spinal disorders such as Scheuermann disease.[27] Third, as opposed to the more "all or none" presentation of

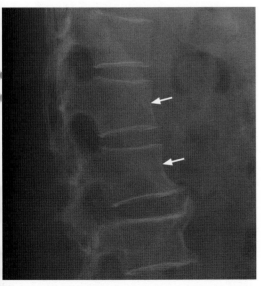

Fig. 1. Lateral radiograph thoracolumbar junction showing mild physiologic anterior wedging of L1 and L2 vertebral bodies (*arrows*). This is a normal appearance not be confused with mild vertebral fracture.

appendicular fracture, vertebral fractures vary considerably in severity, are often incremental in progression (Fig. 2), are often not associated with any discernible radiographic cortical disruption, and often occur in the absence of significant trauma or pain.[28] Fourth, developmental or degenerative scoliosis may lead to radiographic obliquity and side-to-side discrepancy in vertebral body height (Fig. 3). All of these potential pitfalls can usually be sorted out quite adequately by an experienced reader. The current best standard for clinical practice and cross-sectional studies is to use a semiquantitative method of fracture analysis by an experienced reader using standardized radiographs or morphometric x-ray absorptiometry supported by radiographic assessment. Vertebral fracture should be diagnosed when there is greater than 20% loss in vertebral body height compared with an expected normal height for that particular vertebral body (see Fig. 2). True reduction in vertebral body height can only be established on longitudinal follow-up, and as such quantitative morphometric radiography is best undertaken in longitudinal studies supported by semiquantitative radiographic analysis.

As many vertebral fractures are clinically silent, radiologists are best positioned to screen for vertebral fractures.[12] It is imperative that radiologists unambiguously report vertebral "fracture" if present and avoid the unqualified use of more ambiguous terms such as collapse, compression, loss of height, wedging, or wedge deformity in radiology reports. This is also relevant nowadays in the reporting of multidetector computed tomographic (CT) studies of the thorax or abdomen whereby important information regarding the presence of vertebral fracture may be overlooked (Fig. 4). In one such study of male and female subjects older than 55 years undergoing thoracic CT, one-fifth had a moderate or severe thoracic vertebral fracture, although less then one-fifth of these fractures were mentioned in the radiologic report.[29] If diagnosis of a vertebral fracture is in doubt, one should review prior imaging studies, seek a more experienced opinion or, if indicated, proceed to additional imaging such as magnetic resonance (MR) imaging.

Determining the age of a vertebral fracture is sometimes difficult on radiographs in the absence of previous studies. Lack of cortical disruption, the presence of comparable density to adjacent vertebral bodies, and remodeling change such as marginal hyperostosis can favor an old fracture, although often these features may not be present. The best guide to the age of a fracture is the presence of marrow edema on fat-suppressed MR imaging. The presence of marrow edema on

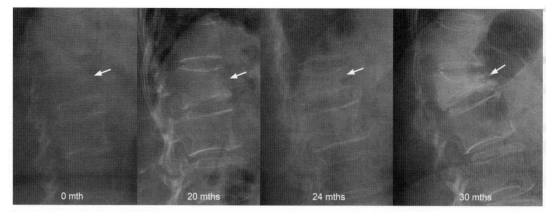

Fig. 2. Lateral radiographs thoracolumbar region showing incremental fracture of T12 vertebral body. Radiographs are obtained at baseline and at 20, 24, and 30 months postbaseline. No fracture is present at baseline (*arrow*), a mild (>20% loss of height) vertebral fracture is present at 20 months (*arrow*), a moderate (>25% loss of height) vertebral fracture is present at 24 months (*arrow*), and a severe (>40% loss of height) vertebral fracture is present at 30 months (*arrow*).

sagittal T2-weighted fat-suppressed MR images is a reliable guide as to the presence of a recent vertebral fracture (**Figs. 5** and **6**). The degree of marrow edema is a reflection of both severity and duration of fracture. Conversely, vertebral fractures that lack marrow edema are not recent fractures, are not likely to respond to percutaneous vertebroplasty, and unlikely to be the cause of patient symptoms.

DIFFERENTIATING OSTEOPOROTIC FROM NONOSTEOPOROTIC NEOPLASTIC FRACTURE

In the acute stage, the marrow cavity of the fractured osteoporotic vertebral body is filled with blood and fluid. This is gradually replaced by a variable degree of granulation tissue and fibroblastic tissue. This reparative tissue is over time reabsorbed, with restoration of normal fatty marrow. It is thus not difficult usually to differentiate a chronic osteoporotic vertebral fracture filled with fatty marrow from a pathologic neoplastic

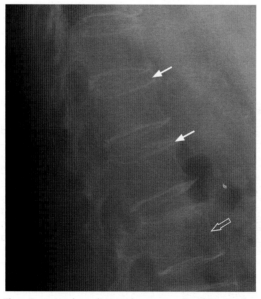

Fig. 3. Lateral radiograph upper lumbar region showing mild obliquity of L1 and L2 vertebral bodies. The superior (*arrows*) and inferior endplates are oval. Diagnosis of mild fracture is more difficult in this setting. There is mild (approximately 15%) loss of height anteriorly of the L3 vertebral body (*open arrow*). This is not of sufficient severity to deem this a fracture.

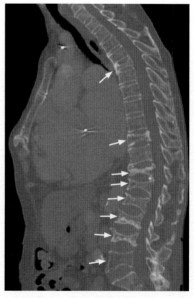

Fig. 4. Sagittal reconstruction of spine in a 64-year-old woman undergoing thoracoabdominal CT examination for abdominal pain. Many severe osteoporotic-type fractures are present in the thoracic and lumbar regions (*arrows*).

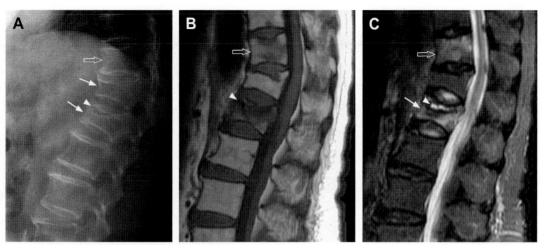

Fig. 5. (A) Lateral radiograph of thoracolumbar region. Moderate fractures of T12 and L1 vertebral bodies (arrows) with a cleft of intravertebral gas in L1 (arrowhead). There is no fracture of T12 (open arrow). (B) T1-weighed sagittal MR image of same region shows osteoporotic-type fractures of T12 and L1 vertebral bodies with fracture of superior endplate of L1 (arrow) and unsuspected fracture T11. (C) T2-weighted fat-suppressed sagittal image shows edema in T11 and L1 vertebral bodies consistent with recent fracture. The T12 vertebral fracture is not recent. Note cleft of fluid in L1 vertebral body (arrowhead) corresponding to gas seen at the same location in (A).

fracture. Difficultly arises when differentiating acute or subacute osteoporotic fracture from neoplastic fracture. The spine is the most common site of skeletal metastases as well as osteoporotic fracture, and both occur in middle-aged and elderly subjects. Up to one-third of vertebral fractures in patients with known malignancies are due to osteoporosis and not malignancy.[30]

Box 1 outlines the most helpful imaging features that are used to make the distinction between osteoporotic and neoplastic fractures. A combination of these signs should be applied when making this distinction, with suitable weighting given to their relative discriminatory power as outlined in **Box 1**. Convexity or bulging of the posterior vertebral cortex on MR or CT imaging is not that useful a discriminatory sign. Although posterior cortical convexity is more common with neoplastic infiltration, it can also be a feature of about 20% of osteoporotic vertebral fractures.[31,32] Lack of pedicle

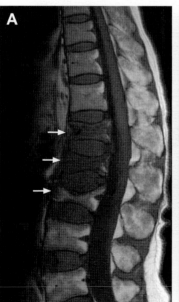

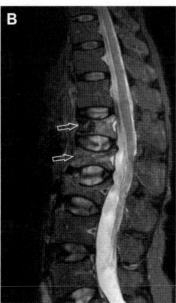

Fig. 6. (A) T1-weighted sagittal images showing severe osteoporotic-type fractures of L1, L2, and L3 vertebral bodies. Note preservation of some fat signal within the vertebral bodies (arrows). (B) T2-weighted fat-suppressed sagittal image shows that only the L1 and L2 fractures are recent with marrow edema (open arrows). Note expansion and edema of intervertebral discs.

Box 1
Useful imaging signs that help distinguish osteoporotic from neoplastic vertebral fracture

1. Preservation of some marrow fat signal within marrow[a] (see **Figs. 5** and **6**).
2. Signal alternation confined to vertebral body with no involvement of pedicles or posterior elements[a] (see **Fig. 8**)
3. Fluid or gas within vertebral body[b] (see **Figs. 5, 8** and **10**)
4. T1-hypointense line within vertebral body (commonly adjacent to fractured endplate) representing primary fracture line[b] (see **Figs. 8** and **11**).
5. Lack of discrete soft tissue mass[a]
6. Minimal or absent paravertebral soft tissue swelling[b]
7. Absence of epidural mass[b]
8. Fracture not involving cervical or upper thoracic (T1-T5) vertebral bodies[a]
9. Posterior located triangular bone area or fracture fragment[c] (**Fig. 7**)
10. Nonconvex posterior cortical border[c]
11. Evidence of metastases elsewhere in spine[c]
12. Near complete fatty marrow of adjacent vertebrae[c]
13. Radiographic evidence of osteopenia[c]
14. Preservation of trabeculae within fractured vertebral body on CT[a]

A known history of malignancy is moderately helpful. If doubt still exists after standard MR imaging, one can proceed to diffusion-weighted imaging or chemical shift imaging.
  [a] Most useful sign.
  [b] Less useful sign.
  [c] Least useful sign.

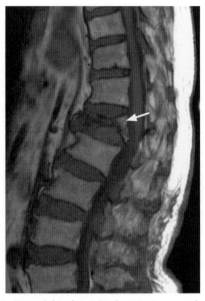

Fig. 7. T1-weighted sagittal MR image showing typical osteoporotic-type fracture of T12 vertebral body with preservation of some marrow fat and triangular area of bone posteriorly (*arrow*).

involvement on MR imaging is usually good evidence of benignity (**Figs. 8** and **9**), although very occasionally pedicle edema can occur in an osteoporotic fracture if fracture extension into a pedicle has occurred.[33] Fluid within the vertebral bone on MR imaging is a helpful sign of osteoporotic fracture, being a feature of about 40% of osteoporotic fractures, although it may also be seen in a small percentage (6%) of neoplastic

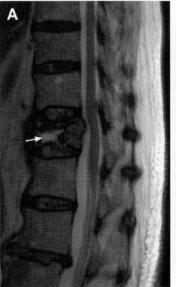
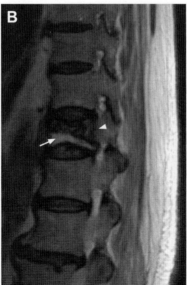

Fig. 8. Central (*A*) and paracentral (*B*) T2-weighted images of the lumbar spine showing a severe osteoporotic fracture of the L2 vertebral body. There is a large fluid-filled cleft centrally and adjacent to the endplates (*arrows*). Note the abrupt transition in signal intensity at the body-pedicle interface (*arrowhead*) often seen in osteoporotic fracture.

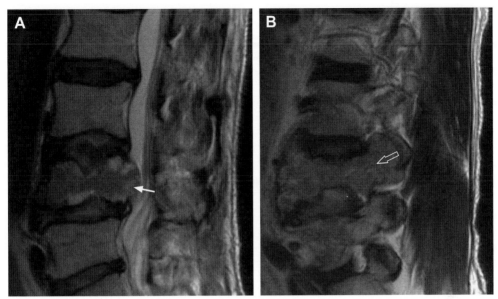

Fig. 9. T2-weighed sagittal (*A*) and parasagittal (*B*) images of lumbar spine showing mild vertebral fracture with metastatic tumor bulging posterior aspect of cortex (*arrow*) and extending into pedicle (*open arrow*). Primary tumor was a carcinoma of lung.

fractures (see **Figs. 5** and **8**).[34] Fluid normally accumulates in a cavity space located anteriorly or adjacent to the endplates of a severely fractured vertebral body and is akin to the vacuum cleft seen occasionally on radiographs (see **Fig. 5**; **Fig. 10**), although it is much more commonly seen on CT. Gas within a vacuum cleft arises from compression/decompression forces leading to the release of nitrogen.[34] Intravertebral gas is generated by flexing or extending the spine, although it is replaced by fluid on resting supine for about 15 minutes (as for MR imaging examination).[34]

Hence, intrabody fluid on MR imaging and intrabody gas on radiographs reflect the same pathology. Both are indicative of a medium-to-large cavity within the vertebral body and thereby quite good evidence that a vertebral body is not filled with neoplastic or other tissue. A standard MR protocol for vertebral fracture assessment should include a (1) T1-weighted sagittal sequence mainly to assess fracture morphology and visibility of marrow fat, (2) T2-weighted fat-suppressed sagittal sequence mainly to assess marrow edema and fluid, and (3) T2-

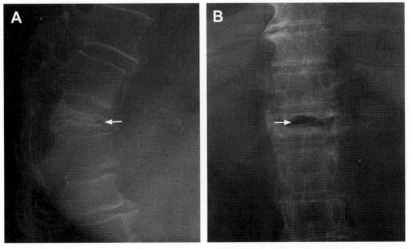

Fig. 10. Lateral (*A*) and anteroposterior (*B*) radiographs of thoracolumbar region showing severe fracture of T12 vertebral body with large intravertebral cleft filled with gas (*arrows*) due to intravertebral vacuum phenomenon.

weighed axial image to assess vertebral and paravertebral soft tissues. If doubt still exists as to the likely cause of fracture, standard MR imaging can be supplemented with diffusion-weighted imaging (DWI) or chemical shift imaging. Intravenous contrast is not generally helpful in differentiating between osteoporotic and neoplastic vertebral fractures. Acute osteoporotic vertebral fractures often enhance quite vividly while reparative tissue in subacute osteoporotic fractures also enhances (**Fig. 11**).

Several studies that have been undertaken to determine the value of diffusion-weighted MR imaging in differentiating osteoporotic from neoplastic vertebral fracture have recently been reviewed.[35,36] DWI is sensitive to water molecule movement, with random motion of water molecules within a varying gradient field resulting in phase dispersion and, as a result, signal attenuation. Extracellular fluid has a much greater capacity to diffuse than intracellular fluid.[37] As osteoporotic fractures contain more extracellular free fluid, they are more prone to signal loss than neoplastic fracture. Osteoporotic fractures tend to become hypointense relative to adjacent vertebrae on DWI (**Fig. 12**).[35,36] Conversely, neoplastic fractures with a higher cellularity and a smaller extracellular fluid component than osteoporotic fractures sustain less signal loss on DWI. Neoplastic fractures tend to become hyperintense relative to adjacent vertebrae on DWI.[35,36]

Fluid-rich tissues with long T2 relaxation time accentuate T2-weighting, which may result in T2 relaxation effects masking the contrast images of DWI. This effect is known as "T2 shine-through." T2 shine-through is prone to occur in osteoporotic fracture and may lead to the fracture appearing hyperintense rather than hypointense on DWI. To help overcome this effect, a quantitative measure of the diffusivity of water molecules within the tissues being studied is applied, known as the apparent diffusion coefficient (ADC). Across independent studies from different institutions, osteoporotic fractures tend to fairly consistently have an ADC value of greater than 1.0×10^{-3} mm^2/s, whereas neoplastic fractures tend to have an ADC value of less than 1.0×10^{-3} mm^2/s.[38–40] DWI overall is considered to be very helpful in the differentiation of vertebral fracture and is a useful adjunct to standard MR imaging if the diagnosis is in doubt.

Chemical shift MR imaging can also be used to differentiate osteoporotic and neoplastic vertebral fracture.[41,42] This technique, also known as in-phase and out-of-phase imaging or opposed-phase imaging, is sensitive in the detection of fat within tissue and is useful in differentiating between malignant and benign lesions. The principle of this technique is based on neoplastic processes replacing the fatty marrow component of the vertebral body, leading to a change in out-of-phase imaging. In general, osteoporotic fractures exhibit a significant signal drop on out-of-phase images and appear hypointense relative to in-phase images, whereas neoplastic lesions show insignificant signal drop on out-of-phase

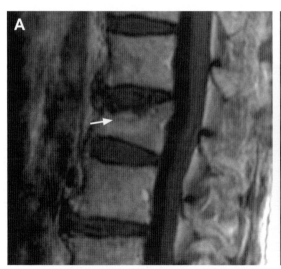
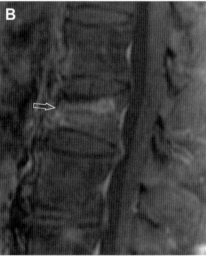

Fig. 11. (*A*) T1-weighted sagittal MR image showing moderate osteoporotic-type anterior wedge fracture of the L1 vertebral body with hypointense fracture line (*arrow*). (*B*) Contrast-enhanced T1-weighted fat-suppressed sagittal MR image showing moderate enhancement of the anterior aspect of the vertebral body due to fracture repair (*open arrow*). This could be wrongly interpreted as being caused by an infiltrative process. Intravenous contrast is generally not helpful in the assessment of vertebral fracture.

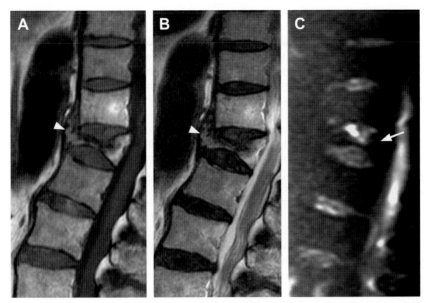

Fig. 12. T1-weighted (*A*), T2-weighted (*B*), and DWI sagittal MR (*C*) images of lumbar spine. Standard images show a severe osteoporotic-type fracture of L1 vertebral body (*arrowheads*). This is supported by DWI, which shows hypointense signal within vertebral body (*arrow*).

images. Quantifying the degree of signal drop on out-of-phase images is necessary to improve the diagnostic accuracy of this technique. Zajick and colleagues[41] proposed a decrease in signal intensity of greater than 20% on out-of-phase images compared with in-phase images as an indictor of osteoporotic fracture. A more recent study proposed a signal drop of greater than 35% on out-of-phase images compared with in-phase images as a threshold value to differentiate osteoporotic from neoplastic vertebral fracture.[42] Using this threshold, the positive predictive value was 100% and the negative predictive value was 95%. Overall, one can usually distinguish accurately between osteoporotic and neoplastic vertebral fracture on imaging (radiography, CT, MR imaging supplemented when necessary by DWI or chemical shift imaging) without the need for percutaneous biopsy.

FDG PET (fluorodeoxyglucose positron emission tomography) imaging can also be helpful in differentiating osteoporotic from neoplastic vertebral fracture if MR imaging or CT findings are equivocal or if there is a contraindication to MR imaging examination (**Fig. 13**). As expected, a higher radioactive uptake is seen in neoplastic

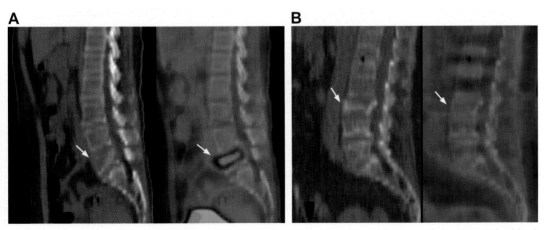

Fig. 13. Sagittal FDG PET-CT images of lumbar spine. (*A*) Severe osteoporotic fracture of the L3 vertebral body with no increased tracer activity at this level. (*B*) Mild metastatic fracture of L5 vertebral body with increased tracer activity at this level. Primary tumor was breast carcinoma.

vertebral fractures (standardized uptake value, 2.2–7.1; mean, 3.99 ± 1.52 [standard deviation]) than in osteoporotic fractures (standardized uptake value, 0.7–4.9; mean, 1.94 ± 0.97).[43] False-positive FDG-PET cases (with benign tumor being incorrectly identified as malignant) may be accentuated by treatment with bone marrow stimulation agents, whereas false-negative cases may occur when metastatic disease is not associated with a high tracer uptake.[43] Preliminary study indicates that the positive predictive value of FDG-PET for detecting malignant vertebral fracture is 71% and the negative predictive value is 91%.[43]

SUMMARY

In conclusion, vertebral fractures are an early manifestation of osteoporosis and when occurring with minimal or no trauma provide indisputable evidence of decreased bone strength irrespective of bone mineral density measurement. Vertebral fractures are often underdiagnosed because they are usually clinically silent and frequently go unreported on radiographs or CT. The recognition of vertebral fracture is important because it provides a warning of further vertebral and nonvertebral osteoporotic fracture and this fracture occurs in a patient group that may benefit from timely anti-osteoporotic treatment. Distinction between osteoporotic and nonosteoporotic vertebral fracture can usually be made accurately on imaging grounds alone without having to resort to percutaneous biopsy.

REFERENCES

1. Siris ES, Miller PD, Barrett-Connor E, et al. Identification and fracture outcomes of undiagnosed low bone mineral density in postmenopausal women: results from the National Osteoporosis Risk Assessment. JAMA 2001;286:2815–22.
2. Sanders KM, Nicholson GC, Watts JJ, et al. Half the burden of fragility fractures in the community occur in women without osteoporosis. When is fracture prevention cost-effective? Bone 2006;38:694–700.
3. Meunier PJ, Delmas PD, Eastell R, et al. Diagnosis and management of osteoporosis in postmenopausal women: clinical guidelines. International Committee for Osteoporosis Clinical Guidelines. Clin Ther 1999;21(6):1025–44.
4. Black DM, Arden NK, Palermo L, et al. Prevalent vertebral deformities predict hip fractures and new vertebral deformities but not wrist fractures. Study of Osteoporotic Fractures Research Group. J Bone Miner Res 1999;14(5):821–8.
5. Lindsay R, Silverman SL, Cooper C, et al. Risk of new vertebral fracture in the year following a fracture. JAMA 2001;285(3):320–3.
6. Lips P, van Schoor NM. Quality of life in patients with osteoporosis. Osteoporos Int 2005;16(5):447–55.
7. Fechtenbaum J, Cropet C, Kolta S, et al. The severity of vertebral fractures and health-related quality of life in osteoporotic postmenopausal women. Osteoporos Int 2005;16(12):2175–9.
8. Kado DM, Browner WS, Palermo L, et al. Vertebral fractures and mortality in older women: a prospective study. Study of Osteoporotic Fractures Research Group. Arch Intern Med 1999;159(11):1215–20.
9. Kado DM, Duong T, Stone KL, et al. Incident vertebral fractures and mortality in older women: a prospective study. Osteoporos Int 2003;14(7):589–94.
10. Briggs AM, Greig AM, Wark JD. The vertebral fracture cascade in osteoporosis: a review of aetiopathogenesis. Osteoporos Int 2007;18(5):575–84.
11. Delmas PD, van de Langerijt L, Watts NB, et al. Underdiagnosis of vertebral fractures is a worldwide problem: the IMPACT study. J Bone Miner Res 2005;20(4):557–63.
12. Lenchik L, Rogers LF, Delmas PD, et al. Diagnosis of osteoporotic vertebral fractures: importance of recognition and description by radiologists. AJR Am J Roentgenol 2004;183(4):949–58.
13. Grigoryan M, Guermazi A, Roemer FW, et al. Recognizing and reporting osteoporotic vertebral fractures. Eur Spine J 2003;12(2):S104–12.
14. Cooper C, Atkinson EJ, O'Fallon WM, et al. Incidence of clinically diagnosed vertebral fractures: a population-based study in Rochester, Minnesota, 1985–1989. J Bone Miner Res 1992;7(2):221–7.
15. Gehlbach SH, Bigelow C, Heimisdottir M, et al. Recognition of vertebral fracture in a clinical setting. Osteoporos Int 2000;11(7):577–82.
16. O'Neill TW, Felsenberg D, Varlow J, et al. The prevalence of vertebral deformity in European men and women: the European Vertebral Osteoporosis Study. J Bone Miner Res 1996;11(7):1010–8.
17. van der Klift M, de Laet CE, McCloskey EV, et al. Risk factors for incident vertebral fractures in men and women: the Rotterdam Study. J Bone Miner Res 2004;19(7):1172–80.
18. Barrett-Connor E, Siris ES, Wehren LE, et al. Osteoporosis and fracture risk in women of different ethnic groups. J Bone Miner Res 2005;20(2):185–94.
19. Banse X, Devogelaer JP, Grynpas M. Patient-specific microarchitecture of vertebral cancellous bone: a peripheral quantitative computed tomographic and histological study. Bone 2002;30(6):829–35.
20. Thomsen JS, Ebbesen EN, Mosekilde LI. Age-related differences between thinning of horizontal and vertical trabeculae in human lumbar bone as

assessed by a new computerized method. Bone 2002;31(1):136–42.

21. Mc Donnell P, Harrison N, Liebschner MA, et al. Simulation of vertebral trabecular bone loss using voxel finite element analysis. J Biomech 2009; 42(16):2789–96.

22. Ito M, Ikeda K, Nishiguchi M, et al. Multi-detector row CT imaging of vertebral microstructure for evaluation of fracture risk. J Bone Miner Res 2005; 20(10):1828–36.

23. Frost HM. The pathomechanics of osteoporoses. Clin Orthop Relat Res 1985;200:198–225.

24. Diamond TH, Clark WA, Kumar SV. Histomorphometric analysis of fracture healing cascade in acute osteoporotic vertebral body fractures. Bone 2007; 40(3):775–80.

25. Ebbesen EN, Thomsen JS, Beck-Nielsen H, et al. Age- and gender-related differences in vertebral bone mass, density, and strength. J Bone Miner Res 1999;14(8):1394–403.

26. Riggs B, Melton Iii L, Robb R, et al. Population-based study of age and sex differences in bone volumetric density, size, geometry, and structure at different skeletal sites. J Bone Miner Res 2004; 19(12):1945–54.

27. Ferrar L, Jiang G, Armbrecht G, et al. Is short vertebral height always an osteoporotic fracture? The Osteoporosis and Ultrasound Study (OPUS). Bone 2007;41(1):5–12.

28. Grados F, Roux C, de Vernejoul MC, et al. Comparison of four morphometric definitions and a semiquantitative consensus reading for assessing prevalent vertebral fractures. Osteoporos Int 2001; 12(9):716–22.

29. Williams AL, Al-Busaidi A, Sparrow PJ, et al. Underreporting of osteoporotic vertebral fractures on computed tomography. Eur J Radiol 2009;69(1): 179–83.

30. Fornasier VL, Czitrom AA. Collapsed vertebrae: a review of 659 autopsies. Clin Orthop Relat Res 1978;131:261–5.

31. Baur A, Stäbler A, Arbogast S, et al. Acute osteoporotic and neoplastic vertebral compression fractures: fluid sign at MR imaging. Radiology 2002;225(3):730–5.

32. Moulopoulos LA, Yoshimitsu K, Johnston DA, et al. MR prediction of benign and malignant vertebral compression fractures. J Magn Reson Imaging 1996;6(4):667–74.

33. Shih TT, Huang KM, Li YW. Solitary vertebral collapse: distinction between benign and malignant causes using MR patterns. J Magn Reson Imaging 1999;9(5):635–42.

34. Malghem J, Maldague B, Labaisse MA, et al. Intravertebral vacuum cleft: changes in content after supine positioning. Radiology 1993;187(2):483–7.

35. Karchevsky M, Babb JS, Schweitzer ME. Can diffusion-weighted imaging be used to differentiate benign from pathologic fractures? A meta-analysis. Skeletal Radiol 2008;37(9):791–5.

36. Raya JG, Dietrich O, Reiser MF, et al. Methods and applications of diffusion imaging of vertebral bone marrow. J Magn Reson Imaging 2006;24(6): 1207–20.

37. Zhou XJ, Leeds NE, McKinnon GC, et al. Characterization of benign and metastatic vertebral compression fractures with quantitative diffusion MR imaging. AJNR Am J Neuroradiol 2002;23(1): 165–70.

38. Balliu E, Vilanova JC, Peláez I, et al. Diagnostic value of apparent diffusion coefficients to differentiate benign from malignant vertebral bone marrow lesions. Eur J Radiol 2009;69(3):560–6.

39. Tang G, Liu Y, Li W, et al. Optimization of b value in diffusion-weighted MRI for the differential diagnosis of benign and malignant vertebral fractures. Skeletal Radiol 2007;36(11):1035–41.

40. Chan JH, Peh WC, Tsui EY, et al. Acute vertebral body compression fractures: discrimination between benign and malignant causes using apparent diffusion coefficients. Br J Radiol 2002; 75(891):207–14.

41. Zajick DC Jr, Morrison WB, Schweitzer ME, et al. Benign and malignant processes: normal values and differentiation with chemical shift MR imaging in vertebral marrow. Radiology 2005;237(2):590–6.

42. Ragab Y, Emad Y, Gheita T, et al. Differentiation of osteoporotic and neoplastic vertebral fractures by chemical shift {in-phase and out-of phase} MR imaging. Eur J Radiol 2009;72(1):125–33.

43. Bredella MA, Essary B, Torriani M, et al. Use of FDG-PET in differentiating benign from malignant compression fractures. Skeletal Radiol 2008;37(5): 405–13.

Radiogrammetry and Radiographic Absorptiometry

Judith E. Adams, MBBS, FRCR, FRCP, FBIR[a,b,*]

KEYWORDS

• Metacarpal index • Osteoporosis • Morphometry
• Radiogrammetry • Digital x-ray radiogrammetry

RADIOGRAPHIC ABSORPTIOMETRY

The photographic density of a bone on a radiograph is approximately proportional to the mass of bone located in the x-ray beam. This was the basis of the oldest quantitative method for measurement of integral (cortical and trabecular) bone mineral density (BMD) in vivo radiographic absorptiometry (RA).[1] The method involved obtaining a radiograph of a peripheral skeleton site (eg, metacarpals, phalanges, radius, ulna, femur, and tibia) simultaneously with a reference step wedge made from an aluminum alloy or hydroxyapatite that has an effective atomic number similar to that of bone (**Fig. 1**). After film processing, the bone and reference step wedge were then evaluated on the radiograph for optical densities with a photodensitometer and BMD expressed as equivalents of step wedge material.[2–4] The method was applied most commonly to the metacarpals and phalanges. The accuracy and precision (coefficient variation [CV]), of RA were reported to be 6% and 1% to 5% respectively.[5,6] With technical advances and automated computer application, precision was reported to improve to 1% to 3.5%.[7–9] RA was found to have similar accuracy, precision, and correlations (r = 0.58–0.9) to more recently developed standard techniques (dual- and single-energy x-ray absorptiometry [DXA/SXA]). RA measurements also predicted low bone mass of the lumbar spine and femoral neck with 90% and 82% sensitivity, respectively.[10,11] The technique was applied in the first National Health and Nutrition Examination Survey Epidemiologic Follow-up Study cohort, in which subjects were followed-up for a maximum of 16 years. RA was a significant predictor of future hip fracture risk (relative risk = 1.8).[12]

RA, however, was labor intensive and operator dependent[11]; was limited by differences in x-ray beam intensity, variable soft tissue thickness, and tissue attenuation coefficients[6,11,13–15]; and was applicable only to peripheral skeletal sites. As a consequence, single-photon absorptiometry was introduced in 1963[14] and displaced RA, although the potential for RA was revived with the advent of computerized image processing.[11]

RADIOGRAPHIC MORPHOMETRY

Methods have been used to standardize skeletal measurements of cortical thickness (CT) (radiogrammetry), trabecular pattern (Singh index) and vertebral deformity (morphometry) from radiographs.

RADIOGRAMMETRY—HISTORICAL ASPECTS

Radiogrammetry was introduced in 1960 and is a quantitative method for assessing cortical bone geometry in tubular bones, in which measurements are made from radiographs with a ruler or, preferably, with fine vernier needle calipers.[16–18] Radiogrammetry has been applied to various

[a] Manchester Royal Infirmary, Central Manchester Universities Hospitals NHS Foundation Trust, Oxford Road, Manchester M13 9WL, UK
[b] Imaging Science and Biomedical Engineering, Stopford Building, Oxford Road, University of Manchester, Manchester M13 9PT, UK
* Manchester Royal Infirmary, Central Manchester Universities Hospitals NHS Foundation Trust, Oxford Road, Manchester M13 9WL, UK.
E-mail address: judith.adams@manchester.ac.uk

Radiol Clin N Am 48 (2010) 531–540
doi:10.1016/j.rcl.2010.03.006
0033-8389/10/$ – see front matter © 2010 Elsevier Inc. All rights reserved.

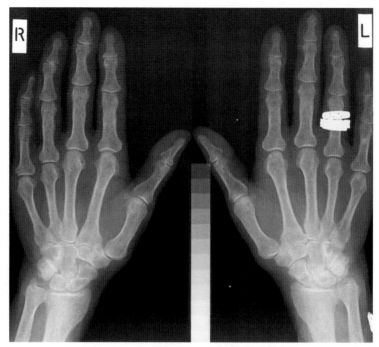

Fig. 1. Radiogrammetry: PA radiograph of the hands, together with an aluminum step wedge. After film processing, the bone and reference step wedge were evaluated on the radiograph for optical densities with a photodensitometer and BMD expressed as equivalents of step wedge material.

bones, including the radius, humerus, clavicle, tibia, and femur. The site to which the method has been most commonly applied, however, is the second metacarpal of the nondominant hand on a posteroanterior (PA) radiograph. Radiogrammetry was, therefore, widely available, inexpensive, and involved a very low dose of ionizing radiation (effective dose equivalent 0.05 to 0.17 microsieverts [μSv]). This equates to less than 1 hour of natural background radiation (2400 μSv per annum; 7 μSv per day),[19,20] so carries negligible risk. Radiographs should be taken with a standardized film focus distance (100 cm) and in longitudinal studies the x-ray equipment, image capture medium, and exposure factors need to be kept consistent.

Measurements

The length of the metacarpal is measured and the midshaft position is identified. At this site, the diaphyseal diameter of the bone (from each periosteal surface) and the medullary cavities (distance between endosteal surfaces) are measured using calipers. A variety of measures and indices have been described, including bone width (BW), CT, medullary width (MW), hand score (HS), metacarpal index (MCI), and

parameters of areal cortical BMD (BMD_a) (g/cm^2) (**Fig. 2**).[21,22]

Calculations

CT = BM − MW
MCI = BW − MW/BW
HS = MCI × 100%

Barnett and Nordin[16] described the MCI and HS in which the sum of the CTs of the radial and ulna side of the second metacarpal, which behave differently metabolically,[23] is divided by the outer diameter width (BW) of the bone, expressed as a ratio or as a percentage.

The cortical area (CA) is calculated assuming that the bone is a cylinder[18,24–26]:

CA = π/4 ($BW^2 - MW^2$)
Percentage CA = $BW^2 - MW^2/BW^2$ × 100
Garn index = $BW^2 - MW^2/BW^2$

Additionally, some measures used bone length (BL) to account for skeletal size, which is pertinent in studies in growing children[27–29]:

CA/surface area (CA/SA) = CA/π × BW × BL or
CA/SA = $BW^2 - MW^2/4L$ × BW

A variation on CA/SA, the Exton-Smith index = $BW^2 - MW^2/BW$ × BL.

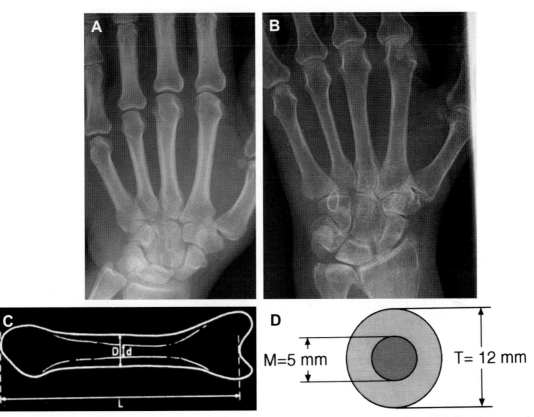

Fig. 2. Second metacarpal radiogrammetry: from a radiograph of the nondominant hand (A) showing normal cortical density and thickness and (B) showing reduced CT and radiographic density in a patient with osteoporosis, (C) the length of the nondominant second metacarpal is measured, and (C) the midshaft defined and the periosteal width (D) and medullary endosteal width (d) measured, optimally with vernier calipers from which (D) are derived various measurements: CT = T − M; 12 − 5 = 7 mm; MCI = T − M/T; 12 − 5/12 = 0.583; Barnett and Nordin index (HS = MCI × 100 = 58.3%). (From Jergas M. Conventional radiographs and basic quantitative methods. In: Grampp S, editor. Radiology of osteoporosis. Berlin Heidelberg: Springer; 2003. p. 61–86; with permission.)

Clinical Outcomes

Reference ranges for various nationalities were published for adults and children. Using metacarpal measurements, it was confirmed that in men and women (1) MW increases with age due to endosteal resorption and (2) BW increases with age due to periosteal apposition; as a consequence, in adults, the fraction of the shaft volume occupied by cortical bone diminishes with advancing age.[30–32] The method also demonstrated that the reduction in CT was greater in women in the early years after menopause.[33] BW increases to a greater extent in boys than girls during puberty and there is some reduction in MW in teenage girls, which may reflect the storing of calcium at the endosteal surface for the requirements of future pregnancy and lactation.

Precision (Reproducibility)

Longitudinal studies using metacarpal radiogrammetry were limited by measurement error of the technique, which may be as large as CV equal to 8% to 11%.[34] As the annual cortical bone loss between 40 and 80 years of age might only be 0.9% for women and 0.4% for men, then many years would be required in longitudinal studies to detect significant changes in individual subjects.[22] The limitations in precision are related principally to the problem of accurate definition of the endosteal margin of the cortex, and this becomes more difficult with bone loss and osteoporosis. For improved consistency, the inner cortical margin should be defined as the border of the solid cortical layer without separate trabeculae in the vicinity.[35] Precision error can be reduced by analyzing 3 metacarpals (second to fourth), and further improvement is feasible if both hands are radiographed and 6 metacarpals measured.[21]

The other limitation of radiogrammetry is that it studies cortical bone, which is 8 times less metabolically active than trabecular bone.

Summary

With the introduction of DXA, which has become the gold standard for defining osteoporosis in terms of bone densitometry (lumbar spine [L1-4], proximal femur [femoral neck and total hip], and distal forearm), in the late 1980s radiogrammetric methods became superseded.[36,37] Metacarpal radiogrammetry, however, was simple to perform, was widely available, used a low radiation dose, and provided useful research, epidemiologic, and clinical information about the skeleton. The reproducibility was limited, however; this old, established technique has been rejuvenated by the application of modern computer vision methods to make it automated (DXR), with great improvement in precision.

DIGITAL X-RAY RADIOGRAMMETRY

In 2001, a new radiogrammetric technique was described, which assumes a physical model of the metacarpal to aim at bridging the gap between radiogrammetry and densitometry[38,39] (Sectra Pronosco Medical Systems, Linkoping, Sweden). The technique provides an estimate of BMD_{DXR} from basic geometric measurements, which are calculated automatically. The metacarpals are identified in the digitized PA hand radiograph using the computer vision algorithm of active shape models (ASMs).[40,41] The ASM algorithm is trained to identify points on the boundaries of the metacarpals. The outer (periosteal) bone edges are defined as points of high curvature and the inner endosteal bone edges are defined as points of high intensity.[38,39]

Technical Aspects

There is automatic segmentation of the cortical and medullary regions of the midshafts of the second, third, and fourth metacarpals (**Fig. 3**). The metacarpal midshaft is identified as the point of minimum width. The automatic segmentation provides the average CT (mm) and average BW (mm) of the bone over the prescribed region of interest.[39] The applied scanning resolution (300 dpi approximately 5.5 lp/mm) allows the average thickness and average width to be accumulated over approximately 118 individual measurements per centimeter along the bone. The length of

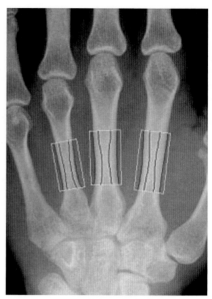

Fig. 3. DXR in an adult: there is automatic segmentation of the cortical and medullary regions of the mid-shafts of the second, third, and fourth metacarpals. The metacarpal midshaft is identified as the point of minimum width. The automatic segmentation provides the average CT (mm) and average BW (mm) of the bone over the prescribed region of interest. The length of bone measured in the second metacarpal is 1.9 cm, the third metacarpal 1.7 cm, and the fourth metacarpal 1.5 cm. From the computed CT and BW of the bone, a compound measurement, VPA, is derived, which is multiplied by a constant to obtain BMD_{DXR}.

bone measured in the second metacarpal is 1.9 cm, the third metacarpal is 1.7 cm, and the fourth metacarpal is 1.5 cm, so the numbers of measurements contributing to the average BWs (118 × lengths) are 450, 400, and 350, respectively. From the computed CT and BW of the bone, a compound measurement called bone volume per area (VPA) is derived. VPA is defined as bone volume per projected area:

VPA = Bone Volume/Area

Assuming that the bone of interest is cylindrical in shape:

$$VPA = \pi \times CT \times (1 - CT/BW)^{39}$$

The VPA formula is modified to take into account the fact that the second metacarpal is not cylindrical but elliptical in shape.[42] The VPA is multiplied then by an appropriate constant (c) to derive BMD_{DXR}. The constant has been determined empirically, such that BMD_{DXR} equates to that of the mid-distal forearm region of the Hologic

QDR-2000 DXA densitometer scanner (Hologic Inc, Bedford, Massachusetts). The constant adapts VPA to the volumetric mineral density of compact cortical bone and the typical shape of the metacarpal bones being measured.[39] Thus, the measurements provided by DXR are mean metacarpal BW, and CT, with an estimate of cortical porosity, VPA, and BMD_{DXR}; MW can be calculated (BW − CT). Original software included measurements of the distal radius and ulna, which are not available on later versions.

Precision

Because the measures are automated and are derived from 3, rather than a single, metacarpal, precision is enhanced. The short-term in vivo precision of BMD_{DXR} is reported to be between 0.60% and 1%.[39] BMD_{DXR} has been found to be closely correlated with DXA BMD_a at the distal forearm ($r = 0.86$, $P<.0001$), as would be expected, taking into account how the DXR measures are derived and calculated. BMD_{DXR} was also correlated to DXA BMD_a at the spine, total hip, and femoral neck ($r = 0.62$, 0.69, and 0.73, respectively; $P<.0001$ for all).[39] In a cohort of 416 women ages 20 to 90 years, the annual decline in BMD_{DXR} was estimated to be 1.05% in the age group 55 to 65 years. Relative to this age-related loss, the reported short-term precision allows for monitoring intervals of 1 year and 1.6 years to detect expected age-related changes with a confidence of 80% and 95%, respectively.[39]

The measurements by DXR seem to be fairly robust to the influence of different image acquisition protocols and operators.[43,44] The BMD_{DXR} calculation was not significantly affected by changes in the method of image capture (film focus distance, exposure level, or film sensitivity/film brand) but was influenced by tube voltage, and different digital image devices had an effect on DXR reproducibility.[43] Different radiographers performing the hand radiograph did not adversely affect precision.[44] Precision was found to be good with double-sided emulsion radiographic film (DF) and single-sided emulsion radiographic film (SF) but better with SF (CV% 0.92 vs 1.12 DF). A significant ($P<.001$) systematic difference was found between BMD_{DXR} measured from DF and SF (mean difference 0.017 g/cm^2). The overall percentage difference between the methods was 2.98% (range 0.18%–5.78%). Correlations between BMD_{DXR} and DXA BMD_a were moderately good ($r = 0.56–0.77$, $P<.001$); with SXA of the forearm, they were excellent ($r = 0.91$, $P<.001$). Relating BMD_{DXR} to the detection of

women with osteopenia by DXA, who had a DXA T score less than −1 (World Health Organization),[37] the sensitivity and specificity of DXR was determined at the spine (area under the curve [AUC] = 0.82), femoral neck (AUC = 0.84), and total hip (AUC = 0.84). Based on femoral neck DXA BMD_a for detection of osteopenia, a DXR T-score threshold of −1.05 was suggested as appropriate for detection of patients who might most appropriately be selected for central DXA measurements.[44]

In a study in Belgium, 221 postmenopausal community-dwelling white women ages 50 to 75 years were recruited.[45] DXA BMD_a was measured at the lumbar spine and total hip. Calcaneus quantitative ultrasound (QUS) and metacarpal and phalangeal BMD_a were estimated by DXR and RA, respectively. Receiver operating characteristic curves were constructed by calculating the specificity and sensitivity of QUS, DXR, and RA at different cutpoint values in discriminating osteoporosis, as defined by a T score below −2.5 at the spine or hip using DXA.[37] The sensitivity for identifying women with osteoporosis was 67.6% using QUS, 76.9% using DXR, and 82.9% using RA. These data suggest that metacarpal DXR and phalangeal RA may be as effective as calcaneus QUS for targeting DXA testing in high-risk postmenopausal women.[45]

In a study to examine precision for the more recently developed direct digital version of DXR, the in vitro precision was tested on 4 different types of x-ray equipment using 31 radiographs of the same phantom.[46] The precision (CV%) ranged from 0.14% to 0.30% and from 0.0012 to 0.0028 g/cm^2 (smallest detectable difference). The precision was correlated to the resolution of the radiographic equipment ($r = 0.95$, $P = .05$). The BMD_{DXR} from 1 type of x-ray equipment differed by 1.1% from the overall mean value. The in vivo mean precision in this study (duplicate hand radiographs, from both hands; n = 39) was CV% = 0.46%; smallest detectable difference = 0.0046 g/cm^2; and least significant change = 1.28%.[47] These results suggest that DXR measurements may differ when obtained on different radiographic equipment, so there should be consistency in the equipment used in longitudinal studies.

In summary, DXR is a robust and highly reproducible quantitative technique to measure changes in metacarpal morphometry.

CLINICAL APPLICATIONS OF DXR

One of the strengths of DXR is that with the original software applicable to hand radiographs, which were digitized, the measurements could be applied retrospectively to longitudinal studies conducted in the past. This has been a particular asset in defining applicability in predicting outcomes in rheumatoid arthritis. The limitations of the method are that it is applicable to a peripheral, non–weight bearing, skeletal site and gives information only on cortical, not trabecular, bone.

In Adults

There are normal reference data available for DXR parameters.[48] These were drawn from 2085 white German patients who were prospectively enrolled (954 women and 1131 men) from a data pool of 11,915 patients who had radiographs of the nondominant hand. DXR measurements were made of BMD, CT, BW, and the MCI. These data showed a continuous age-related increase of the DXR parameters to peak bone mass (PBM), followed by a continuous decline beyond PBM, with accentuated age-related cortical bone loss in women. PBM in this cross-sectional study occurred at approximately 30 to 34 years in women and 45 to 49 years in men. Men had a significantly higher BMD_{DXR} (mean +12.8%) compared with woman, in all age groups.[48]

Fracture Prediction

In the United States, hand radiographs and DXA at the forearm and hip were performed on 832 women (20–79 years).[49] PBM for BMD_{DXR} occurred at age 38 (mean = 0.598 g/cm^2, SD = 0.034 g/cm^2). The correlation between BMD_{DXR} and DXA BMD_a was 0.90 at the wrist and 0.61 at the hip. The relationship of BMD_{DXR} to reported history of fracture was of similar magnitude to that for DXA at the wrist and hip.

The Study of Osteoporotic Fracture is a case-cohort study within a prospective study of 9704 community-dwelling elderly women. BMD_{DXR} and DXA BMD_a (radius, calcaneus, femoral neck, and lumbar spine) were studied in women who subsequently suffered a wrist, hip, or vertebral fracture and in controls from the same cohort (n = 392–398). BMD_{DXR} performed as well as other peripheral BMD_a measurements for prediction of wrist, hip, and vertebral fractures, with a relative hazard of 1.5 to 1.9 for a 1SD reduction in BMD_a.[50]

In the Danish third Copenhagen City Heart Study, a large population-based study, 1370 postmenopausal women had BMD_{DXR}.[51] Follow-up time was 6.1 years and 245 women suffered a fracture. Age, fracture, and smoking were negatively correlated with BMD_{DXR}, whereas body mass index, age at menopause, hormone replacement therapy, physical fitness, and muscle strength were positively correlated with BMD_{DXR}. Odds ratios (ORs) per 1 SD decline in BMD_{DXR} were statistically significant for fracture of wrist, proximal humerus, and vertebrae. In the hip fracture group, the P value almost reached significance (0.052). The highest ORs (2.4) were found for fractures of the proximal humerus and vertebrae (2.0).[51]

Based on these reports, metacarpal BMD_{DXR} seems to predict later osteoporotic fracture in the wrist, humerus, and vertebrae, although femoral neck DXA BMD_a remains the best predictor of hip fracture.

Application in Rheumatoid Arthritis

Because of the high reproducibility (precision) of BMD_{DXR}, the technique has acquired an important and increasing application in assessing prediction of severity and outcomes in rheumatoid arthritis.[52,53] In a retrospective study commenced in 1978, 152 consecutive patients with rheumatoid arthritis (78% women, mean disease duration 14.2 years) were enrolled and hand radiographs were available in 108 patients. Low BMD_{DXR} predicted overall mortality in age- and gender-adjusted analyses, which supports DXR as a valid prognostic measurement of disease activity or damage.[52] DXR was performed in a small longitudinal study (n = 24; hand radiographs at baseline and 12, 24, and 48 months) in which radiographic scores and other markers of disease activity were measured. BMD_{DXR} decreased significantly throughout the study and change in BMD_{DXR} at 1 year was very specific (100%) and highly sensitive (63%) in predicting the development of erosions or increased severity of erosive change. These results showed the potential of DXR as a method of determining disease severity, which could be relevant in targeting patients who might require more aggressive and expensive therapy.[53]

DXR and DXA were applied to measure bone density in the hand in 72 patients with inflammatory arthritis (n = 51; 21 unclassified inflammatory arthritis). BMD_{DXR} decreased significantly in patients with rheumatoid arthritis from month 6 and was associated with mean disease activity. DXA BMD_a did not change, suggesting that DXR is superior to DXA BMD_a for detecting and monitoring osteopenia related to disease severity.[54] This greater sensitivity of DXR to demonstrate reduction in BMD_a, when compared with DXA of the hand and at central skeletal sites, has also been demonstrated in other studies.[55,56] More recent studies have confirmed that loss of hand bone measured by DXR is an independent predictor of longer term radiological joint damage, which it precedes.[57,58]

DXR measurements have also been applied in therapeutic trials in rheumatoid arthritis.[59–61] The combination of adalimumab and methotrexate arrested hand bone loss (DXR-MCI) less effectively than radiographic joint damage; quantitative measures of osteoporosis may, therefore, be a more sensitive tool for assessing inflammatory bone involvement in rheumatoid arthritis.[61] Disease-related loss of hand bone density, measured by DXR, in rheumatoid arthritis can be diminished by prednisolone, suggesting that the deleterious effect of prednisolone on bone may be counterbalanced by its beneficial anti-inflammatory effect.[59]

These studies confirm that DXR parameters are sensitive to bone loss associated with rheumatoid arthritis, can predict long-term outcomes and is a quantitative tool applicable to therapeutic trials.

In Children

Although the ASMs have been trained to recognize metacarpals on adult hand radiographs, DXR has been applied to research studies in children (Fig. 4).[62–66] A radiograph of the nondominant hand is a frequently performed examination in children in clinical practice for assessment of bone age. This x-ray examination uses an extremely low dose of ionizing radiation (0.05 to 0.17 μSv)[19,20] with negligible risk. DXR fails in approximately 4% of children's hand radiographs[62]; this is mostly in younger children (6 years and under) in whom the metacarpals are small but is also related to inadequate contrast difference between bone and soft tissue or under- or overexposure of the radiographic film.[66]

Some normal reference data are available.[62,66] In the study from the Netherlands (n = 535),[62] the short-term precision of DXR was CV of 0.59%. Significant differences were found in BMD$_{DXR}$ between boys and girls for the ages of 11, 12, 16, 17, and 18 years. There were also significant differences in sequential Tanner stages. For 88 subjects, repeat longitudinal radiographs were available (mean interval 1.8 years) and in all there was an increase in BMD$_{DXR}$. In a small subgroup (n = 20) of children with disease, girls with inflammatory bowel disease, juvenile chronic arthritis, or a history of forearm fractures and boys with inflammatory bowel disease showed a significantly lower BMD$_{DXR}$ compared with healthy controls. DXR is, therefore, applicable in children, and in a small subpopulation it was possible to discriminate children with a high risk of low BMD.[62]

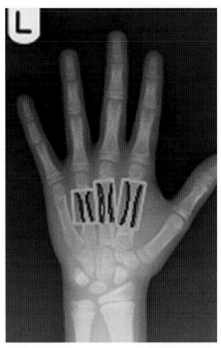

Fig. 4. DXR in a child: although the ASMs have been trained to recognize metacarpals in adult hand radiographs, DXR has been applied to research studies in children. DXR fails in approximately 4% of children's hand radiographs; this is mostly in younger children (6 years and under) in whom the metacarpals are small. (*Data from* van Rijn RR, Grootfaam DS, Lequin MH, et al. Digital radiogrammetry of the hand in a pediatric and adolescent Dutch Caucasian population: normative data and measurements in children with inflammatory bowel disease and juvenile chronic arthritis. Calcif Tissue Int 2004;74(4):342–50.)

In a study from Germany (n = 200 healthy white children [120 boys and 80 girls, ages 4–18 y]) BMD$_{DXR}$ increased with age from 0.40 g/cm^2 to 0.62 g/cm^2 in boys and from 0.39 g/cm^2 to 0.54 g/cm^2 in girls. Girls (ages 11–12 y) had a higher BMD$_{DXR}$ than boys, corresponding to the earlier entry to puberty of girls. DXR-MCI increased with age from 0.36 to 0.47 for boys and from 0.34 to 0.49 for girls, with a maximum SD of 0.6.[66]

SUMMARY

Metacarpal radiogrammetry and morphometry are the longest established quantitative methods of assessment of the skeleton, having been available for more than 70 years. Much useful research and epidemiologic information was acquired in children and adults. Poor reproducibility, however, limited longitudinal studies. The methods were superseded initially by single- and dual-photon absorptiometry and in the 1980s by SXA and

DXA, which are now the most widely used and available quantitative methods for assessment of BMD. The application of modern computer vision techniques (ASMs) and automation, however, has enabled rejuvenation of metacarpal morphometry since 2000 with the introduction of DXR.

DXR is quick and simple to perform, having potential for application in a variety of settings as analysis can be performed in a central unit, with radiographs taken in sites over a wide geographic area. The Sectra company (Sectra Pronosco Medical Systems, Linkoping, Sweden) now offers central analysis on line (dxr@dxr-online.com). Retrospective analysis can also be performed (eg, on radiographs taken to monitor rheumatoid arthritis). DXR has been shown to have high reproducibility, the ability to predict future fracture, and to reflect activity and predict outcomes in rheumatoid arthritis. A hand radiograph requires a low radiation dose, a particular advantage in children, and DXR has also been found to be applicable in studies of normal children and those with diseases that adversely affect bone health. DXR has the potential to provide a simple, widely available and inexpensive method to assess patients at risk of osteopenia or osteoporosis who might appropriately be referred for central DXA. This may be particularly relevant to patients who suffer low-trauma fractures and attend accident and emergency or fracture clinics, where investigation for osteoporosis is often neglected.

REFERENCES

1. Mack PB, O'Brien AT, Smith JM, et al. A method for estimating the degree of mineralization of bones from tracings of roentgenograms. Science 1939; 89(2316):467.
2. Meema HE, Harris CK, Porrett RE. A method for determination of bone-salt content of cortical bone. Radiology 1964;82:986–97.
3. Morgan DB, Spiers FW, Pulvertaft CN, et al. The amount of bone in the metacarpal and the phalanx according to age and sex. Clin Radiol 1967;18(1):101–8.
4. Ose GP. Estimation of changes in bone calcium content by radiographic densitometry. Radiology 1969;93(4):841–4.
5. Mack PB, Vogt FB. Roentgenographic bone density changes in astronauts during representative Apollo space flight. Am J Roentgenol Radium Ther Nucl Med 1971;113(4):621–33.
6. Tothill P. Methods of bone mineral measurement. Phys Med Biol 1989;34(5):543–72.
7. Meema HE, Meema S. Cortical bone mineral density versus cortical thickness in the diagnosis of osteoporosis: a roentgenologic-densitometric study. J Am Geriatr Soc 1969;17(2):120–41.
8. Trouerbach WT, Birkenhäger JC, Collette BJ, et al. A study on the phalanx bone mineral content in 273 normal pre- and post-menopausal females (transverse study of age-dependent bone loss). Bone Miner 1987;3(1):53–62.
9. Hayashi Y, Yamamoto K, Fukunaga M, et al. Assessment of bone mass by image analysis of metacarpal bone roentgenograms: a quantitative digital image processing (DIP) method. Radiat Med 1990;8(5):173–8.
10. Cosman F, Herrington B, Himmelstein S, et al. Radiographic absorptiometry: a simple method for determination of bone mass. Osteoporos Int 1991;2(1):34–8.
11. Yates AJ, Ross PD, Lydick E, et al. Radiographic absorptiometry in the diagnosis of osteoporosis. Am J Med 1995;98(2A):41S–7S.
12. Mussolino ME, Looker AC, Madans JH, et al. Phalangeal bone density and hip fracture risk. Arch Intern Med 1997;157(4):433–8.
13. Cameron JR, Mazess RB, Sorenson JA. Precision and accuracy of bone mineral determination by direct photon absorptiometry. Invest Radiol 1968; 3(3):141–50.
14. Cameron JR, Sorenson J. Measurement of bone mineral in vivo: an improved method. Science 1963;11(142):230–2.
15. West RR, Reed GW. The measurement of bone mineral in vivo by photon beam scanning. Br J Radiol 1970;43(516):886–93.
16. Barnett E, Nordin BE. The radiological diagnosis of osteoporosis: a new approach. Clin Radiol 1960; 11:166–74.
17. Virtama P, Mahonen H. Thickness of the cortical layer as an estimate of mineral content of human finger bones. Br J Radiol 1960;33:60–2.
18. Garn SM. The earlier gain and the later loss of cortical bone in nutritional perspectives. Springfield (IL): Charles C Thomas; 1970.
19. Okkalides D, Fotakis M. Patient effective dose resulting from radiographic examinations. Br J Radiol 1994;67(798):564–72.
20. Huda W, Gkanatsios NA. Radiation dosimetry for extremity radiographs. Health Phys 1998;75(5):492–9.
21. Nielsen SP. The metacarpal index revisited: a brief overview. J Clin Densitom 2001;4(3):199–207.
22. Dequeker J. Quantitative radiology: radiogrammetry of cortical bone. Br J Radiol 1976;49(587):912–20.
23. Fox KM, Kimura S, Powell-Threets K, et al. Radial and ulnar cortical thickness of the second metacarpal. J Bone Miner Res 1995;10(12):1930–4.
24. Horsman A, Kirby PA. Geometric properties of the second metacarpal. Calcif Tissue Res 1972;10(4) 289–301.
25. Garn SM. An annotated bibliography on bone densitometry. Am J Clin Nutr 1962;10:59–67.

26. Garn SM, Poznanski AK, Nagy JM. Bone measurement in the differential diagnosis of osteopenia and osteoporosis. Radiology 1971;100(3):509–18.

27. Gryfe CI, Exton-Smith AN, Payne PR, et al. Pattern of development of bone in childhood and adolescence. Lancet 1971;1(7698):523–6.

28. Exton-Smith AN, Millard PH, Payne PR, et al. Method for measuring quantity of bone. Lancet 1969; 2(7631):1153–4.

29. Exton-Smith AN, Millard PH, Payne PR, et al. Pattern of development and loss of bone with age. Lancet 1969;2(7631):1154–7.

30. Meema HE. The occurrence of cortical bone atrophy in old age and in osteoporosis. J Can Assoc Radiol 1962;13:27–32.

31. Adams P, Davies GT, Sweetnam P. Osteoporosis and the effects of ageing on bone mass in elderly men and women. Q J Med 1970;39(156):601–15.

32. Adams P, Davies GT. Sweetnam P Cortical bone-loss with age. Lancet 1971;2(7735):1201–2.

33. Horsman A, Simpson M, Kirby PA, et al. Non-linear bone loss in oophorectomized women. Br J Radiol 1977;50(595):504–7.

34. Adams P, Davies GT, Sweetnam PM. Observer error and measurements of the metacarpal. Br J Radiol 1969;42(495):192–7.

35. Virtama P, Helelä T. Radiographic measurements of cortical bone. Variations in a normal population between 1 and 90 years of age. Acta Radiol Suppl 1969;293.

36. Blake GM, Fogelman I. The clinical role of dual energy X-ray absorptiometry. Eur J Radiol 2009; 71(3):406–14.

37. World Health Organisation Study Group. Assessment of fracture risk and its application to screening for postmenopausal osteoporosis. Geneva (Switzerland): World Health Organisation; 1994. (WHO Technical Report Series 843).

38. Jørgensen JT, Andersen PB, Rosholm A, et al. Digital X-ray radiogrammetry: a new appendicular bone densitometric method with high precision. Clin Physiol 2000;20(5):330–5.

39. Rosholm A, Hyldstrup L, Backsgaard L, et al. Estimation of bone mineral density by digital X-ray radiogrammetry: theoretical background and clinical testing. Osteoporos Int 2001;12(11):961–9.

40. Cootes T, Hill A, Taylor CJ, et al. Use of active shape models for locating structure in medical images. Image Vis Comput 1994;12(6):355–65.

41. Hill A, Cootes TF, Taylor CJ, et al. Medical image interpretation: a generic approach using deformable templates. Med Inform (Lond) 1994;19(1):47–59.

42. Lazenby R. Brief communication: non-circular geometry and radiogrammetry of the second metacarpal. Am J Phys Anthropol 1995;97(3):323–7.

43. Böttcher J, Pfeil A, Rosholm A, et al. Influence of image-capturing parameters on digital X-ray radiogrammetry. J Clin Densitom 2005;8(1):87–94.

44. Ward KA, Cotton J, Adams JE. A technical and clinical evaluation of digital X-ray radiogrammetry. Osteoporos Int 2003;14(5):389–95.

45. Boonen S, Nijs J, Borghs H, et al. Identifying postmenopausal women with osteoporosis by calcaneal ultrasound, metacarpal digital X-ray radiogrammetry and phalangeal radiographic absorptiometry: a comparative study. Osteoporos Int 2005;16(1):93–100.

46. Hoff M, Dhainaut A, Kvien TK, et al. Short-time in vitro and in vivo precision of direct digital X-ray radiogrammetry. J Clin Densitom 2009;12(1):17–21.

47. Glüer CC. Monitoring skeletal changes by radiological techniques. J Bone Miner Res 1999;14(11): 1952–62.

48. Böttcher J, Pfeil A, Schäfer ML, et al. Normative data for digital X-ray radiogrammetry from a female and male German cohort. J Clin Densitom 2006;9(3): 341–50.

49. Black DM, Palermo L, Sørensen T, et al. A normative reference database study for Pronosco X-posure System. J Clin Densitom 2001;4(1):5–12.

50. Bouxsein ML, Palermo L, Yeung C, et al. Digital X-ray radiogrammetry predicts hip, wrist and vertebral fracture risk in elderly women: a prospective analysis from the study of osteoporotic fractures. Osteoporos Int 2000;13(5):358–65.

51. Bach-Mortensen P, Hyldstrup L, Appleyard M, et al. Digital x-ray radiogrammetry identifies women at risk of osteoporotic fracture: results from a prospective study. Calcif Tissue Int 2006;79(1):1–6.

52. Book C, Algulin J, Nilsson JA, et al. Bone mineral density in the hand as a predictor for mortality in patients with rheumatoid arthritis. Rheumatology (Oxford) 2009;48(9):1088–91.

53. Stewart A, Mackenzie LM, Black AJ, et al. Predicting erosive disease in rheumatoid arthritis. A longitudinal study of changes in bone density using digital X-ray radiogrammetry: a pilot study. Rheumatology (Oxford) 2004;43(12):1561–4.

54. Jensen T, Klarlund M, Hansen M, et al. TIRA Group. Bone loss in unclassified polyarthritis and early rheumatoid arthritis is better detected by digital X-ray radiogrammetry than dual X-ray absorptiometry: relationship with disease activity and radiographic outcome. Ann Rheum Dis 2004; 63(1):15–22.

55. Hoff M, Haugeberg G, Kvien TK. Hand bone loss as an outcome measure in established rheumatoid arthritis: 2-year observational study comparing cortical and total bone loss. Arthritis Res Ther 2007;9(4):R81.

56. Böttcher J, Malich A, Pfeil A, et al. Potential clinical relevance of digital radiogrammetry for quantification of periarticular bone demineralization in patients suffering from rheumatoid arthritis depending on severity and compared with DXA. Eur Radiol 2004; 14(4):631–7.

57. Forslind K, Boonen A, Albertsson K, et al. Barfot Study Group Hand bone loss measured by digital X-ray radiogrammetry is a predictor of joint damage in early rheumatoid arthritis. Scand J Rheumatol 2009;38(6):431–8.

58. Böttcher J, Pfeil A. Diagnosis of periarticular osteoporosis in rheumatoid arthritis using digital X-ray radiogrammetry. Arthritis Res Ther 2008; 10(1):103.

59. Haugeberg G, Strand A, Kvien TK, et al. Reduced loss of hand bone density with prednisolone in early rheumatoid arthritis: results from a randomized placebo-controlled trial. Arch Intern Med 2005; 165(11):1293–7.

60. Pfeil A, Lippold J, Eidner T, et al. Effects of leflunomide and methotrexate in rheumatoid arthritis detected by digital X-ray radiogrammetry and computer-aided joint space analysis. Rheumatol Int 2009;29(3):287–95.

61. Hoff M, Kvien TK, Kälvesten J, et al. Adalimumab therapy reduces hand bone loss in early rheumatoid arthritis: explorative analyses from the PREMIER study. Ann Rheum Dis 2009;68(7):1171–6.

62. van Rijn RR, Grootfaam DS, Lequin MH, et al. Digital radiogrammetry of the hand in a pediatric and adolescent Dutch Caucasian population: normative data and measurements in children with inflammatory bowel disease and juvenile chronic arthritis. Calcif Tissue Int 2004;74(4):342–50.

63. Mentzel HJ, John U, Boettcher J, et al. Evaluation of bone-mineral density by digital X-ray radiogrammetry (DXR) in pediatric renal transplant recipients. Pediatr Radiol 2005;35(5):489–94.

64. van Rijn RR, Boot A, Wittenberg R, et al. Direct X-ray radiogrammetry versus dual-energy X-ray absorptiometry: assessment of bone density in children treated for acute lymphoblastic leukaemia and growth hormone deficiency. Pediatr Radiol 2006; 36(3):227–32.

65. Mentzel HJ, Blume J, Boettcher J, et al. The potential of digital X-ray radiogrammetry (DXR) in the assessment of osteopenia in children with chronic inflammatory bowel disease. Pediatr Radiol 2006;36(5): 415–20.

66. Malich A, Freesmeyer MG, Mentzel HJ, et al. Normative values of bone parameters of children and adolescents using digital computer-assisted radiogrammetry (DXR). J Clin Densitom 2003; 6(2):103–11.

Dual X-ray Absorptiometry in Today's Clinical Practice

Lance G. Dasher, MD, Christopher D. Newton, MD,
Leon Lenchik, MD*

KEYWORDS

• DXA • Absorptiometry • Osteoporosis • FRAX

Osteoporosis is a common but treatable disease that is increasingly recognized by the general public and health care providers. Before fracture, osteoporosis is usually diagnosed with dual x-ray absorptiometry (DXA). This technique allows for noninvasive measurement of bone mineral density (BMD), which approximates overall bone strength with a reasonable degree of accuracy and precision. DXA is not only used for diagnosis of osteoporosis, but is used to help assess fracture risk, to help select patients for pharmacologic therapy, and to help monitor therapy or disease progression. Although other densitometric methods including quantitative ultrasonography[1] and quantitative computed tomography[2] have seen clinical utility, central DXA has been the most widely used method.[3] This is partly because DXA is relatively inexpensive, widely available, has short scan times, and generates little radiation exposure.[3–10] Most importantly, there is a long-standing, broad consensus on how central DXA results should be interpreted.[11–14] This article describes the current approach to and recent advances in the clinical use of central DXA.

TECHNICAL ASPECTS OF CENTRAL DXA

Before DXA there were single photon absorptiometry (SPA) and dual photon absorptiometry (DPA); both are no longer in use. SPA measures the transmission of photons through the mid-radius or calcaneus. Iodine-125 source is used to generate 27.3 keV photons and a scintillator crystal is used to detect them.[8,9] In contrast, DPA measures the transmission of 2 distinct photons, allowing for the separation of soft tissue from bone density in the spine and hip.[8,9]

In 1987, DXA scanners became available for clinical use. Instead of the radionuclide source used in SPA and DPA, DXA uses an x-ray source composed of 2 distinct energies. By using computer analysis, the soft tissue contribution to the measured density is eliminated, allowing for measurement of BMD. Compared with DPA, DXA has much faster scanning, reducing the problems inherent with patient motion, greater image resolution, because of smaller focal spot, improved collimation, and lower radiation dose.[8–10]

DXA manufacturers use various methods for generating the high- and low-energy x-ray photons as well as for detecting them. To produce the dual energies, either voltage switching (Hologic, Bedford, MA, USA) or K-edge filtering (General Electric, Milwaukee, WI, USA) is used. Regardless of what method is used to produce dual energies, the measurement of bone relies on the K-absorption edge of soft tissue. The K-edge is the energy level at which the maximum amount of photons is absorbed by a particular tissue. Using an x-ray with the energy level just above the K-edge of soft tissue generates maximal absorption of x-rays, which can be analyzed using the absorption

Department of Radiology, Wake Forest University Baptist Medical Center, Medical Center Boulevard, Winston-Salem, NC 27157, USA
* Corresponding author.
E-mail address: llenchik@wfubmc.edu

Radiol Clin N Am 48 (2010) 541–560
doi:10.1016/j.rcl.2010.02.019
0033-8389/10/$ – see front matter © 2010 Elsevier Inc. All rights reserved.

of a concurrent higher energy level of x-rays. Using high- and low-energy x-rays allows the soft tissue and bone contributions to measured density to be differentiated.[8–10]

When measuring BMD, different DXA manufacturers use slightly different anatomic regions of interest (ROIs), edge detection algorithms, and calibration methods. Although early DXA systems were mainly pencil beam, most current systems are fan beam, allowing for faster scanning (**Fig. 1**). Some systems have a rotating gantry, allowing for supine lateral scanning. Although clinical utility is not affected by the different techniques, comparison of individual patient studies should be performed on similar scanners.

The 2 main performance measures traditionally used in bone densitometry are accuracy[15–17] and precision.[17–21] Accuracy is usually assessed by comparing results of DXA scan to ash mineral content of a cadaveric specimen. Precision is usually assessed by repeated measurements of a phantom or a group of subjects. Central DXA accuracy ranges from 5% to 7%.[15] Central DXA precision is better than accuracy, ranges between 1% and 3%, is site dependent, and is usually better at the spine than the hip.[21] Recently, slightly different nomenclature has been introduced, with the term "trueness" replacing accuracy and the term "accuracy" encompassing both trueness and precision. This is described in great detail in a recent article by Engelke and Glüer.[22]

Perhaps a more useful way to assess DXA performance is to determine if BMD measured by DXA actually predicts bone strength and bone fractures. This has been accomplished in laboratory studies, where there is good correlation between BMD and the force required to fracture the bone,[23] and in population studies, where BMD predicts fractures.[24–27] There have been several large meta analyses[24,25] of epidemiologic

studies showing that for every standard deviation decrease in BMD, fracture risk approximately doubles. In the United States the largest such trial was the Study of Osteoporotic Fractures.[26,27]

The radiation dose of central DXA is site dependent but ranges from 1 to 6 mrem.[5–7] These doses are low enough that the DXA examination rooms do not require lead shielding. The low radiation dose has contributed to the rapid proliferation of this technology outside of traditional radiology departments to many types of outpatient settings, under the direction of many different types of health care providers.

CLINICAL DXA TECHNIQUE

One of the primary BMD measurement sites for DXA is the lumbar spine. This is because the spine contains a high proportion of trabecular bone, allowing for early detection of patients with high bone turnover and because the spine measurement has good precision, allowing for patient monitoring. Unfortunately in patients with spinal degenerative changes, the utility of spine measurement is more limited.

For spine DXA scan, the patient is positioned supine on the scanner table, centered on the table, with the spine aligned with the long axis of the scanner table. The patient's hips and knees are flexed using a positioning block, which helps straighten the normal lumbar lordosis and allows for more reproducible results on subsequent examinations (**Fig. 2**). The x-ray beam is directed in a posterior to anterior (PA) direction. When the patient is properly positioned, the DXA image should show the spine as straight as possible, with an equal amount of soft tissue on both sides and should include the superior margin of both iliac crests, the middle of the T12 vertebral body, and the middle of the L5 vertebral body (**Fig. 3**).

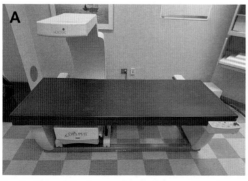 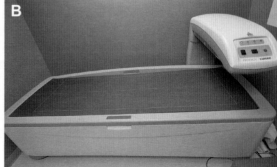

Fig. 1. Central dual x-ray absorptiometry (DXA) scanners. (*A*) Hologic's Delphi fan-beam scanner. (*B*) General Electric's Prodigy fan-beam scanner.

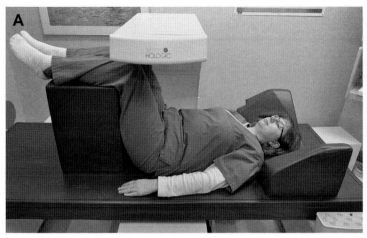
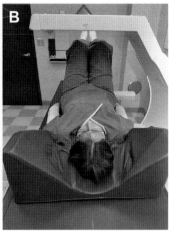

Fig. 2. Correct patient positioning for DXA scan of posterior-anterior (PA) spine. (*A*) Lateral photograph shows the positioning block under the subject's feet. (*B*) Frontal photograph shows the subject is centered on the scanner table and aligned with the scanner's long axis.

Spine BMD measurement is obtained in various ROIs including total lumbar spine (L1–L4), individual vertebral levels, and various combinations of vertebral levels.

Another common site for BMD measurement by DXA is the hip. This is because the proximal femur BMD is the best predictor of hip fracture, the fracture with the highest morbidity and mortality of all osteoporotic fractures, accounting for the largest proportion of economic costs associated with osteoporosis.

For hip DXA scan, the patient is positioned supine on the scanner table, centered on the table, with the long axis of the femoral diaphysis aligned with the long axis of the scanner table. A positioning device is used to place the femur in internal rotation, to elongate the femoral neck and allow for more reproducible results on subsequent examinations (**Fig. 4**). When the patient is properly positioned, the DXA image should show the femoral shaft aligned with the long axis of the scanner and the lesser trochanter should be small or not seen,

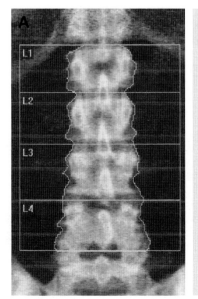
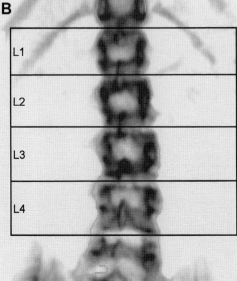

Fig. 3. DXA images of the spine with correct patient positioning. (*A*) Hologic image shows the spine is centered on the scanner table and aligned with the scanner's long axis. (*B*) General Electric image shows the scan extends from T12 to L5 vertebrae.

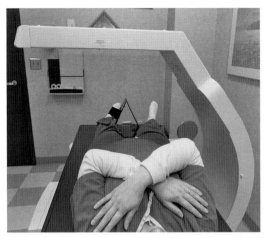

Fig. 4. Correct patient positioning for DXA scan of left hip. Note the positioning device bringing the subject's left hip into internal rotation.

indicating sufficient internal rotation (**Fig. 5**). Hip BMD measurement is obtained for various ROIs including the femoral neck, trochanter, Ward's area, intertrochanteric region, and total hip.

The third site used for BMD measurement by DXA in the forearm. This measurement is useful for patients in whom the spine or the hip is either not measurable or not interpretable, such as in patients with severe degenerative disease or with extensive surgical instrumentation. Because it contains a large proportion of cortical bone, forearm measurement is also useful in patients with hyperparathyroidism.

For forearm DXA scan, the patient is positioned sitting in a chair adjacent to the scanner table. A positioning device is used to align the forearm with the scanner table and allow for more reproducible results on subsequent examinations (**Fig. 6**). Ideally the nondominant forearm should be measured. The ROIs in the forearm are defined relative to the length of the ulna. When the patient is properly positioned, the DXA image should show the distal cortex of the radius and ulna and the diaphyses of both bones aligned with the long axis of the image (**Fig. 7**). Forearm BMD measurement is obtained for various ROIs including the mid-radius and mid-ulna (33% or one-third) and ultra distal-radius and distal-ulna (UD).

When evaluating the skeletal health of children, the whole-body BMD measurement is most often used.[28] This is because accounting for longitudinal growth is somewhat easier using whole body rather than spine or femur and because the reproducibility of whole-body measurement is quite good.[28]

For whole-body DXA scan, the patient is positioned centered and aligned with the scanner table, arms at sides separated slightly from the trunk (**Fig. 8**). The positioning of the feet varies according to manufacturer. BMD measurement is obtained for the whole body as well as smaller ROIs, including left upper extremity, right upper extremity, left thorax, right thorax, thoracic spine, lumbar spine, pelvis, left lower extremity, right lower extremity, and head. It is important to use

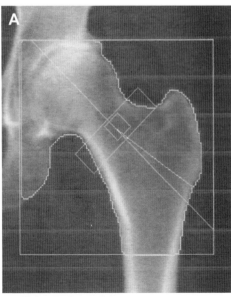

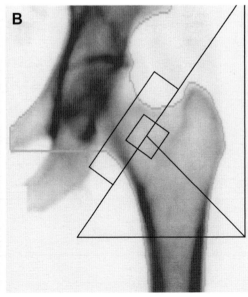

Fig. 5. DXA images of left hip with correct patient positioning. (*A*) Hologic image shows the proximal femur is aligned with the scanner's long axis. (*B*) General Electric image shows proper internal rotation of the femur with lesser trochanter not seen in profile.

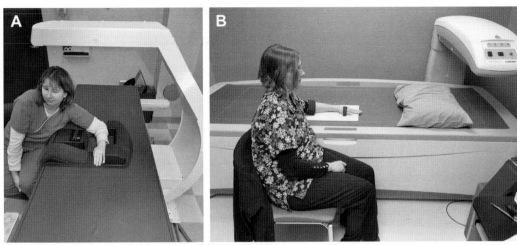

Fig. 6. Correct patient positioning for DXA scan of left forearm. (*A*) A subject properly positioned for Hologic forearm scan. Note the subject sitting on a chair adjacent to scanner. Note the positioning device aligning the forearm with scanner table. (*B*) A subject properly positioned for General Electric forearm scan.

dedicated pediatric software as adult software algorithms may overestimate BMD in children.[28]

DIAGNOSIS OF OSTEOPOROSIS USING DXA

The value of DXA in helping clinicians make the diagnosis of osteoporosis in patients before they fracture cannot be overstated. There is great diversity among health care providers who see patients with osteoporosis. They include radiologists and clinicians, primary care providers and specialists, gerontologists and pediatricians, rheumatologists and endocrinologists, internists and orthopedists, nephrologists, pulmonologists, gynecologists, and others. With so many specialties involved in the care of one disease it is actually surprising that there is considerable agreement on how to use central DXA to help diagnose patients with osteoporosis, to help assess their fracture risk, and to help select high-risk patients for pharmacologic therapy.[29–42] That is not to say that there have not been significant controversies. But that

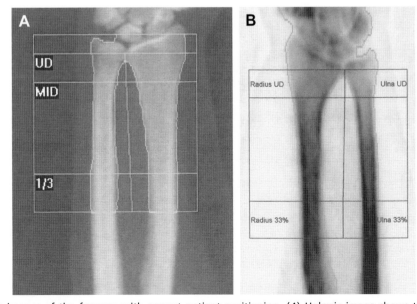

Fig. 7. DXA images of the forearm with correct patient positioning. (*A*) Hologic image shows the forearm is aligned with the scanner's long axis. (*B*) General Electric image shows the forearm is aligned with the scanner's long axis.

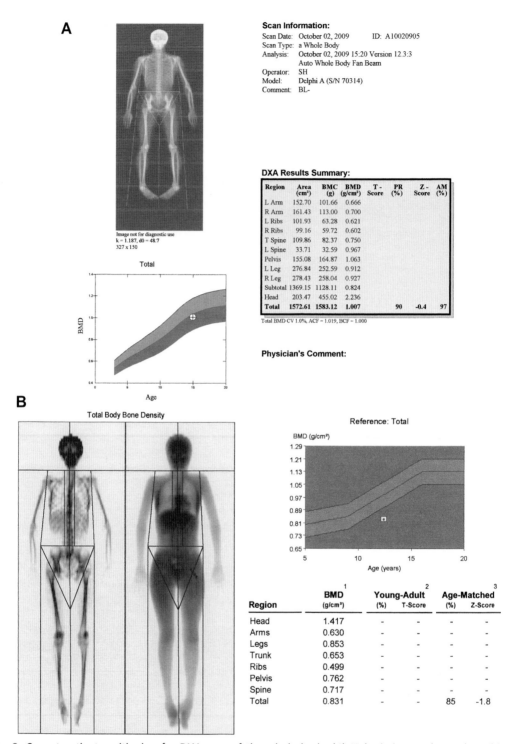

A

Scan Information:

Scan Date: October 02, 2009   ID: A10020905
Scan Type: a Whole Body
Analysis: October 02, 2009 15:20 Version 12.3:3
    Auto Whole Body Fan Beam
Operator: SH
Model: Delphi A (S/N 70314)
Comment: BL-

Image not for diagnostic use
k = 1.187, d0 = 48.7
327 x 150

DXA Results Summary:

Region	Area (cm²)	BMC (g)	BMD (g/cm²)	T-Score	PR (%)	Z-Score	AM (%)
L Arm	152.70	101.66	0.666				
R Arm	161.43	113.00	0.700				
L Ribs	101.93	63.28	0.621				
R Ribs	99.16	59.72	0.602				
T Spine	109.86	82.37	0.750				
L Spine	33.71	32.59	0.967				
Pelvis	155.08	164.87	1.063				
L Leg	276.84	252.59	0.912				
R Leg	278.43	258.04	0.927				
Subtotal	1369.15	1128.11	0.824				
Head	203.47	455.02	2.236				
Total	**1572.61**	**1583.12**	**1.007**		90	-0.4	97

Total BMD CV 1.0%, ACF = 1.019, BCF = 1.000

Physician's Comment:

Total

BMD

Age

B

Total Body Bone Density

Reference: Total

BMD (g/cm²)

Age (years)

Region	BMD¹ (g/cm²)	Young-Adult² (%) T-Score	Age-Matched³ (%) Z-Score
Head	1.417	-	-	-	-
Arms	0.630	-	-	-	-
Legs	0.853	-	-	-	-
Trunk	0.653	-	-	-	-
Ribs	0.499	-	-	-	-
Pelvis	0.762	-	-	-	-
Spine	0.717	-	-	-	-
Total	0.831	-	-	85	-1.8

Fig. 8. Correct patient positioning for DXA scan of the whole body. (*A*) Hologic image shows the subject is centered on the scanner table, heels are shoulder-width apart, and toes are together. (*B*) General Electric image shows the subject is centered on the scanner table, heels and toes are together.

too is a good sign, indicating that the field is not stagnant, that there is continued innovation that might settle current controversies while undoubtedly creating new ones.

In current clinical practice, when the diagnosis of osteoporosis is made based on DXA results, the raw BMD values (in grams per square centimeter) are not used. Instead, T-scores or Z-scores are used. T-scores and Z-scores compare the patient's BMD values with average BMD values of large population controls. The main function of standardized scores (T and Z) is to allow for patient diagnosis that is not dependent on the manufacturer of the DXA scanner. Although DXA scanners from different manufacturers often provide slightly different BMD values for the same patient, the T-score and Z-scores are similar.

The T-score is the number of standard deviations that the patient's BMD is above or below the mean BMD of a control group of young adults. Therefore, the normal BMD for a healthy young adult is defined as a T-score of zero with positive and negative values defining standard deviation from the mean. For example, a T-score of –1.0 would represent a patient with a BMD 1 standard deviation below the mean BMD of a young healthy adult. There are different reference standards for men and women as well as for different races.

The Z-score is the number of standard deviations that the patient's BMD is above or below the mean of age-matched controls. Just like the T-score, a normal Z-score is defined as zero with positive and negative values defining the number of standard deviations from the mean. For example, a Z-score of –1.0 would represent a patient with a BMD 1 standard deviation below the mean BMD for controls of the same age. As with T-score, there are different reference standards for men and women as well as for different races. For calculating T- and Z-scores at the hip, the National Health and Nutrition Examination Survey III (NHANES III) database is usually used, whereas for spine, forearm, and whole-body scores manufacturers use their own reference data.

In postmenopausal women and elderly men, the T-score is used to stratify patients into one of the following categories: normal, osteopenia (low bone mass), and osteoporosis. Normal is defined as a T-score of –1.0 or greater. Osteopenia is defined as a T-score of –1.0 to –2.5. Osteoporosis is defined as a T-score of –2.5 or lower. The World Health Organization (WHO) defined osteoporosis as a T-score of –2.5 so that approximately 30% of postmenopausal women would be classified as osteoporotic.[29] This percentage approximates the lifetime risk of osteoporotic fracture of the spine, hip, or forearm in postmenopausal women.[43,44] The Z-score has less clinical utility in postmenopausal women. Because the Z-score is age matched, if these values were used to define osteoporosis, there would be no increase in the prevalence of osteoporosis with advancing age.

In evaluating skeletal health of premenopausal women, younger men, and children, T-scores are not used.[45] Instead, Z-scores are used to define BMD relative to BMD of age-matched controls. Based on DXA measurement, the patients are placed into 1 of 2 categories: (1) normal BMD for age and (2) low BMD for age. Normal BMD is defined as Z-score higher than –2.0, whereas low BMD for age is defined as Z-score of –2.0 or lower.[45] However, densitometric criteria alone should not be used for the diagnosis of osteoporosis in these patient populations.[45] Thorough clinical evaluation should always be used in combination with DXA results to allow for appropriate clinical management of these patients.

DETERMINING FRACTURE RISK USING DXA

Although DXA-measured BMD has been shown to be predictive of absolute risk, relative risk, and lifetime risk of all types of osteoporotic fracture, for many years it was unclear on how to apply such epidemiologic data to clinical practice. Recently, the clinical assessment of fracture risk has been standardized using the fracture risk assessment tool (FRAX).[46–50]

Released in 2008, FRAX was developed to combine BMD with other risk factors to provide a 10-year probability of hip fracture and a 10-year probability of major osteoporotic fracture.[46–49] The populations intended for use with the FRAX include previously untreated postmenopausal women and older men. Children, premenopausal women, and younger men should not be evaluated using the FRAX algorithm.[49]

The FRAX algorithm is based on a number of different risk factors including age, sex, weight, height, previous fracture (occurring in adult life that was spontaneous or would not have occurred in a healthy young adult), paternal or maternal history of hip fracture, smoking, oral glucocorticoids for longer than 3 months, diagnosis of rheumatoid arthritis, underlying disorder strongly associated with osteoporosis (eg, type 1 diabetes mellitus), and 3 or more units of alcohol per day.[49]

Although, the FRAX algorithm can be used with or without BMD measurement, in the United States it is usually used as an adjunct to central DXA measurement, especially in patients who are osteopenic.[50] This is because in patients who are osteoporotic or have normal BMD based on DXA measurement, FRAX results are unlikely to change patient management. In patients with normal BMD, regardless of FRAX results, there is little evidence that pharmacologic therapy would reduce fracture risk. In osteoporotic patients, regardless of FRAX results, therapy is usually indicated.

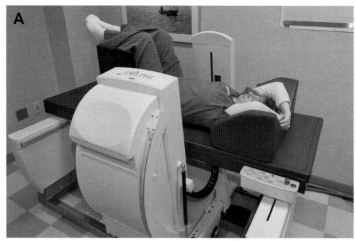
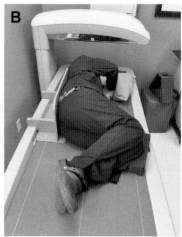

Fig. 9. Correct patient positioning for DXA scan for lateral vertebral assessment (LVA). (*A*) A Hologic scanner with a rotating gantry shows the subject is placed supine with arms over her head. (*B*) A General Electric scanner with a stationary gantry shows the subject is placed in a decubitus position using a positioning device.

The femoral neck BMD is currently used in the calculations of risk assessment. It is possible that patients who have low BMD in the spine but not hip will have their fracture risk underestimated by FRAX.[50] So the introduction of FRAX has not been without controversy. That said, FRAX is an important first step in helping clinicians quantify fracture risk in individual patients using DXA.

MONITORING BMD USING DXA

Follow-up DXA scans are important for the monitoring of BMD in both treated and untreated patients.[51,52] Decrease in BMD over time is associated with an increased risk of fractures for both treated and untreated patients. In patients who are not already on osteoporosis therapy, a follow-up DXA scan with a statistically significant decrease in BMD should prompt an investigation into secondary causes of osteoporosis or medical noncompliance.

On follow-up DXA scans it is important to reproduce all the parameters of the original scan as much as possible.[51,52] Ideally, the patient should be followed on the exact same DXA scanner and using the same software as the original examination. Unless cross-calibration has been performed, studies from different institutions or different scanners from the same institution should not be directly compared. On follow-up DXA scans, patient positioning and scan analysis should be the same as on the original scan. DXA images should be evaluated for changes in the visualized bones and soft tissues, including interval fractures, increasing degenerative changes, new hardware, or other new artifacts. On follow-up DXA scans

large changes in measured area (in cm²) should raise concern and the DXA images should be reexamined for technical factors (ie, patient positioning, scan analysis, and artifacts) that may explain the difference.

When monitoring patients using DXA, it is important to compare the BMD values rather than the T-score or Z-score. T-score and Z-score are not used because they are based on the reference

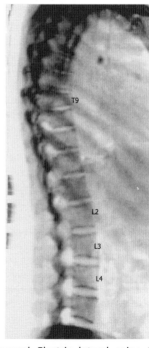

Fig. 10. General Electric lateral spine DXA image shows a T9 wedge fracture.

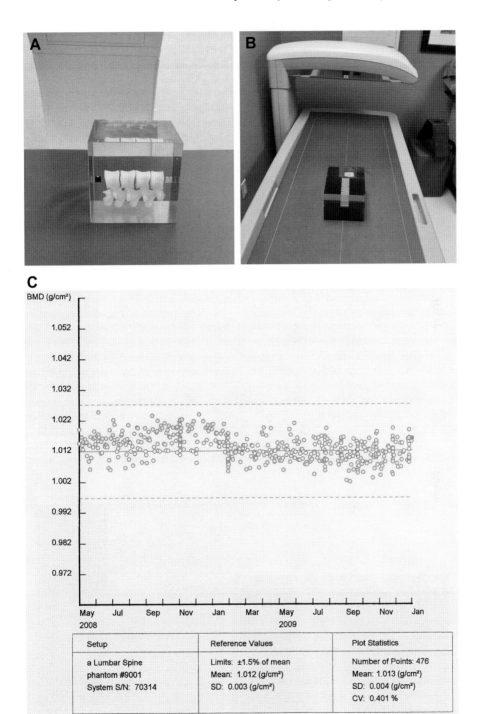

Fig. 11. Central DXA phantoms and calibration plots. (*A*) Hologic spine phantom. (*B*) General Electric spine phantom. (*C*) Hologic spine phantom BMD plot.

data that may change with upgrades in scanner software. Many scanners include software that can calculate changes in BMD, percent change in BMD, or annual change in BMD.

Each DXA facility has measurement inconsistencies relating to scanner, technologist, and patient. To monitor patients using DXA, each DXA facility should determine the precision error of its equipment and from that calculate the least significant change (LSC). A change of BMD greater than the LSC constitutes a significant change.[52]

Each center should conduct a precision error analysis rather than using the provided precision error of the DXA manufacturer. The precision study is performed by having a technologist measure 15 patients 3 times or 30 patients 2 times with repositioning of the patient between each scan. A precision error calculator is then used to determine the root mean square standard deviation. The LSC is calculated by multiplying the precision error by 2.77.[52]

On follow-up scans, the BMD from the original scan is subtracted from the BMD of the follow-up scan, and that value is compared with the LSC. If the change in BMD is greater than the LSC, then the change is considered statistically significant. Conversely, change in BMD that is less than the LSC does not represent statistically significant change.

The time between follow-up examinations varies from patient to patient based on a variety of clinical factors including osteoporosis therapy, glucocorticoid use, and underlying secondary causes of osteoporosis. Ideally, follow-up DXA examinations should be performed when the expected change in BMD would exceed the LSC at that center. In general, postmenopausal women and elderly men without glucocorticoid use or secondary causes of osteoporosis are followed at 1- to 2-year intervals. In general, patients on glucocorticoids or with secondary causes of osteoporosis are followed at 6- to 12-month intervals.[52]

The preferred site for monitoring change in BMD is the PA spine. In patients without degenerative disease, it has the best precision and shows the greatest changes owing to high proportion of metabolically active cancellous bone. In patients with spinal degenerative disease, the hip BMD is used for monitoring, with the total hip ROI preferred over the femoral neck ROI.

LATERAL VERTEBRAL ASSESSMENT

Increasing numbers of centers are using DXA to diagnose vertebral fractures. On modern fan-beam DXA systems, lateral images of the lower thoracic and lumbar spine are obtained in less than 10 seconds. On scanners with a rotating gantry, the patients are scanned supine, whereas on scanners where the gantry does not rotate, decubitus lateral positioning is used (**Fig. 9**). These low-dose images are used to screen for vertebral fractures usually following the routine BMD measurement (**Fig. 10**).

The lateral vertebral assessment (LVA) images are lower resolution than standard radiographs and are of limited use in evaluation of mild fractures and fractures of the upper thoracic spine.[53,54] Upper thoracic spine, however, is an uncommon region for osteoporotic fracture. Studies have shown that for the 90% of vertebrae that can be seen with LVA, sensitivity and

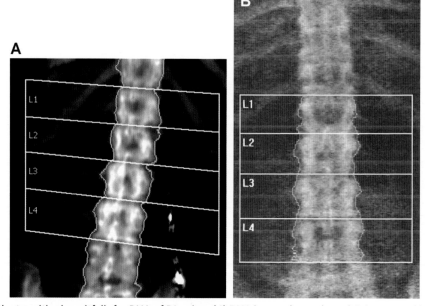

Fig. 12. Patient positioning pitfalls for DXA of PA spine. (*A*) DXA image shows the pelvis is centered but the spine is off center. Also noted is contrast in the colon. (*B*) DXA image shows the scan extends from T11 to L4, instead of T12 to L5 vertebrae.

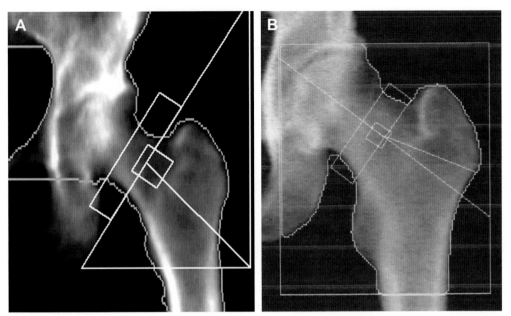

Fig. 13. Patient positioning pitfalls for DXA of the hip. (*A*) DXA image shows the proximal femur is abducted. (*B*) DXA image shows the proximal femur is externally rotated with too much lesser trochanter visible.

specificity for detection of moderate to severe fractures, the most clinically relevant ones, exceed 90%.[53,54] Because many elderly patients have asymptomatic vertebral fractures and the presence of such fractures may indicate a need for pharmacologic treatment regardless of BMD, adding LVA to quantitative BMD measurements is an easy way to improve patient care.

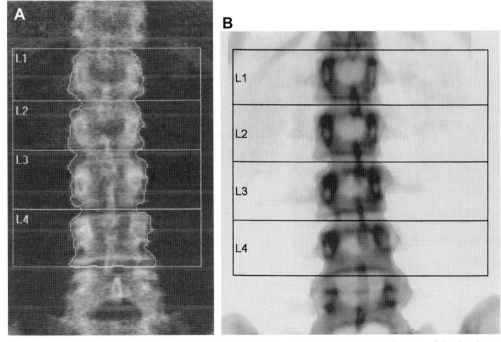

Fig. 14. Correct analysis of PA spine scan. (*A*) Hologic spine image shows correct numbering of the lumbar vertebrae, correct placement of intervertebral lines, and correct bone edge detection. (*B*) General Electric spine image shows correct analysis of PA spine scan.

PITFALLS OF DXA INTERPRETATION

All centers involved in clinical DXA scanning and interpretation should pay careful attention to pitfalls in interpretation related to the scanner and its software, the technologist and his or her positioning of patient and analysis of scans, and various patient-related artifacts.[55–57] These pitfalls may lead to errors in interpretation; both false positive and false negative results are common.

A

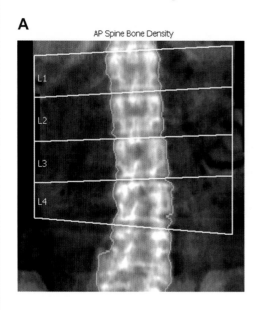

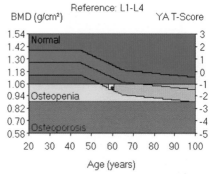

Region	BMD (g/cm²)	Young-Adult (%)	T-Score	Age-Matched (%)	Z-Score
L1	0.996	88	-1.1	93	-0.6
L2	1.025	85	-1.5	90	-1.0
L3	1.066	89	-1.1	93	-0.6
L4	1.040	87	-1.3	91	-0.9
L1-L2	1.011	88	-1.2	92	-0.7
L1-L3	1.029	88	-1.2	92	-0.7
L1-L4	1.032	87	-1.2	92	-0.8
L2-L3	1.045	87	-1.3	91	-0.8
L2-L4	1.043	87	-1.3	91	-0.8
L3-L4	1.051	88	-1.2	92	-0.8

B

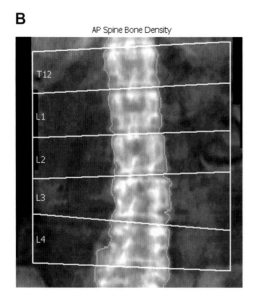

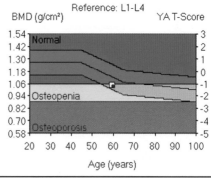

Region	BMD (g/cm²)	Young-Adult (%)	T-Score	Age-Matched (%)	Z-Score
L1	1.025	91	-0.9	96	-0.4
L2	1.066	89	-1.1	93	-0.6
L3	1.040	87	-1.3	91	-0.9
L4	1.043	87	-1.3	91	-0.8
L1-L2	1.045	91	-0.9	96	-0.4
L1-L3	1.043	89	-1.1	94	-0.6
L1-L4	1.043	88	-1.1	93	-0.7
L2-L3	1.051	88	-1.2	92	-0.8
L2-L4	1.048	87	-1.3	92	-0.8
L3-L4	1.041	87	-1.3	91	-0.8

Fig. 15. Analysis pitfalls of PA spine scan. (*A*) Spine image shows incorrect numbering of the vertebrae. (*B*) Spine image shows corrected numbering. (*C*) Spine image shows the bone edges were not properly recognized. (*D*) Spine image shows the corrected bone edges.

C

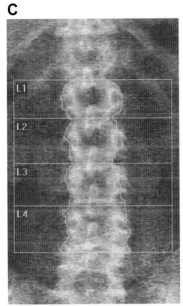

Image not for diagnostic use
k = 1.136, d0 = 42.8
116 x 123

Scan Information:

Scan Date: January 05, 2010   ID: A01051004
Scan Type: a Lumbar Spine
Analysis: January 05, 2010 10:01 Version 12.3:3
Lumbar Spine
Operator: SH
Model: Delphi A (S/N 70314)
Comment: BL-

DXA Results Summary:

Region	Area (cm²)	BMC (g)	BMD (g/cm²)	T-Score	PR (%)	Z-Score	AM (%)
L1	10.78	8.17	0.758	-1.5	82	0.1	102
L2	11.11	8.51	0.766	-2.4	74	-0.6	92
L3	11.55	9.52	0.824	-2.4	76	-0.5	94
L4	15.49	13.80	0.890	-2.1	80	-0.1	99
Total	**48.93**	**40.00**	**0.817**	**-2.1**	**78**	**-0.3**	**97**

D

Image not for diagnostic use
k = 1.136, d0 = 42.8
116 x 123

Scan Information:

Scan Date: January 05, 2010   ID: A01051004
Scan Type: a Lumbar Spine
Analysis: January 05, 2010 10:33 Version 12.3:3
Lumbar Spine
Operator: SH
Model: Delphi A (S/N 70314)
Comment: BL-

DXA Results Summary:

Region	Area (cm²)	BMC (g)	BMD (g/cm²)	T-Score	PR (%)	Z-Score	AM (%)
L1	10.78	8.17	0.758	-1.5	82	0.1	102
L2	12.73	9.44	0.741	-2.6	72	-0.8	89
L3	12.64	10.21	0.808	-2.5	74	-0.6	92
L4	15.49	13.80	0.890	-2.1	80	-0.1	99
Total	**51.65**	**41.62**	**0.806**	**-2.2**	**77**	**-0.4**	**95**

Fig. 15. (continued)

To minimize scanner-related pitfalls, proper calibration should be performed. Phantoms should be scanned per the manufacture's guidelines, typically, at least weekly. Phantom data should be plotted and reviewed to ensure consistency (**Fig. 11**). If there are significant shifts or drifts in phantom data, the scanner should be serviced before scanning any patients.

All DXA images should be carefully assessed for patient positioning, scan analysis, and artifacts before reporting any given BMD, T-score, or Z-score.[55–57] An interpreting physician should treat

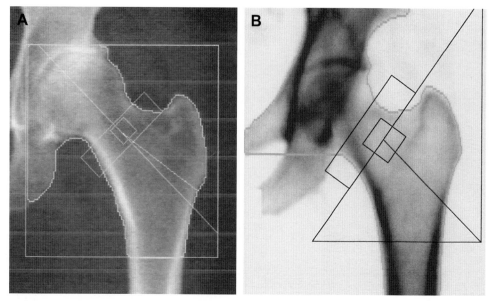

Fig. 16. Correct analysis of hip DXA scan. (*A*) Hologic hip shows femoral neck region of interest properly anchored on the greater trochanter. (*B*) General Electric image shows femoral neck region of interest in the middle of the femoral neck.

the DXA image with the same attention given to any other x-ray image.

Common pitfalls in patient positioning include improper centering of the lumbar spine (**Fig. 12**) and abduction or external rotation of the hip (**Fig. 13**). In the spine, common analytic pitfalls relate to numbering of the vertebrae, placement of intervertebral markers, and detection of bone edges (**Figs. 14** and **15**). In the hip, analytic pitfalls relate to placement of femoral ROIs and detection of bone edges (**Figs. 16** and **17**).

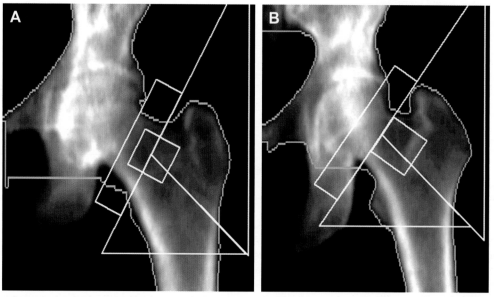

Fig. 17. Analysis pitfall of hip DXA scan. (*A*) DXA image shows the bone edge of the medial femoral neck is not detected. (*B*) DXA image shows femoral neck region of interest is positioned too high including portions of the femoral neck and ischium.

A

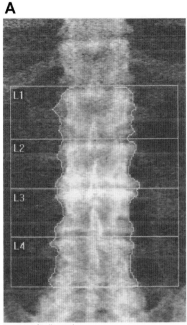

Image not for diagnostic use
k = 1.133, d0 = 42.7
116 x 134

Scan Information:

Scan Date: October 28, 2009 ID: A10280907
Scan Type: a Lumbar Spine
Analysis: October 28, 2009 11:43 Version 12.3:3
Lumbar Spine
Operator: SH
Model: Delphi A (S/N 70314)
Comment: BL-

DXA Results Summary:

Region	Area (cm²)	BMC (g)	BMD (g/cm²)	T - Score	PR (%)	Z - Score	AM (%)
L1	17.41	19.59	1.125	1.1	112	2.0	124
L2	16.85	25.98	1.542	4.1	141	5.1	156
L3	16.27	26.15	1.607	4.6	146	5.6	162
L4	18.64	24.80	1.330	1.7	116	2.7	129
Total	**69.17**	**96.52**	**1.395**	**2.8**	**128**	**3.7**	**142**

B

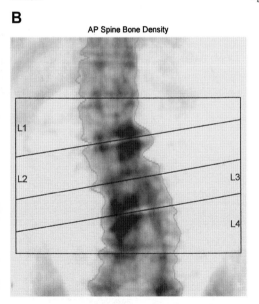

AP Spine Bone Density

Reference: L1-L4

Region	BMD[1] (g/cm²)	Young-Adult[2] (%)	T-Score	Age-Matched[3] (%)	Z-Score
L1	1.315	116	1.5	135	2.8
L2	1.623	135	3.5	156	4.8
L3	1.739	145	4.5	167	5.8
L4	1.609	134	3.4	154	4.7
L1-L4	1.570	133	3.3	153	4.6

Fig. 18. Common artifacts seen on DXA scans. (*A*) Degenerative disease, most prominent at L3-L4 disk level. (*B*) Scoliosis and degenerative disease. (*C*) L1 vertebral fracture. (*D*) Spinal instrumentation involving L4 and L5 vertebrae. (*E*) Barium in the colon. (*F*) Hip osteoarthritis.

Common anatomic artifacts found on DXA images of the lumbar spine include degenerative disc disease, compression fractures, postsurgical defects, and overlying atherosclerotic calcifications (**Fig. 18**). Other artifacts include implantable devices such as stents and vena cava filters, overlying gastrointestinal contrast, lumbar hardware, vertebroplasty cement, and external objects such as piercings, bra clips, and metallic buttons. Care should be made to identify patient motion that results in blurring or irregular contour of the bone margins on the DXA images. Anatomic artifacts found on DXA images of the hip include osteoarthritis, heterotopic ossification, and large

C

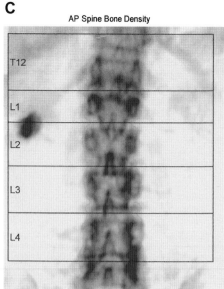

AP Spine Bone Density

T12
L1
L2
L3
L4

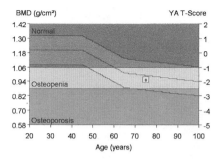

Reference: L1-L4

		BMC¹	Young-Adult²		Age-Matched³	
Region	BMD (g/cm²)		(%)	T-Score	(%)	Z-Score
L1	0.943		83	-1.6	100	0.0
L2	0.865		72	-2.8	86	-1.2
L3	1.021		85	-1.5	101	0.1
L4	0.992		83	-1.7	98	-0.2
L1-L4	0.960		81	-1.8	97	-0.3

Scan Information:

Scan Date: December 21, 2009   ID: A1221090F
Scan Type: a Lumbar Spine
Analysis: December 21, 2009 14:52 Version 12.3:3
          Lumbar Spine
Operator: SH
Model: Delphi A (S/N 70314)
Comment: BL-

D

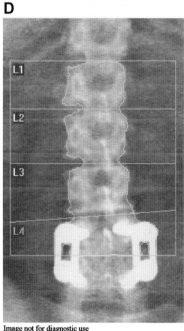

L1
L2
L3
L4

Image not for diagnostic use
k = 1.141 d0 = 45.0

DXA Results Summary:

Region	Area (cm²)	BMC (g)	BMD (g/cm²)	T-Score	PR (%)	Z-Score	AM (%)
L1	11.88	8.21	0.691	-2.1	75	-1.1	86
L2	13.81	11.30	0.818	-1.9	80	-0.7	91
L3	14.30	13.29	0.929	-1.4	86	-0.1	98
Total	**39.99**	**32.79**	**0.820**	**-1.8**	**81**	**-0.6**	**92**

Fig. 18. (*continued*)

panniculus (see **Fig. 18**). Additional artifacts including wallets, keys, coins, surgical hardware, and motion may be seen.

CENTRAL DXA REPORTING

Although there is broad consensus on clinical DXA interpretation, DXA reporting varies widely across different facilities.[58] The International Society for Clinical Densitometry (ISCD) has made recommendations on reporting that serve as basis for our approach. Consistent, concise, and clear reporting is essential to ensure relevant data are conveyed to the referring clinicians. Demographic data should include age, race, sex, menopausal status, risk factors, and osteoporosis therapy. The DXA scanner type should be included for future comparisons. The measured BMD, T-score,

E

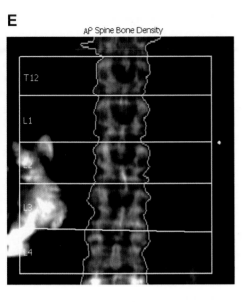

AP Spine Bone Density

T12

L1

L2

L3

L4

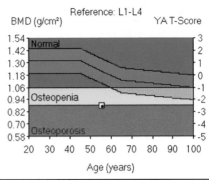

Reference: L1-L4

BMD (g/cm²)   YA T-Score

Region	BMD (g/cm²)	Young-Adult (%)	T-Score	Age-Matched (%)	Z-Score
L1	0.766	68	-3.0	66	-3.3
L2	0.911	76	-2.4	74	-2.7
L3	0.880	73	-2.7	71	-3.0
L4	0.967	81	-1.9	78	-2.3
L1-L2	0.836	73	-2.6	71	-2.9
L1-L3	0.852	73	-2.6	71	-2.9
L1-L4	0.884	75	-2.5	73	-2.8
L2-L3	0.894	75	-2.5	72	-2.9
L2-L4	0.920	77	-2.3	74	-2.6
L3-L4	0.924	77	-2.3	75	-2.6

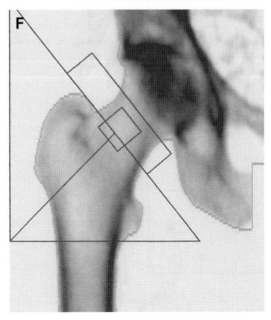

F

Fig. 18. (continued)

and Z-score should be clearly included. Finally, diagnostic assessment and treatment recommendations should be listed (**Box 1**).

CLINICAL CONTEXT FOR DXA MEASUREMENT

There are many organizations dedicated to proper diagnosis and management of patients with osteoporosis. The ISCD,[12] the United States Preventative Services Task Force (USPSTF),[34] and the National Osteoporosis Foundation (NOF)[59] recommend that all women older than 65 should have their BMD measured.

Several risk assessment tools have been developed to identify those at higher risk for osteoporosis. These include the Simple Calculated

<table>
<tr><td>

Box 1
Template of our DXA report

BONE DENSITOMETRY (DXA)

CLINICAL HISTORY:

   Age:

   Race:

   Gender:

   Menopausal Status:

   Risk Factors:

   Osteoporosis Therapy:

TECHNIQUE

   The study was performed using a GE Lunar Prodigy bone densitometer.

RESULTS:

   PA Lumbar Spine:

   BMD measured in [ ] region of interest is [ ] g/cm^2.

   T-score:

   Z-score:

   Comments:

PROXIMAL FEMUR:

   BMD measured in [ ] region of interest is [ ] g/cm^2.

   T-score:

   Z-score:

   Comments:

CONCLUSIONS:

   1. Diagnosis:

   2. Fracture Risk:

   3. Monitoring:

   4. Treatment recommendations:

   5. Follow up DXA:

</td></tr>
</table>

Osteoporosis Risk Estimation (SCORE); the Osteoporosis Risk Assessment Instrument (ORAI); the Osteoporosis Index of Risk (OSIRIS); Age, Body, Size, No Estrogen (ABONE); and the Osteoporosis Self-Assessment Tool (OST).[60,61] In general, these tools rely on common clinical risk factors for low BMD including height loss, low body weight, advanced age, late age of menarche, menopausal, smoking, alcohol use, and low dietary calcium.[60] The introduction of FRAX has led to a more uniform approach to incorporating non–BMD-related risk factors into clinical practice.

Although the treatments for primary osteoporosis are focused on restoring BMD, it is important to identify any potential secondary causes so that treatment can be tailored to correct the underlying disorder. There are many causes for secondary osteoporosis including lifestyle factors (eg, alcohol use, vitamin deficiency, smoking, inadequate physical activity), genetic factors (eg, family of osteoporosis, cystic fibrosis, Marfan's syndrome), endocrine disorders (eg, hypogonadal states, hyperparathyroidism), gastrointestinal disorders, hematologic disorders, autoimmune conditions, and medications (eg, glucocorticoids). In a study of 173 healthy women, Tannenbaum and colleagues[62] found that 32% had disorders that affect BMD. The most common disorders were hypercalciuria, malabsorption, hyperparathyroidism, and vitamin D deficiency.[62] On central DXA, there is no way to differentiate primary from secondary osteoporosis. For this reason, laboratory evaluation to exclude secondary causes of osteoporosis should complement BMD measurement.

SUMMARY

Central DXA is rapid, reliable, and the most commonly used method of measuring bone mineral density in clinical practice. Although interpretation of clinical DXA scans is generally straightforward, it is important for the interpreting physician to be aware of common pitfalls and to maintain rigorous quality assurance. A firm understanding of the clinical utility of DXA allows the interpreting physician to provide valuable recommendations to treating clinicians, thereby improving the care of patients with osteoporosis.

REFERENCES

1. Guglielmi G, de Terlizzi F. Quantitative ultrasound in the assessment of osteoporosis. Eur J Radiol 2009; 71:425–31.
2. Adams JE. Quantitative computed tomography. Eur J Radiol 2009;71:415–24.
3. Blake GM, Fogelman I. The clinical role of dual energy X-ray absorptiometry. Eur J Radiol 2009;71: 406–14.
4. Grampp S, Genant HK, Mathur A, et al. Comparisons of noninvasive bone mineral measurements in assessing age-related loss, fracture discrimination, and diagnostic classification. J Bone Miner Res 1997;12:697–711.
5. Lewis MK, Blake GM, Fogelman I. Patient dose in dual x-ray absorptiometry. Osteoporos Int 1994;4: 11–5.
6. Njeh CF, Fuerst T, Hans D, et al. Radiation exposure in bone mineral density assessment. Appl Radiat Isot 1999;50:215–36.

7. Blake GM, Naeem M, Boutros M. Comparison of effective dose to children and adults from dual X-ray absorptiometry examinations. Bone 2006;38: 935–42.

8. Guglielmi G, Gluer CC, Majumdar S, et al. Current methods and advances in bone densitometry. Eur Radiol 1995;5:129–39.

9. Grampp S, Jergas M, Glüer CC, et al. Radiologic diagnosis of osteoporosis. Current methods and perspectives. Radiol Clin North Am 1993;31: 1133–45.

10. Blake GM, Fogelman I. Technical principles of dual energy x-ray absorptiometry. Semin Nucl Med 1997;27:210–28.

11. Lewiecki EM, Gordon CM, Baim S, et al. International Society for Clinical Densitometry 2007 adult and pediatric official positions. Bone 2008;43: 1115–21.

12. Binkley N, Bilezikian JP, Kendler DL, et al. Official positions of the International Society for Clinical Densitometry and executive summary of the 2005 position development conference. J Clin Densitom 2006;9:4–14.

13. Lenchik L, Leib ES, Hamdy RC, et al. International Society for Clinical Densitometry Position Development Panel and Scientific Advisory Committee. Executive summary International Society for Clinical Densitometry position development conference Denver, Colorado July 20–22, 2001. J Clin Densitom 2002;5(Suppl):S1–3.

14. Miller PD, Bonnick SL, Rosen CJ, et al. Clinical utility of bone mass measurements in adults: consensus of an international panel. The Society for Clinical Densitometry. Semin Arthritis Rheum 1996;25:361–72.

15. Svendsen OL, Hassager C, Skodt V, et al. Impact of soft tissue on in vivo accuracy of bone mineral measurements in the spine, hip and forearm: a human cadaver study. J Bone Miner Res 1995; 10:868–73.

16. Blake GM, Fogelman I. How important are BMD accuracy errors for the clinical interpretation of DXA scans? J Bone Miner Res 2008;23:457–62.

17. Tothill P, Hannan J. Precision and accuracy errors of measuring changes in bone mineral density by dual-energy X-ray absorptiometry. Osteoporos Int 2007; 18:1515–23.

18. Bonnick SL, Johnston CC, Kleerekoper M, et al. Importance of precision in bone density measurements. J Clin Densitom 2001;4:105–10.

19. Kiebzak GM, Faulkner KG, Wacker W, et al. Effect of precision error on T-scores and diagnostic classification of bone status. J Clin Densitom 2007;10: 239–43.

20. Blake GM, Herd RJM, Fogelman I. A longitudinal study of supine lateral DXA of the lumbar spine: a comparison with posteroanterior spine, hip and total body DXA. Osteoporos Int 1996;16:462–70.

21. Patel R, Blake GM, Rymer J, et al. Long-term precision of DXA scanning assessed over seven years in forty postmenopausal women. Osteoporos Int 2000; 11:68–75.

22. Engelke K, Glüer CC. Quality and performance measures in bone densitometry: part 1: errors and diagnosis. Osteoporos Int 2006;17:1283–92.

23. Courtney AC, Wachtel EF, Myers ER, et al. Age-related reductions in the strength of the femur tested in a fall-loading configuration. J Bone Joint Surg Am 1995;77:387–95.

24. Marshall D, Johnell O, Wedel H. Meta-analysis of how well measures of bone mineral density predict occurrence of osteoporotic fractures. BMJ 1996; 312:1254–9.

25. Johnell O, Kanis JA, Oden A, et al. Predictive value of BMD for hip and other fractures. J Bone Miner Res 2005;20:1185–94.

26. Cummings SR, Black DM, Nevitt MC, et al. Bone density at various sites for prediction of hip fractures. Lancet 1993;341:72–5.

27. Stone KL, Seeley DG, Lui LY, et al. BMD at multiple sites and risk of fracture of multiple types: long-term results from the Study of Osteoporotic Fractures. J Bone Miner Res 2003;18:1947–54.

28. Binkovitz LA, Henwood MJ, Sparke P. Pediatric dual-energy X-ray absorptiometry: technique, interpretation, and clinical applications. Semin Nucl Med 2007;37:303–13.

29. Kanis JA, Melton L III, Christiansen C, et al. The diagnosis of osteoporosis. J Bone Miner Res 1994; 9:1137–41.

30. Kanis JA, Delmas P, Burckhardt P, et al. Guidelines for diagnosis and treatment of osteoporosis. Osteoporos Int 1997;7:390–406.

31. Genant HK, Cooper C, Poor G, et al. Interim report and recommendations of the World Health Organization task-force for osteoporosis. Osteoporos Int 1999;10:259–64.

32. Kanis JA, Gluer CC. An update on the diagnosis and assessment of osteoporosis with densitometry: committee of scientific advisors, International Osteoporosis Foundation. Osteoporos Int 2000;11: 192–202.

33. Rosen CJ. Issues facing bone densitometry in the new century: reflections from the National Institutes of Health consensus development conference on osteoporosis. Clin Densitom 2000;3:211–3.

34. US Preventive Services Task Force. Screening for osteoporosis in postmenopausal women: recommendations and rationale. Ann Intern Med. 2002; 137:526–8.

35. Hodgson SF, Watts NB, Bilezikian JP, et al. AACE osteoporosis task force. American Association of Clinical Endocrinologists medical guidelines for clinical practice for the prevention and treatment of postmenopausal osteoporosis: 2001 edition, with

selected updates for 2003. Endocr Pract 2003;9: 544–64.

36. Compston J. US and UK guidelines for glucocorti-coid-induced osteoporosis: similarities and differences. Curr Rheumatol Rep 2004;6:66–9.

37. Kornbluth A, Hayes M, Feldman S, et al. Do guidelines matter? Implementation of the ACG and AGA osteoporosis screening guidelines in inflammatory bowel disease (IBD) patients who meet the guidelines' criteria. Am J Gastroenterol 2006;101:1546–50.

38. Baddoura R, Awada H, Okais J, et al. An audit of bone densitometry practice with reference to ISCD, IOF and NOF guidelines. Osteoporos Int 2006;17:1111–5.

39. Zethraeus N, Borgstrom F, Strom O, et al. Cost-effectiveness of the treatment and prevention of osteoporosis—a review of the literature and a reference model. Osteoporos Int 2007;18:9–23.

40. Liu H, Paige NM, Goldzweig CL, et al. Screening for osteoporosis in men: a systematic review for an American College of Physicians guideline. Ann Intern Med 2008;148:685–701.

41. Lim LS, Hoeksema LJ, Sherin K, ACPM prevention practice committee. Screening for osteoporosis in the adult US population: ACPM position statement on preventive practice. Am J Prev Med 2009;36:366–75.

42. Dawson-Hughes B, Looker AC, Tosteson AN, et al. The potential impact of new National Osteoporosis Foundation guidance on treatment patterns. Osteoporos Int 2010;21:41–52.

43. Melton LJ, Chrischilles EA, Cooper C, et al. How many women have osteoporosis? J Bone Miner Res 1992;7:1005–10.

44. Melton LJ. The prevalence of osteoporosis. J Bone Miner Res 1997;12:1769–71.

45. Baim S, Leonard MB, Bianchi ML, et al. Official positions of the International Society for Clinical Densitometry and executive summary of the 2007 ISCD pediatric position development conference. J Clin Densitom 2008;11:6–21.

46. Kanis JA, Johnell O, Oden A, et al. Ten-year probabilities of osteoporotic fractures according to BMD and diagnostic thresholds. Osteoporos Int 2001;12: 989–95.

47. Kanis JA, Oden A, Johnell O, et al. The use of clinical risk factors enhances the performance of BMD in the prediction of hip and osteoporotic fractures in men and women. Osteoporos Int 2007;18:1033–46.

48. Borgstrom F, Johnell O, Kanis JA, et al. At what hip fracture risk is it cost effective to treat? International intervention thresholds for the treatment of osteoporosis. Osteoporos Int 2006;17:1459–71.

49. Kanis J, Oden A, Johansson H, et al. FRAX and its applications to clinical practice. Bone 2009;44: 734–43.

50. Watts N, Lewieki E, Miller P, et al. National Osteoporosis Foundation 2008 clinician's guide to prevention and treatment of osteoporosis and the World Health Organization fracture risk assessment tool (FRAX): what they mean to the bone densitometrist and bone technologist. J Clin Densitom 2008;11: 473–7.

51. El Maghraoui A, Achemlal L, Bezza A. Monitoring of dual-energy X-ray absorptiometry measurement in clinical practice. J Clin Densitom 2006;9:281–6.

52. Lenchik L, Kiebzak GM, Blunt BA. International Society for Clinical Densitometry position development panel and scientific advisory committee. What is the role of serial bone mineral density measurements in patient management? J Clin Densitom 2002;5(Suppl):S29–38.

53. Schousboe JT, Vokes T, Broy SB, et al. Vertebral fracture assessment: the 2007 ISCD official positions. J Clin Densitom 2008;11:92–108.

54. Fuerst T, Wu C, Genant HK, et al. Evaluation of vertebral fracture assessment by dual X-ray absorptiometry in a multicenter setting. Osteoporos Int 2009;20: 1199–205.

55. El Maghroui A, Roux C. DXA scanning in clinical practice. QJM 2008;101:605–17.

56. Lenchik L, Rochmis P, Sartoris DJ. Optimized interpretation and reporting of dual X-ray absorptiometry (DXA) scans. AJR Am J Roentgenol 1998;171: 1509–20.

57. Watts NB. Fundamentals and pitfalls of bone densitometry using dual-energy X-ray absorptiometry (DXA). Osteoporos Int 2004;15:847–54.

58. Lentle BC, Prior JC. Osteoporosis: what a clinician expects to learn from a patient's bone density examination. Radiology 2003;228:620–8.

59. National Osteoporosis Foundation. Clinician's guide to prevention and treatment of osteoporosis. Washington, DC: National Osteoporosis Foundation; 2008.

60. Weinstein L, Ullery B. Identification of at-risk women for osteoporosis screening. Am J Obstet Gynecol 2000;183:547–9.

61. Ribot C, Tremollieres F, Pouilles JM. Can we detect women with low bone mass using clinical risk factors? Am J Med 1995;98:52s–5s.

62. Tannenbaum C, Clark J, Schwartzman K, et al. Yield of laboratory testing to identify secondary contributors to osteoporosis in otherwise healthy women. J Clin Endocrinol Metab 2002;87:4431–7.

Vertebral Morphometry

Daniele Diacinti, MD[a], Giuseppe Guglielmi, MD[b],*

KEYWORDS

- Osteoporotic vertebral fractures
- Semiquantitative vertebral assessment
- Vertebral morphometric x-ray radiography
- Dual x-ray absorptiometry
- Morphometric x-ray absorptiometry
- Vertebral fracture assessment

Vertebral fractures are the hallmark of osteoporosis. Vertebral fractures are the most common of all osteoporotic fractures, occurring in 15% of women 50 to 59 years old and in 50% of women 85 years or older.[1–5] The majority of osteoporotic vertebral fractures are mild vertebral deformities, with a reduction in height of not more than 20% to 25%, and they are asymptomatic and occur in absence of specific trauma.[6] Even these mild vertebral deformities could have clinical consequences for the patient because of the increased, approximately fivefold, risk of future fractures that may be symptomatic.[7–10] Multiple vertebral fractures are associated with an increased mortality rate[11,12] and impaired quality of life.[13–17] For these reasons the prevention of incident vertebral fractures in patients with mild and asymptomatic vertebral fractures has been considered the end point in clinical osteoporosis therapy trials.[18–23]

Therefore, it is in the accurate classification of vertebral deformities as mild vertebral fractures that radiologists make perhaps the most significant contribution to osteoporotic patient care.

VERTEBRAL FRACTURE OR VERTEBRAL DEFORMITY?
Algorithm-Based Qualitative Method

The diagnosis of vertebral fractures is usually based on the presence of a deformation of vertebral body on lateral spinal radiographs, but a vertebral deformity is not always a vertebral fracture.[24]

Because there is no consensus on the exact definition of a vertebral fracture, it may sometimes be difficult to discriminate the prevalent vertebral fracture from a normal variant of vertebral shape or from a vertebral deformation that may have occurred long ago, especially in mild cases. The conventional approach for diagnosis of osteoporotic vertebral fracture is regarded as subjective and therefore may lead to disagreement, especially when performed by inexperienced observers.[25,26] For example, the distinction between a fractured endplate and the deformity associated with Schmorl nodes can only be made visually by an experienced observer, as is the case for the diagnosis of the wedge-shaped appearance caused by remodeling of the vertebral bodies in degenerative disc disease.[27]

To improve the visual identification of prevalent vertebral fractures, an algorithm-based qualitative (ABQ) method has been developed.[28] The ABQ method assumes that all osteoporotic vertebral fractures initially involve concave depression of the center of the endplate within the vertebral ring, that is, the weakest area. Thus by definition, wedge and crush fractures are initially concave fractures. If the vertebral ring is displaced with fracture of the lateral or anterior cortex of the vertebral body, there will be wedge or crush fracture. There is some evidence to support this model of vertebral fracture. Anterior, but not middle vertebral height, was found to be significantly shorter in subjects with osteoarthritis.[29] Also,

[a] Department of Radiology, University "Sapienza", Policlinico Umberto I, Viale Regina Elena 324, 00161 Rome, Italy
[b] Department of Radiology, University of Foggia, Scientific Institute Hospital "Casa Sollievo della Sofferenza", San Giovanni Rotondo, Viale Luigi Pinto, 71100 Foggia, Italy
* Corresponding author.
E-mail address: guglielmi.g@unifg.it

Radiol Clin N Am 48 (2010) 561–575
doi:10.1016/j.rcl.2010.02.018
0033-8389/10/$ – see front matter © 2010 Published by Elsevier Inc.

wedge deformities involving an apparent reduction in anterior height alone have a weaker association with low bone density compared with concave or biconcave deformities.[30,31] The nonfracture deformity with apparent "reduction" in vertebral height of approximately greater than 15%, without endplate depression, is categorized as nonosteoporotic short vertebral height (SVH). Therefore according to the visual ABQ method, the expert reader classifies the vertebrae into 1 of 3 outcomes: (1) normal, (2) osteoporotic fracture, or (3) short vertebral height (SVH), which include normal variation in height, developmental abnormalities (eg, "balloon disc" or "steplike" endplates), degenerative change (narrowed disc spaces, sclerotic endplates, osteophytes), Scheuermann disease, large Schmorl nodes, scoliosis, or kyphosis (**Fig. 1**).

Visual Semiquantitative Method

The semiquantitative (SQ) method previously described by Genant and colleagues[32] is based on evaluation of conventional radiographs by radiologists or experienced clinicians to identify and then classify vertebral fractures. Vertebrae T4 to L4 are graded by visual inspection and without direct vertebral measurement as *normal* (grade 0), *mild* but "definite" fracture (grade 1 with approximately 20%–25% reduction in anterior, middle, and/or posterior height and 10%–20% reduction in area), *moderate* fracture (grade 2 with approximately 25%–40% reduction in any height and 20%–40% reduction in area), and *severe* fracture (grade 3 with approximately 40% or grater reduction in any height and area). In addition, a grade 0.5 is used to designate a borderline deformed vertebra that is not considered to be a definite fracture (**Fig. 2**). Incident fractures are defined as those vertebrae that show a higher deformity grade on the follow-up with respect to baseline radiographs.

The SQ method represents a simple but standardized approach that provides reasonable reproducibility, sensitivity, and specificity, allowing excellent agreement (97%; $\kappa = 0.89$) for the diagnosis of prevalent and incident vertebral fractures to be achieved among trained observers.[32] Accurate diagnosis of prevalent fractures, which requires assessment of normal variations and degenerative changes and distinguishing them from true fractures, still depends on the experience of the observer. Thus, although the SQ method is simple and accessible to all physicians, it has a learning curve. If used by trained and experienced observers, the SQ method is considered

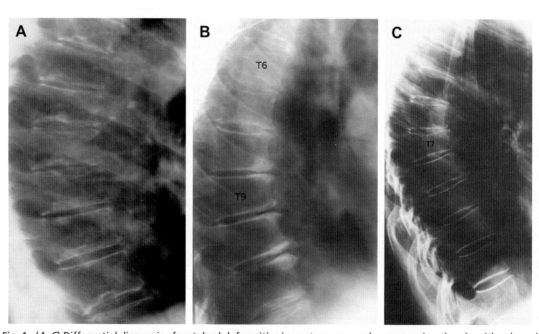

Fig. 1. (*A–C*) Differential diagnosis of vertebral deformities in postmenopausal women using the algorithm-based qualitative method (ABQ). (*A*) Scheuermann disease: short anterior height (SVH) identified by ABQ at vertebrae T5 through T7. Several vertebrae are wedged-shaped and elongated with irregular endplates, Schmorl nodes, kyphosis, and narrowed disc paces. (*B*) Degenerative changes at vertebrae T6 through T11. SVH at vertebra T9: the anterior height is shorter than normal in relation to posterior height due to overgrowth of the anterior vertebral border. Mild concave central depression at the superior endplate of T6 is a mild osteoporotic concave fracture. (*C*) Osteoporotic fracture of T7: evident concave depression of the central endplate.

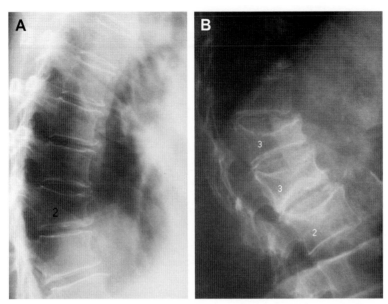

Fig. 2. (*A, B*) Visual semiquantitative (SQ) assessment for vertebral fractures. (*A*) Moderate (grade 2) wedge fracture of T10. (*B*) Moderate (grade 2) biconcave fracture of L2, and severe (grade 3) fractures of L1 (biconcave) and T12 (wedge).

a gold standard for the assessment of vertebral fractures, and therefore it is currently most widely used in multicenter clinical trials.

However, to assess subtle deformities such as mild wedgelike deformities in the midthoracic region and bowed endplates in the lumbar region, the distinction between borderline deformity (grade 0.5) and definite mild (grade 1) fractures can be difficult and sometimes arbitrary. Therefore in these cases, it is necessary to measure vertebral dimensions to accurately establish grade of vertebral deformity (**Fig. 3**).

VERTEBRAL MORPHOMETRY

Vertebral morphometry is a quantitative method to identify osteoporotic vertebral fractures based on the measurement of vertebral heights. Vertebral morphometry may be performed on conventional spinal radiographs (MRX: morphometric x-ray radiography) or on images obtained from dual x-ray absorptiometry (DXA) scans (MXA: morphometric x-ray absorptiometry).

Morphometric X-Ray Radiography

This technique was introduced as early as 1960 by Barnett and Nordin,[33] who used a transparent ruler to measure vertebral heights on conventional lateral radiographs of the thoracolumbar spine. Before performing the vertebral heights measurement the radiologist has to identify the vertebral levels; to make this easier, T12 and L1 should be

visualized on both the lateral thoracic and lumbar radiographs. Identification of vertebral levels on radiographs of lumbar and thoracic spine may be difficult at times (eg, anatomic variants of the lumbosacral transition or the thoracolumbar junction). The vertebral bodies should be marked so that they can be more easily identified in other reading sessions or when compared with follow-up radiographs. On lateral radiographs, with 6-point placement—the most widely used technique[34]—the 4 corner points of each vertebral body from T4 to L4 and additional point in the middle of the upper and lower endplates are manually marked. The manual point placement is done according to Hurxthal,[35] who proposed excluding the uncinate process at the posterosuperior border of the thoracic vertebrae and the Schmorl nodes and osteophytes from vertebral height measurement (**Fig. 4**). When the outer contours of the endplate are not superimposed (incorrect patient positioning or severe scoliosis), the middle points are placed in the center between the upper and the lower contour. Vertebral morphometry should be performed by trained observers, resulting in good interobserver measurement precision (intraoperator coefficient of variation [CV] 1.2%; interoperator CV 1.9%).[36]

Spine Radiographic Technique

The accuracy and precision of SQ and morphometric methods are heavily influenced by the quality of the spinal radiographs. Optimal

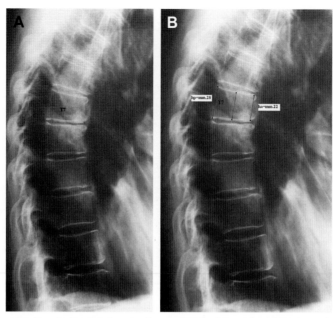

Fig. 3. (*A, B*) T7, defined as "borderline" deformity (grade 0.5) by SQ method (*A*), shows by vertebral morphometry (MRX) mild wedging with 20% of reduction in anterior height with respect to posterior height (Ha/Hp <80%) (*B*).

radiographs can be achieved by training x-ray technologists and making sure that they are aware of the difference between radiographs for osteoporotic vertebral assessment and those for routine clinical practice, by using a standardized radiographic technique,[37] which includes both patient positioning and the choice of radiographic parameters. Because the lateral views of the thoracic and lumbar spine are the most important views for the assessment of osteoporotic deformity, time and attention should be taken in correctly positioning the patient and in properly exposing the films. However, for the baseline identification of prevalent vertebral fractures, anteroposterior (AP) spinal views are also required to detect nonfracture vertebral deformities and to accurately define the number of vertebrae present. So the identification of the vertebral levels is easier on the lateral spinal views. At present, T4 to L4 are routinely used for vertebral morphometry, because of limitations in visualizing T1 to T3 due to overlying shoulders and L5 due to overlying pelvis. In a patient with marked scoliosis of the thoracic or lumbar spine (Cobb angle >15° on the AP view), it is unlikely that vertebral morphometry can be performed because of the difficulty of positioning the spine parallel to the x-ray table. The obliquity of the vertebrae can also be observed at the periphery of the radiographs due to the effect of parallax, which is caused by the divergence of the cone-beam of x-rays. The obliquity causes false appearance of biconcavity, thus affecting the diagnosis of vertebral deformity. If positioning of the patient and centering of the x-ray beam (eg, T7 and L3) has been correctly performed, the vertebral endplates should be superimposed and

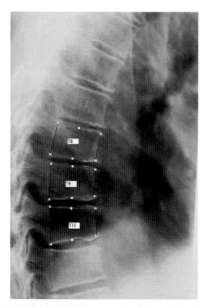

Fig. 4. MRX. Manual placement of 6 vertebral points according to Hurxthal. (*Data from* Hurxthal LM. Measurement of vertebral heights. AJR Am J Roentgenol 1968;103:635–44.)

the intervertebral disc spaces clearly seen throughout the length of the spine.

Computerized Morphometric X-Ray Radiography

Manual point placement represents a source of error in the measurement of the vertebral body because the placement can vary widely between various operators. The need to reduce these operator-dependent errors led to the development more than a decade ago of a computer-assisted system.[38–40] The procedure is based on an algorithm that automatically locates the vertebral body contour in the digitized x-ray image with the 6-point placement, which is then checked by the operator for accuracy. Correction is possible through operator intervention at any time by moving the calipers along a vertical line joining the vertebral endplates. The x- and y-coordinates of each point are stored in the computer, which calculates the posterior, middle, and anterior heights (Hp, Hm, Ha) of each vertebra, from T4 to L5, and specific indices derived from height measurements for defining vertebral deformities. The system also performs additional geometric calculations, enhancing the diagnostic capability of quantitative vertebral morphometry. Postprocessing of the digital images can highlight the endplate and the 4 corners of vertebral bodies, allowing points to be placed more precisely. There are many advantages in performing digital morphometry: magnification of the images to a specific level; selection of the contrast and brightness levels for optimum visibility of the cortical bone, a capability that is especially valuable when the film is of less than optimal quality; the images may be stored on optical disks, CD or DVD, and can be measured on multiple occasions; finally, measurement data can be captured directly from the images into a database, eliminating the need for data entry. Therefore, digital morphometry with computer assistance represents a useful tool to evaluate a large number of cases, allowing centralization of images for a large-scale clinical trial.

A new digital technique for vertebral morphometry has been introduced recently in clinical practice using an instrument called MorphoXpress (Procter & Gamble Pharmaceuticals, Rusham Park, Egham, UK). MorphoXpress is a statistical model–based vision system to digitize and analyze plain film vertebral X-rays for semiautomated morphometric assessment. This system is based on a new technology that represents the next generation of statistical model–based techniques. To the authors' knowledge, MorphoXpress is the first automated 6-point morphometric system to operate on digitized plain film radiographic images, as opposed to DXA. Furthermore, unlike DXA, radiographs of the spine are still the only approved modality for diagnosis of vertebral fracture by the US Food and Drug administration (FDA). This system works as follows. Having defined a patient record, original lateral spine radiographs are digitized using a flatbed scanner connected to the personal computer that hosts the MorphoXpress software application, and analysis is initialized by the manual indication of the centers of the upper and lower vertebrae to be analyzed. The software then automatically finds the positions of the contours of the vertebrae, including the double endplate contours and part of vertebral process. This annotation is then used to determine landmarks for a standard 6-point morphometry measurement, providing an optional confidence measure of correct registration for each vertebra. The software allows these points to be moved by the operator, if necessary, before the points are confirmed as being correctly positioned. The positions of the confirmed points are then used by the software to calculate anterior, medial, and posterior vertebral heights, and these heights may also be used for the determination of a deformity metric (**Fig. 5**). Reproducibility of this semiautomatic method results in a high (1.68%) CV. Another advantage of this approach is given by the improvement of the workflow and in the overall positive results in terms of accuracy for diagnosing vertebral fractures.[41,42] More recently another automated software tool for vertebral shape analysis has been reported (Optasia Medical, Cheadle, UK). The mean accuracy error associated with this technique is 1.06 mm, with almost 95% of errors less than 3.0 mm in magnitude, which is the threshold morphometric of vertebral body height loss for defining incident vertebral fractures.[43]

MORPHOMETRIC DEFINITION OF VERTEBRAL FRACTURES

There is no gold standard for osteoporotic fracture. Definition of vertebral fracture is based on the differences in anterior, middle, or posterior vertebral heights within a vertebra, or between adjacent vertebrae.[44,45]

However, there is variation in vertebral body (VB) size and shape at different levels of the spine for the construction of thoracolumbar curvatures, which reduce bending moments created by upright posture and so provide stability during motion.[46] The VB is anteriorly wedged from T1 through L2 (peak at T7), nonwedged at L3, and

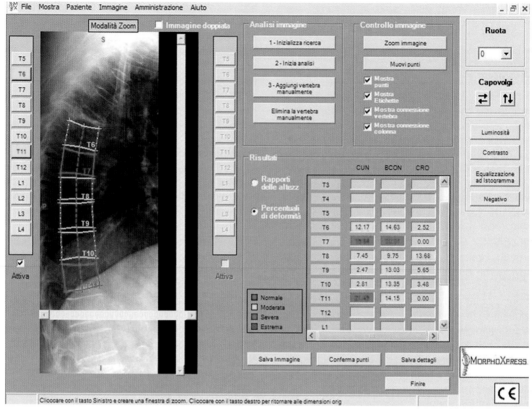

Fig. 5. Analysis of a digitized radiograph using the MorphoXpress technique with localization of the morphometric points.

posteriorly wedged at L4 to L5 (peak at L5).[47] Vertebral size also varies between individuals: large people tend to have larger vertebrae.[48,49] For this reason reference ranges for VB heights should be established in the population under study. Some investigators obtained means and standard deviations (SD) from premenopausal women, assuming that the prevalence of vertebral fractures is zero.[50] This approach may not be feasible for many studies because it involves radiation exposure for fertile women. Moreover, it has been demonstrated that vertebral heights change significantly with age, showing rates of loss of 1.2 to 1.3 mm/y in cross-sectional studies[51–53] and rate of height loss of 0.9 mm/y in a longitudinal study.[54] Age-related decrease of vertebral heights influences the definition of the normal range of vertebral shape, because a deformity that may be in excess of 2 SD from the mean in younger subjects may be well within this limit 20 years later. Therefore, other investigators derived reference values from postmenopausal women with and without vertebral fractures, using a fixed trimming procedure that removed the tails of the distribution of vertebral heights normally distributed.[55,56] The

derivation of reference data from populations with a high prevalence of vertebral fracture is problematic. To reduce the variation caused by the larger number of deformities, the use of medians and percentiles[57] or the use of a modified quantitative approach based on the calculation of standardized vertebral height, referred to as standardized quantitative morphometry (SQM), have been recommended.[58] There is still disagreement about establishing a threshold of height reduction, which would allow unequivocal discrimination between vertebral fractures, deformities, and normal shape.[59] Various morphometric algorithms to define vertebral fractures have therefore been developed by comparison within a vertebra (comparing the anterior or middle height to the posterior height) and with the adjacent vertebrae (comparing the posterior height to the posterior height of the vertebra above or below).[44,45,55] Thus, it is not possible to evaluate accurately the true- and false-positive rates of various morphometric definitions of vertebral fractures because there is no gold standard for defining a vertebral fracture. In fact, results vary widely between studies on the prevalence and on the incidence of postmenopausal vertebral fractures.[60–64] In particular, less stringent criteria (eg, 2 SD) result in too many false-positive results, because they identify as fractures some deformities that may represent developmental abnormalities. By contrast, a more stringent cutoff level, such as 4 SD, results in a higher false-negative rate.[65]

Overall, by MRX a prevalent vertebral fracture is defined on the baseline radiograph if any of the 3 ratios Ha/Hp, Hm/Hp,Hp/Hp^{+1}, or Hp/Hp^{-1}, is less than 3 SD from the corresponding normal reference ratio obtained from a population of normal fertile women. An incident vertebral fracture is defined by a decrease of 20% or more and of least 4 mm in any vertebral height of one or more vertebrae between follow-up and baseline radiographs.[66]

COMPARISON OF SQ AND MRX FOR THE IDENTIFICATION OF VERTEBRAL FRACTURES IN OSTEOPOROSIS

Some comparative studies[67–69] found a high concordance between different MRX approaches and the visual SQ method in the evaluation of prevalent vertebral fractures defined as moderate or severe (Fig. 6). In these cases there was a strong association with clinical parameters (bone mineral density, height loss, back pain, incidence of subsequent deformities). There were discrepancies between SQ and quantitative morphometry approaches in the detection of mild fractures as classified by an experienced radiologist.[70] A comparative study between ABQ and MRX on 904 postmenopausal women demonstrated that all the prevalent vertebral fractures identified by MRX but not by the ABQ method were classified as SVH and were mainly mild thoracic wedge deformities.[71] Another comparative study between the ABQ approach, SQ method, and MRX for the identification of vertebral fracture in a population of elderly men demonstrated that most of the men with vertebral fractures identified by SQ or MRX but not by ABQ were classified as having a SVH by ABQ. In these comparative studies, both women and men with SVH had bone mineral density (BMD) mean values similar to those among normal subjects. The investigators speculated that mild wedge deformity (SVH) in a vertebra without osteoporotic depression of the central endplate is possibly the greatest source of misclassification of vertebral fracture. It was recommended that differential diagnosis of morphometric vertebral deformities be conducted by an expert reader to rule out nonosteoporotic deformities with SVH.[72]

VERTEBRAL FRACTURE ASSESSMENT BY DUAL-ENERGY X-RAY ABSORPTIOMETRY

Vertebral fracture assessment (VFA) is the correct term for designating the assessment of lateral spine views acquired by DXA to detect vertebral fractures, using new-generation densitometers of 2 major manufacturers: Hologic, Inc (Bedford, MA, USA) and GE Medical

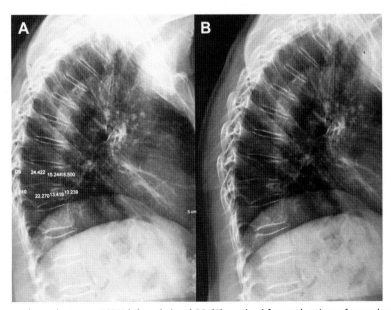

Fig. 6. (A, B) Concordance between MRX (A) and visual SQ (B) method for evaluation of prevalent vertebral fractures: severe wedging of T9 and mild concavity of T10.

Systems (Lunar, Madison, WI, USA). DXA scan of the spine is performed either by using a rotating arm (Hologic QDR 4500A, QDR Delphi, GE-Lunar Expert) with the patient lying supine or by placing the patient on in the left decubitus position similar to standard spinal radiographs (GE-Lunar Prodigy and i-DXA). Despite the difficulties in obtaining correct positioning, there are no significant differences between the lateral decubitus (Prodigy) and supine position (Expert) in measuring vertebral dimensions and in identifying vertebral fractures.[73] In patients with inadequate thoracic vertebral visualization in the left decubitus, a reverse image can be made by repositioning the patients on the right side.[74] In Hologic systems, 2 views of the thoracic and lumbar spine are acquired: a posteroanterior (PA) scan and a lateral scan. The PA image is acquired to visualize spinal anatomy such as scoliosis, to determine the centerline of the spine. This information is used in subsequent lateral scans to maintain a constant distance between the center of the spine and the x-ray tube for all subjects at all visits, regardless of patient position or degree of scoliosis, thus eliminating the geometric distortion. Each lateral scan covers a distance of 46 cm, imaging the area from L4 to T4.[75]

The GE/Lunar scanner determines the starting position of the lateral spine scan by positioning a laser spot 1 cm above the iliac crest. The scan range for the GE-Lunar systems is determined by measuring the length between the iliac crest and the armpit. The lateral scan can be acquired using a rapid (10-second) single-energy imaging mode during suspended respiration, allowing visualization of a substantial proportion of the vertebrae.[76] However, the analysis may be affected by soft tissue artifacts in the image caused by prominent lung structures. These artifacts are absent in the dual-energy scans, which, however, take between 6 minutes (array mode) and 12 minutes (fast and high definition modes).

After the scan, the program can automatically perform vertebral morphometry, namely MXA. The software automatically places 6 points in each VB from L4 to T4 to calculate the vertebral heights, their ratios, and average height. The operator analyzes all scans to manually reposition point placements that are not correct.

To guide the operator during image analysis of follow-up scans, the vertebral endplate markers from the previous scan are superimposed on the current scan, improving long-term precision. After the analysis is finished, a final report is displayed. This display gives information on the measured VB heights and their ratios, and includes an assessment of the patient's fracture status based on normative data and different models for fracture assessment using quantitative morphometry (Fig. 7).

Because the 6-point placement technique is time consuming and might not completely describe vertebral shape, Smyth and colleagues[77] have developed a technique based on use of an active shape model (ASM) or active appearance model (AAM). An AAM is a statistical model to locate and measure the shapes of variable objects in images, applied to the measurement of vertebral shape on lateral spine DXA scans from L4 up to T7. The AAM technique obtained entire shape information, with accuracy as good as that with manual methods for vertebral assessment on DXA images. However, the AAM can be performed more easily and rapidly, and with better precision than by a manual method.[78]

COMPARISON BETWEEN CONVENTIONAL RADIOGRAPHY AND DXA IMAGES

The main attraction of DXA is that the effective dose-equivalent to the patient is considerably lower (42 μSv) than for conventional radiography (500 μSv).[79,80] When using the scanning fan-beam geometry of DXA devices, the X-ray beam is parallel to the endplates, instead of being fan-shaped as during conventional radiography, which eliminates problems related to image amplification and geometric distortion.[81] Whereas the DXA technique is able to acquire the entire spine in a single image, in conventional radiography radiographs of the lumbar and thoracic spine have to be performed separately, so the identification of the vertebral levels to perform MRX may be difficult at times. In a single session, a single DXA machine supplies the 2 fundamental data to the diagnosis and prognosis of osteoporosis, namely, BMD and VFA. If the DXA scanner has a "C" arm, the lateral spine images can be obtained in the supine position without repositioning the patient into lateral decubitus position. Conventional radiology, with its superior image quality, has the potential for qualitative reading of the radiographs to aid the differential diagnosis. In fact, although it is recognized that the visual interpretation of radiographs is subjective, it is also true that an expert eye can better distinguish between true fractures and vertebral anomalies than can quantitative morphometry. On the other hand, DXA images have a limited spatial resolution so a large proportion of vertebrae are not visualized sufficiently for analysis on scans, and this reduces the number

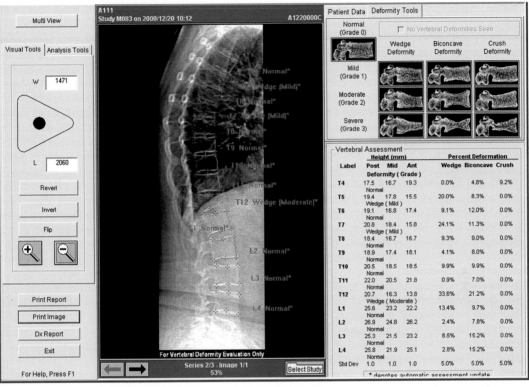

Fig. 7. Morphometric analysis of DXA spine image (MXA) in a postmenopausal (65-year-old) woman shows two vertebral fractures: mild wedging of T5 and moderate wedging of T12.

of vertebral fractures identified, particularly in the upper thoracic spine (T4–T5).[82]

CLINICAL APPLICATIONS OF VFA

To identify vertebral fractures on DXA images the visual SQ method and vertebral morphometry (MXA) are used, as on radiographs.

Several studies have been performed to compare the DXA images to the gold standard lateral spine radiographs for the detection of vertebral fracture. First, in a large study it has been demonstrated that reference ranges of vertebral heights derived from standard radiographs could not be applied to VFA on DXA images, in view of the observed differences between their MXA mean vertebral heights values when compared with MRX values reported in earlier studies.[83] The differences observed led to a tendency for lower MXA critical values for detection of vertebral deformities, suggesting the use of technique-specific reference ranges. Although densitometer manufacturers provide reference data for MXA, these values do not take into account the variability of VB heights due to racial differences. Therefore, some studies have been published that give normative MXA data derived from a local

population.[84–86] The preliminary report of an Italian multicenter study showed that vertebral heights of 569 normal Italian women measured from T4 to L4 using VFA on Lunar Prodigy (GE Healthcare) densitometers in all vertebrae were significantly smaller than the existing values collected from normal American women.[87] Rea and colleagues[88] found in 161 postmenopausal women a good agreement ($\kappa = 0.81$) between visual VFA with visual SQ on lateral radiographs. Comparing visual VFA and radiographic vertebral fracture assessment using the ABQ method in postmenopausal women, agreement resulted ($\kappa = 0.62$ and 0.81) in populations at low and high risk of fracture, respectively.[89] When quantitative morphometric techniques, MXA and MRX, were compared, agreement was lower ($\kappa = 0.79–0.70$), with sensitivity of 74% and specificity of 98% for MXA,[90] suggesting that the use of the visual VFA method would be preferable. Both MRX and MXA, when compared with SQ assessment of radiographs, showed poor agreement in a normal population ($\kappa = 0.47$) and a moderate agreement in an osteoporotic population ($\kappa = 0.71$).[91] In a successive study, Ferrar and colleagues[92] reported a better sensitivity of VFA (91.9%) in the identification of moderate/severe SQ deformities, and an excellent negative predictive value (98%) to distinguish subjects with very low risk of vertebral fractures from those with possible fractures. VFA and SQ methods disagree in the identification of mild deformities, particularly in the upper thoracic vertebrae that were not visualized sufficiently by DXA because of the poor image quality. Although some vertebral fractures were missed by VFA, all patients with prevalent vertebral fractures were identified; therefore, for the identification of patients with fracture, visual assessment of DXA scans had 100% sensitivity and specificity.[93] This result means that if VFA had been used as a diagnostic prescreening tool at the first assessment, all the patients with prevalent vertebral fracture would have been correctly referred for radiography to confirm the diagnosis (**Fig. 8**). The "normal" subjects can then be excluded before performing conventional radiographs and further time-consuming and costly methods of vertebral deformity assessment such as SQ by an experienced radiologist, and/or quantitative morphometry. More recently, VFA has been applied in a clinical population of 1168 men referred for BMD measurements, visualizing 93% of vertebral bodies from T8 to L5.[94] However, VFA cannot be performed in patients with severe scoliosis or osteoarthritis with multilevel degenerative disc disease.[95] Also, with its low radiation and good precision, VFA could be used to identify vertebral fractures in populations affected by conditions different from osteoporosis but with high vertebral fracture risk, that is, liver or kidney transplant patients.[96,97] Moreover, in patients with ankylosing spondylitis quantitative morphometric techniques, MXA and MRX, showed insufficient agreement ($\kappa = 0.79$–0.70) in measuring global vertebral wedging, expressed as (mean) AP-ratio. However, as the negative predictive value was high, the investigators suggest that VFA could be of clinical value to select patients for further evaluation by radiography to assess vertebral fractures.[98]

In clinical practice, VFA may be a tool to detect previously unrecognized vertebral fractures in asymptomatic women and in men with no known fractures having T-score values less than −1. If all vertebrae are visualized adequately by lateral DXA images and classified as normal by VFA or MXA, the patient could be classified as normal. If all vertebrae are not visualized by DXA and if one or more deformities are detected by VFA or MXA, it will be necessary to acquire conventional radiographs to check for further prevalent deformities and to identify the nature of the deformity.

CAN VERTEBRAL MORPHOMETRY PREDICT A VERTEBRAL FRACTURE?

The aim of osteoporosis treatment is to decrease the risk of fracture, particularly in individuals at high risk. Although bone mass is an important determinant of the risk of fracture, other factors contribute to skeletal fragility. There are several clinical factors (age, prior fragility fracture, smoking, excess alcohol, family history of hip fracture, rheumatoid arthritis, and the use of oral glucocorticoids) that, in conjunction with BMD, can be integrated to provide estimates of 10-year fracture probability using a new algorithm, FRAX.[99] Moreover, evidence from the literature suggests that bone quality parameters, particularly trabecular microarchitecture, and spinal properties, including vertebral macroarchitecture, intervertebral disc integrity, and spinal curvature, contribute to the "vertebral fracture cascade" in osteoporosis.[100]

Vertebral morphometry, in calculating the deformity of overall thoracic and lumbar spine, may supply useful data about the vertebral fracture risk.

Minne and colleagues[101] and Sauer and colleagues[61] developed the Spinal Deformity Index (SDI) to quantify spinal deformity and assess progression of vertebral deformation during follow-up. Irregularity in the curvature of the spine can be quantified as the integrated average of the ratios of the anterior to posterior vertebral heights of adjacent vertebrae. This Spinal Curvature Irregularity Index (SCII) is a measure of the "smoothness" of the spinal curvature, and a large SCII is

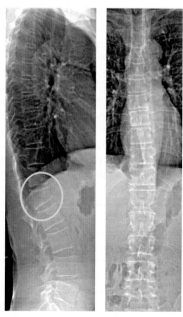

Fig. 8. VFA on DXA image shows, according to SQ method, a moderate fracture of L1.

correlated with the presence of vertebral deformities.[102] Summing the fracture grades by SQ assessment of the 13 vertebrae from T4 to L4 gives the SDI (**Fig. 9**). An increase in SDI could occur either due to a new vertebral fracture or due to worsening of mild or moderate prevalent vertebral fractures. Patients with greater baseline SDI have greater future risk for vertebral fractures: each 1-point increase in the baseline SDI is associated with a 5% increase in the 3-year vertebral fracture risk.[103] The SDI allows assessment of the effect of the osteoporotic therapies on the vertebral fracture risk.[104] The number and the severity of vertebral fractures are associated with the outcome independent of BMD values.[105] Patients with grade 3 vertebral fractures have more severe bone microarchitecture alterations.[106] Other investigators[107] using MRX developed new morphometric indices to quantify the spinal deformity, namely, sums of anterior, middle, and posterior heights (AHS, MHS, PHS) of the respective 14 VB heights from T4 to L5. A strong correlation ($r = 0.9$) between these indices and the lumbar bone mineral density (L-BMD) has been found. In a recent longitudinal study, the same investigators have demonstrated that the morphometric index, AHS, has better performance than BMD in predicting incident fractures. Therefore they suggest that radiologists reading spine radiographs in subjects with suspected osteoporosis should also include AHS measurement,

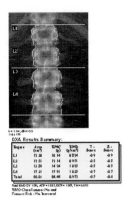
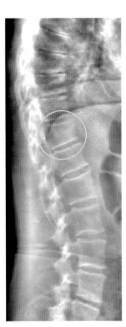

Fig. 10. A new approach to improve the diagnosis rate of vertebral fracture: combining BMD measurement and VFA. A postmenopausal (55-year-old) woman with normal BMD in whom VFA detected a mild wedge fracture of T11.

reporting low AHS values as an index for high risk of vertebral fracture.[108]

SUMMARY

For epidemiologic studies and clinical drug trials in osteoporosis research, and to minimize subjective biases intrinsic to qualitative readings and homogenize data analysis, visual SQ assessment of the radiographs by a trained and experienced observer is the gold standard method to detect vertebral fractures.[109,110] In clinical practice, the preferred method is also radiographic SQ assessment, because an expert eye can better distinguish between true fractures and vertebral anomalies than can quantitative morphometry.

Therefore, vertebral morphometry should not be conducted alone but as a complementary technique, to objectively graduate vertebral fractures already identified by the SQ method. However, vertebral morphometry, in calculating predictive indexes for vertebral fractures, could have clinical relevance by selecting among the nonfractured those patients at high risk for vertebral fractures.

The availability of advanced fan-beam DXA devices allows performance of VFA during routine densitometry, identifying by visual or morphometric method most osteoporotic vertebral fractures, even those that are asymptomatic. The

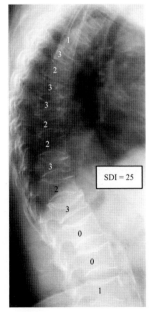

Fig. 9. Spine Deformity Index (SDI), calculated by summarizing the semiquantitative grades of all vertebrae from T4 to L4.

routine use of VFA is recommended as a practical means for integrated assessment of BMD and vertebral fracture status (**Fig. 10**), improving the selection of candidates for therapeutic intervention.[111]

REFERENCES

1. Cooper C. Epidemiology of vertebral fractures in western populations. State of art reviews. Spine 1995;8:1–11.
2. Davies KM, Stegman MR, Heaney RP, et al. Prevalence and severity of vertebral fracture: the Saunders County Bone Quality Study. Osteoporos Int 1996;6:160–5.
3. O'Neill TW, Felsenberg D, Varlow J, et al. The prevalence of vertebral deformity in European men and women: the European Vertebral Osteoporosis Study. J Bone Miner Res 1996;11:1010–8.
4. Jackson SA, Tenenhouse A, Robertson L. Vertebral fracture definition from population-based data: preliminary results from the Canadian Multicenter Osteoporosis Study (CaMos). CaMos Study Group. Osteoporos Int 2000;11:680–7.
5. Cummings SR, Melton LJ. Epidemiology and outcomes of osteoporotic fractures. Lancet 2002; 359:1761–7.
6. Cauley JA, Palermo L, Vogt M, et al. Prevalent vertebral fractures in black women and white women. J Bone Miner Res 2008;23:1458–67.
7. Pongchaiyakul C, Nguyen ND, Jones G, et al. Asymptomatic vertebral deformity as a major risk factor for subsequent fractures and mortality: a long-term prospective study. J Bone Miner Res 2005;20:1349–55.
8. Lindsay R, Pack S, Li Z. Longitudinal progression of fracture prevalence through a population of postmenopausal women with osteoporosis. Osteoporos Int 2005;16:306–12.
9. Roux C, Fechtenbaum J, Kolta S, et al. Mild prevalent and incident vertebral fractures are risk factors for new fractures. Osteoporos Int 2007; 18:1617–24.
10. Cauley JA, Hochberg MC, Lui LY, et al. Long term risk of incident vertebral fractures. JAMA 2007; 298:2761–7.
11. Kado DM, Duong T, Stone KL, et al. Incident vertebral fractures and mortality in older women: a prospective study. Osteoporos Int 2003;14: 589–94.
12. Center JR, Nguyen TV, Schneider D, et al. Mortality after all major types of osteoporotic fractures in men and women: an observational study. Lancet 1999;353:878–82.
13. Schlaich C, Minne HW, Bruckner T, et al. Reduced pulmonary function in patient with spinal osteoporotic fractures. Osteoporos Int 1998;8:261–7.
14. Fink HA, Ensrud KE, Nelson DB, et al. Disability after clinical fracture in postmenopausal women with low bone density: The Fracture Intervention Trial (FIT). Osteoporos Int 2003;14:69–76.
15. Burger H, Van Daele PLA, Gashuis K, et al. Vertebral deformities and functional impairment in men and women. J Bone Miner Res 1997;12:152–7.
16. Nevitt MC, Ettinger B, Black DM, et al. The association of radiographically detected vertebral fractures with back pain and function: a prospective study. Ann Intern Med 1998;128:793–800.
17. Hasserius R, Karlsson MK, Jonsson B, et al. Long-term morbidity and mortality after a clinically diagnosed vertebral fracture in the elderly—a 12- and 22-year follow-up of 257 patients. Calcif Tissue Int 2005;76:235–42.
18. Liberman UA, Weiss SR, Broll J, et al. Effect of oral alendronate on bone mineral density and the incidence of fractures in postmenopausal osteoporosis. N Engl J Med 1995;333:1437–43.
19. Ettinger B, Black DM, Mitlak BH, et al. Reduction of vertebral fracture risk in postmenopausal women with osteoporosis treated with raloxifene: results from a 3-year randomised clinical trial—Multiple Outcomes of Raloxifene Evaluation (MORE) Investigators. JAMA 1999;282:637–45.
20. Reid DM, Hughes RA, Laan RFJM, et al. Efficacy and safety of daily risedronate in the treatment of corticosteroid-induced osteoporosis in men and women: a randomized trial. European Corticosteroid-Induced Osteoporosis Treatment Study. J Bone Miner Res 2000;15:1006–13.
21. Chesnut IC, Skag A, Christiansen C, et al. Effects of oral ibandronate administered daily or intermittently on fracture risk in postmenopausal osteoporosis. J Bone Miner Res 2004;19:1241–9.
22. Neer RM, Arnaud CD, Zanchetta JR, et al. Effect of parathyroid hormone (1-34) on fractures and bone mineral density in postmenopausal women with osteoporosis. N Engl J Med 2001;344: 1434–41.
23. Black DM, Delmas PD, Eastell R, et al. Once-yearly zoledronic acid for treatment of postmenopausal osteoporosis. N Engl J Med 2007;356: 1809–22.
24. Kleerekoper M, Nelson DA. Vertebral fracture or vertebral deformity? Calcif Tissue Int 1992;50:5–6.
25. Fink AH, Milavetz DL, Palermo L, et al. What proportion of incident radiographic vertebral deformities is clinically diagnosed and vice versa? J Bone Miner Res 2005;20:1216–22.
26. Delmas PD, van de Langerijt L, Watts NB, et al. Underdiagnosis of vertebral fractures is a worldwide problem: the IMPACT study. J Bone Miner Res 2005;20:557–63.
27. Lenchik LL, Rogers LF, Delmas PD, et al. Diagnosis of osteoporotic vertebral fractures: importance of

recognition and description by radiologists. AJR Am J Roentgenol 2004;183:949–58.

28. Jiang G, Eastell R, Barrington NA, et al. Comparison of methods for the visual identification of prevalent vertebral fractures in osteoporosis. Osteoporos Int 2004;15:887–96.

29. Abdel-Hamid OA, Bassiouni H, Koutri R, et al. Aging of the thoracic spine: distinction between wedging in osteoarthritis and fracture in osteoporosis: a cross-sectional and longitudinal study. Bone 1994;15:437–42.

30. Ismail AA, Cooper C, Felsenberg D, et al. Number and type of vertebral deformities: epidemiological characteristics and relation to back pain and height loss. European Vertebral Osteoporosis Study Group. Osteoporos Int 1999;9:206–13.

31. Jones G, White C, Nguyen T, et al. Prevalent vertebral deformities: relationship to bone mineral density and spinal osteophytosis in elderly men and women. Osteoporos Int 1996;6:233–9.

32. Genant HK, Wu CY, van Kuijk C, et al. Vertebral fracture assessment using a semiquantitative technique. J Bone Miner Res 1993;8:1137–48.

33. Barnett E, Nordin BEC. Radiographic diagnosis of osteoporosis: new approach. Clin Radiol 1960;11:166–74.

34. Jergas M, San Valentin R. Techniques for the assessment of vertebral dimensions in quantitative morphometry. In: Genant HK, Jergas M, van Juijk C, editors. Vertebral fracture in osteoporosis. San Francisco (CA): University of California Osteoporosis Research Group; 1995. p. 163–88.

35. Hurxthal LM. Measurement of vertebral heights. AJR Am J Roentgenol 1968;103:635–44.

36. Gardner JC, von Ingersleben G, Heyano SL, et al. An interactive tutorial-based training technique for vertebral morphometry. Osteoporos Int 2001;12:63–70.

37. Banks LM, van Juijk C, Genant HK. Radiographic technique for assessing osteoporotic vertebral fracture. In: Genant HK, Jergas M, van Juijk C, editors. Vertebral fracture in osteoporosis. San Francisco (CA): University of California Osteoporosis Research Group; 1995. p. 131–47.

38. Diacinti D, Acca M, Tomei E. Metodica di radiologia digitale per la valutazione dell'osteoporosi vertebrale. Radiol Med 1995;91:1–5 [in Italian].

39. Nicholson PHF, Haddaway MJ, Davie MWJ, et al. A computerized technique for vertebral morphometry. Physiol Meas 1993;14:195–204.

40. Kalidis L, Felsenberg D, Kalender WA, et al. Morphometric analysis of digitized radiographs: description of automatic evaluation. In: Ring EFJ, editor. Current research in osteoporosis and bone mineral measurement II. London: British Institute of Radiology; 1992. p. 14–6.

41. Guglielmi G, Stoppino LP, Placentino MG, et al. Reproducibility of a semiautomatic method for 6-point vertebral morphometry in a multicentre trial. Eur J Radiol 2009;69:173–8.

42. Guglielmi G, Calmieri F, Placentino MG, et al. Assessment of osteoporotic vertebral fractures using specialized workflow software for six point morphometry. Eur J Radiol 2009;70:142–8.

43. Brett A, Miller CG, Curtis W, et al. Development of a clinical workflow tool to enhance the detection of vertebral fractures. Spine 2009;34:2437–43.

44. Eastell R, Cedel SL, Wahner H, et al. Classification of vertebral fractures. J Bone Miner Res 1991;6:207–15.

45. Mc Closkey EV, Spector TD, Eyres KS, et al. The assessment of vertebral deformity: a method for use in population studies and clinical trials. Osteoporos Int 1993;3:138–47.

46. Putz R, Muller-Gerbl M. The vertebral column—a phylogenetic failure? Clin Anat 1996;9:205–12.

47. Masharawi Y, Salame K, Mirovsky Y, et al. Vertebral body shape variation in the thoracic and lumbar spine: characterization of its asymmetry and wedging. Clin Anat 2008;21:46–54.

48. O'Neill TW, Varlow J, Felsenberg D, et al. Variation in vertebral heights ratios in population studies. J Bone Miner Res 1994;9:1895–907.

49. Johnell O, O'Neill T, Felsenberg D, et al. Anthropometric measurements and vertebral deformities. European Vertebral Osteoporosis Study (EVOS) Group. Am J Epidemiol 1997;146:287–93.

50. Smith-Bindman R, Cummings SR, Steiger P, et al. A comparison of morphometric definitions of vertebral fracture. J Bone Miner Res 1991;6:25–34.

51. Cline MG, Meredith KE, Boyer JT, et al. Decline in height with age in adults in a general population sample: estimating maximum height and distinguishing birth cohort effect from actual loss of stature with aging. Hum Biol 1989;61:415–25.

52. Nicholson PHF, Haddaway MJ, Davie MWJ, et al. Vertebral deformity, bone mineral density, back pain and height loss in unscreened women over 50 years. Osteoporos Int 1993;3:300–7.

53. Diacinti D, Acca M, D'Erasmo E, et al. Aging changes in vertebral morphometry. Calcif Tissue Int 1995;57:426–9.

54. Masunari N, Fujiwara S, Nakata Y, et al. Historical height loss, vertebral deformity, and health-related quality of life in Hiroshima cohort study. Osteoporos Int 2007;18:1493–9.

55. Melton LJ III, Kan SH, Frye MA, et al. Epidemiology of vertebral fractures in women. Am J Epidemiol 1989;129:1000–10.

56. Black DM, Cummings SR, Stone K, et al. A new approach to defining normal vertebral dimensions. J Bone Miner Res 1991;6:883–92.

57. Zebaze Djoumessi RM, Maalouf G, Wehbe J, et al. The varying distribution of intra- and intervertebral height ratios determines the prevalence of vertebral fractures. Bone 2004;35:348–56.

58. Jingo G, Ferrar L, Barrington NA, et al. Standardised quantitative morphometry: a modified approach for quantitative identification of prevalent vertebral deformities. Osteoporos Int 2007;18:1411–9.

59. Ziegler R, Scheidt-Nave C, Leidig-Bruckner G. What is a vertebral fracture? Bone 1996;18:169–77.

60. Genant HK, Jergas M. Assessment of prevalent and incident vertebral fractures in osteoporosis research. Osteoporos Int 2003;14(S3):S43–55.

61. Sauer P, Leidig G, Minne HW, et al. Spine Deformity Index (SDI) versus other objective procedures of vertebral fracture identification in patients with osteoporosis: a comparative study. J Bone Miner Res 1991;6:227–38.

62. Nevitt MC, Ross PD, Palermo L, et al. Association of prevalent vertebral fractures, bone density, and alendronate treatment with incident vertebral fractures: effect of number and spinal location of fractures. Bone 1999;25:613–9.

63. Lunt M, Ismail AA, Felsenberg D, et al. Defining incident vertebral deformities in population studies: a comparison of morphometric criteria. Osteoporos Int 2002;13:809–15.

64. Hochberg MC, Ross PD, Black D, et al. Larger increases in bone mineral density during alendronate therapy are associated with a lower risk of new vertebral fractures in women with postmenopausal osteoporosis. Fracture Interventional Trial Research Group. Arthritis Rheum 1999;42:1246–54.

65. Melton LJ III, Egan KS, O'Fallon WM, et al. Influence of fracture criteria on the outcome of a randomized trial of therapy. Osteoporos Int 1998;8:184–91.

66. Melton LJ III, Lane AW, Cooper C, et al. Prevalence and incidence of vertebral deformities. Osteoporos Int 1993;3:113–9.

67. Black DM, Palermo L, Nevitt MC, et al. Comparison of methods for defining prevalent vertebral deformities: the study of osteoporotic fractures. J Bone Miner Res 1995;10:890–902.

68. Genant HK, Jergas M, Palermo L, et al. Comparison of semiquantitative visual and quantitative morphometric assessment of prevalent and incident vertebral fractures in osteoporosis. J Bone Miner Res 1996;11:984–96.

69. Wu C, van Kuijk C, Jiang Y, et al. Comparison of digitized images with original radiography for semiquantitative assessment of osteoporotic fractures. Osteoporos Int 2000;11:25–30.

70. Grados F, Roux C, de Vernejoul MC, et al. Comparison of four morphometric definitions and a semiquantitative consensus reading for assessing prevalent vertebral fractures. Osteoporos Int 2001;12:716–22.

71. Ferrar L, Jiang G, Ambrecht G, et al. Is short vertebral height always an osteoporotic fracture? The Osteoporosis and Ultrasound Study (OPUS). Bone 2007;41:5–12.

72. Ferrar L, Jiang G, Cawthon PM, et al. Identification of vertebral fracture and non-osteoporotic short vertebral height in men: the MrOS study. J Bone Miner Res 2007;22:1434–41.

73. Pearson D, Horton B, Green DJ, et al. Vertebral morphometry by DXA: a comparison of supine lateral and decubitus lateral densitometers. J Clin Densitom 2006;9:295–301.

74. Vallarta-Ast N, Krueger D, Binkley N. Addition of right lateral decubitus positioning improves vertebral visualization with VFA in selected patients. J Clin Densitom 2006;9:375–9.

75. Blake JM, Jagathesan T, Herd RJM, et al. Dual x-ray absorptiometry of the lumbar spine: the precision of paired anteroposterior/lateral studies. Br J Radiol 1994;67:624–30.

76. Crabtree N, Wright J, Walgrove A, et al. Vertebral morphometry: repeat scan precision using the Lunar Expert-XL and the Hologic 4500A. A study for the 'WISDOM' RCT of hormone replacement therapy. Osteoporos Int 2000;11:537–43.

77. Smyth PP, Taylor CJ, Adams JE. Vertebral shape: automatic measurement with active shape models. Radiology 1999;211:571–8.

78. Roberts M, Cootes TF, Adams JE. Vertebral morphometry. Semiautomatic determination of detailed shape from dual-energy X-ray absorptiometry images using active appearance models. Invest Radiol 2006;41:849–59.

79. Lewis MK, Blake GM. Patient dose in morphometric x-ray absorptiometry [letter]. Osteoporos Int 1995;5:281–2.

80. Njeh CF, Fuerst T, Hans D, et al. Radiation exposure in bone mineral density assessment. Appl Radiat Isot 1999;50:215–36.

81. Kalender WA, Eidloth H. Determination of geometric parameters and osteoporosis indices for lumbar vertebrae from lateral QCT localizer radiographs. Osteoporos Int 1991;1:197–200.

82. Adams JE. Single and dual energy X-ray absorptiometry. Eur Radiol 1997;7(Suppl 2):S20–31.

83. Rea JA, Steiger P, Blake GM, et al. Morphometry X-ray absorptiometry: reference data for vertebral dimensions. J Bone Miner Res 1998;13:464–74.

84. Bagur A, Solis F, Di Gregorio S, et al. Reference data of vertebral morphometry (MXA) in Argentine women. Calcif Tissue Int 2000;66:259–62.

85. Salimzadeh A, Moghaddassi M, Alishiri GH, et al. Vertebral morphometry reference data by X-ray absorptiometry (MXA) in Iranian women. Clin Rheumatol 2007;26:704–9.

86. Bianco AC, Malvestiti LF, Gouveia CHA, et al. Morphometric dual-energy X-ray absorptiometry of the spine: report of a large series and correlation with axial bone mineral density. J Bone Miner Res 1999;14:1605–13.

87. Diacinti D, Francucci C, Fiore C, et al. Italian preliminary reference data of normal vertebral dimensions for Morphometric X-ray Absorptiometry (MXA): Normal Morphometric Dexa (NORMO-DEXA) Study. Bone 2005;36(Suppl 2):S351.

88. Rea JA, Li J, Blake GM, et al. Visual assessment of vertebral deformity by X-ray absorptiometry: a highly predictive method to exclude vertebral deformity. Osteoporos Int 2000;11:660–8.

89. Ferrar L, Jiang G, Clowes JA, et al. Comparison of densitometric and radiographic vertebral fracture assessment using the algorithm-based qualitative (ABQ) method in postmenopausal women at low and high risk of fracture. J Bone Miner Res 2008; 23:103–11.

90. Rea JA, Chen MB, Li J, et al. Morphometry X-ray absorptiometry and morphometric radiography of the spine: a comparison of prevalent vertebral deformity identification. J Bone Miner Res 2000;15:564–74.

91. Ferrar L, Jiang G, Barrington NA, et al. Identification of vertebral deformities in women: comparison of radiological assessment and quantitative morphometry using morphometric radiography and morphometric X-ray absorptiometry. J Bone Miner Res 2000;15:575–85.

92. Ferrar L, Jiang G, Eastell R, et al. Visual identification of vertebral fractures in osteoporosis using morphometric x-ray absorptiometry. J Bone Miner Res 2003;18:933–8.

93. Binkley N, Krueger D, Gangnon R, et al. Lateral vertebral assessment: a valuable technique to detect clinically significant vertebral fractures. Osteoporos Int 2005;16:1513–8.

94. Vallarta–Ast N, Krueger D, Wrase C, et al. An evaluation of densitometric vertebral fracture assessment in men. Osteoporos Int 2007;18:1405–10.

95. Schousboe TJ, DeBold RC. Reliability and accuracy of vertebral fracture assessment with densitometry compared to radiography in clinical practice. Osteoporos Int 2006;17:281–9.

96. Giannini S, Nobile M, Dalle Carbonare L, et al. Vertebral morphometry by x-ray absorptiometry before and after liver transplant: a cross-sectional study. Eur J Gastroenterol Hepatol 2001;13:1201–7.

97. Mazzaferro S, Diacinti D, Proietti E, et al. Morphometric x-ray absorptiometry in the assessment of vertebral fractures in renal transplant patients. Nephrol Dial Transplant 2006;21:466–71.

98. Vosse D, Heijckmann C, Landewé R, et al. Comparing morphometric X-ray absorptiometry and radiography in defining vertebral wedge fractures in patients with ankylosing spondylitis. Rheumatology 2007;46:1667–71.

99. Kanis JA, Mc Closkey EV, Johansson H, et al. Case finding for the management of osteoporosis with FRAX-assessment and intervention thresholds for the UK. Osteoporos Int 2008;19:1395–408.

100. Briggs AM, Greig AM, Wark JD. The vertebral fracture cascade in osteoporosis: a review of aetiopathogenesis. Osteoporos Int 2007;18:575–84.

101. Minne HW, Leidig C, Wuster CHR, et al. A newly developed spine deformity index (SDI) to quantitative vertebral crush fractures in patients with osteoporosis. Bone Miner 1988;3:335–49.

102. Zebaze R, Maalouf G, Maalouf N, et al. Loss of regularity in the curvature of the thoracolumbar spine: a measure of structural failure. J Bone Miner Res 2004;19:1099–104.

103. Crans GG, Genant HK, Krege JH. Prognostic utility of a semiquantitative spinal deformity index. Bone 2005;37:175–9.

104. Genant HK, Siris E, Crans GG, et al. Reduction in vertebral fracture risk in teriparatide-treated postmenopausal women as assessed by spinal deformity index. Bone 2005;37:170–4.

105. Siris ES, Genant HK, Laster AJ, et al. Enhanced prediction of fracture risk combining vertebral status and BMD. Osteoporos Int 2007;18:761–70.

106. Genant HK, Delmas PD, Chen P, et al. Severity of vertebral fracture reflects deterioration of bone microarchitecture. Osteoporos Int 2007; 18:69–76.

107. Mazzuoli GF, Diacinti D, Acca M, et al. Relationship between spine bone mineral density and vertebral body heights. Calcif Tissue Int 1998; 62:486–90.

108. Diacinti D, Pisani D, Barone-Adesi F, et al. A new predictive index for vertebral fractures: the sum of the anterior vertebral body heights. Bone 2009;10.1016/j.bone.2009.10.033.

109. National Osteoporosis Foundation. Osteoporosis: review of the evidence for prevention, diagnosis and treatment and cost-effectiveness analysis. Osteoporos Int 1998;8(Suppl 4):S1–85.

110. Kanis JA, Burlet N, Cooper C, et al. European guidance for the diagnosis and management of osteoporosis in postmenopausal women. Osteoporos Int 2008;19:399–428.

111. Schousboe JT, Vokes T, Broy SB, et al. Vertebral fracture assessment: the 2007 ISCD official positions. J Clin Densitom 2008;11(1):92–108.

Quantitative Ultrasound in Osteoporosis and Bone Metabolism Pathologies

Giuseppe Guglielmi, MD[a,b],*, Giacomo Scalzo, MD[b],
Francesca de Terlizzi, MSc[c],
Wilfred C.G. Peh, MD, FRCPG, FRCPE, FRCR[d,e]

KEYWORDS

- Quantitative ultrasound • Speed of sound
- Broadband ultrasound attenuation
- Amplitude dependent speed of sound
- Stiffness • Quantitative ultrasound index
- Bone quality • Osteoporosis

Among the techniques used to investigate bone tissue, quantitative bone ultrasound (QUS) was introduced approximately 10 years ago, to deepen the information on the material characteristics of the tissue, especially with regard to postmenopausal osteoporosis.[1–3] The technique has been studied to better understand the mechanism of action of the ultrasound wave with bone tissue without decisive results,[1] but from the clinical point of view several studies have confirmed that the method is able to identify the changes in bone tissue connected with menopause, with increased bone fragility, and hence, with fracture risk from osteoporosis.[4–7] The best results have been obtained in the clinical research, even in medical fields different from osteoporosis; in fact, QUS has also been applied in the study of various pathologies of mineral metabolism[8–14] and in the investigation of populations other than those involving women who are postmenopausal (male population,[15,16] centenarian population,[17] pediatric population,[18–21]

newborns,[22] preterms,[23–26] and so forth). For this reason, the use of the QUS technique has been extended to other medical conditions, especially in those situations where only an apparatus of this kind (noninvasive, not using ionizing radiation, and so forth) can enable assessment of the state of the bone tissue and supply data to complete the clinical picture of patients under examination. The major example of this is in pediatrics and neonatology.[21,26]

Today, quantitative bone ultrasound represents an effective alternative method for studying bone tissue, and managing patients presenting from a variety of medical specialties who need assessment of the condition of bone tissue in relation to pathologies, consequences of treatments, growth evaluation, and so forth.

The aim of this article is to review the latest available literature on the ultrasound method, to detect and describe the main technological developments achieved through in vitro and in vivo study,

[a] Department of Radiology, University of Foggia, Viale L Pinto, 71100 Foggia, Italy
[b] Scientific Institute 'Casa Sollievo della Sofferenza' Hospital, San Giovanni Rotondo 71013, Italy
[c] MSc Medical Office, IGEA srl, Via Parmenide 10/A 41012 Carpi (MO), Italy
[d] Yong Loo Lin School of Medicine, National University of Singapore, Singapore
[e] Department of Diagnostic Radiology, Alexandra Hospital, Singapore
* Corresponding author. Department of Radiology, University of Foggia, Viale L Pinto, 71100 Foggia, Italy.
E-mail address: g.guglielmi@unifg.it

Radiol Clin N Am 48 (2010) 577–588
doi:10.1016/j.rcl.2010.02.013
0033-8389/10/$ – see front matter © 2010 Elsevier Inc. All rights reserved.

and the possibilities of application on patients and in clinical practice.

PHYSICAL PRINCIPLES

Ultrasound is a mechanical wave characterized by a frequency exceeding the threshold of audibility of the human ear (>20 kHz). The frequency range employed in quantitative bone ultrasound lies between 200 kHz and 1.5 MHz. The QUS method involves generating ultrasound impulses that are transmitted (transversally or longitudinally) through the bone of study. The ultrasound wave is produced in the form of a sinusoid impulse by special piezoelectric probes, and is detected once it has passed through the medium; there are two distinct probes (emitting and receiving) and the skeletal segment for evaluation is placed between them.[1]

The first ultrasound parameters employed for characterizing the bone tissue are speed of sound (SoS) and broadband ultrasound attenuation (BUA). More complex parameters have been developed from combination of the aforementioned: amplitude dependent speed of sound (AD-SoS); stiffness; and quantitative ultrasound index (QUI).[3] In the diagnosis of osteoporosis, these latter parameters have proved to be more useful in identifying subjects with low bone mineral density and therefore at high risk for fracture.[4,7] In recent years, a new approach to the study of the interaction between ultrasound and bone tissue has been made possible by the availability of data additional and complementary to those provided by densitometry techniques. This approach has led to important results for the investigation not only of osteoporosis but also, and above all, of metabolic pathologies affecting the skeleton, with significant alterations not only in the density but also in the elasticity and structure.[8,11,13,27]

MEASUREMENT SITE

The skeletal sites currently studied by QUS techniques are the distal metaphysis of the phalanx, the calcaneus, the radius, and the tibia. All sites are peripheral.

The phalanx is a long bone consisting of a trabecular component and a cortical component, the principal determinant of the mechanical resistance of the bone. This site is strongly predictive of the condition of the bone tissue throughout the skeletal system, and also predictive of osteoporotic-type, vertebral, hip, and forearm fractures. The phalanx is measured with QUS at the metaphyseal level, where the trabecular bone (at about 40%) and cortical bone are present. The metaphysis of the phalanx is characterized by a high bone turnover and is a site extremely sensitive to changes regarding the skeleton, whether natural (growth and ageing); caused by metabolic disease (hyperparathyroidism); or drug induced (treatment with glucocorticoids).[28]

The calcaneus is made up almost entirely of trabecular bone and has the advantage of featuring two flat, parallel surfaces that are very useful for optimizing the geometry of transmission of the ultrasound band through it. Several studies have confirmed the high predictive ability of the calcaneus in identifying osteoporotic-type fractures, especially in the elderly female population (more than 65–70 years of age).[4–6] Although numerous devices for QUS measurement of calcaneus are available on the market, few of these have been studied in depth and have attained an acceptable level of scientific validation with regard to the prediction of fracture risk from osteoporosis.

Tibia and radius are other peripheral skeletal sites studied by longitudinal transmission of ultrasound. Propagation occurs mainly along the external surface of the bone, and thus, provides indications mostly on the cortical bone tissue. Investigation of the tibia and radius are sensitive to phenomena of endosteal reabsorption.[29]

Other skeletal sites (metacarpus, humerus, tibia and radius) have been suggested for evaluation of bone tissue in newborns and preterm infants.

QUALITY ASSURANCE PROCEDURES

One of the most important requirements for medical devices in the study of bone tissue is an adequate reproducibility of the measurement, which involves the reproducibility of measurements performed by different operators with the same device and the reproducibility of the measurement performed with different devices of the same model. To limit all possible sources of errors, quality assurance procedures have been developed for QUS devices.

Ultrasound technique demands constant check of the calibration of the apparatus in the ultrasound signal emitted and the determination of the speed of propagation of the impulse emitted by the probes (ie, a check of correct functioning of the probes).

Testing the correct working of probes and calibration is an operation commonly requested by all devices on the market. Each device has its own calibration procedure and uses its own calibration phantom; the latter is mainly composed of plastic material or of plexiglass.[30] The procedure is generally capable of detecting errors or malfunctioning of the device, and of signaling every kind of problem. Some devices may exhibit dependence of the measurement on environmental conditions. For example, calcaneus devices that use water as the coupling medium between probes and measurement site are sensitive to variations in the temperature of the water itself, as observed by Paggiosi and colleagues[31] and Krieg and colleagues,[32] though the variations connected with the temperature are more evident in the measurement on the phantom than on that in vivo. Various attempts at quality control on the calcaneus devices for longitudinal studies, however, have turned out to be laborious, complex, and poorly suited to clinical practice.[33,34]

The additional problem of cross calibration of devices assumes determining importance in the case of multicenter clinical studies involving the use of several instruments of the same model where data are to be collected in different places. A first attempt at control of the ultrasound devices in a European multicenter clinical study was proposed by Glüer and colleagues[35] in the osteoporosis and ultrasound (OPUS) study. This control was achieved by using a single specific phantom for all the devices and a monitor subject, who underwent periodic tests at all the centers involved in the study, subjected to measurements to check the agreement and calculate the error of reproducibility among the devices.

Although much progress has been made in the control and reliability of some devices, it must be emphasized that, as yet, there is no procedure for standardizing the QUS devices currently in use, not even in those that perform measurements on the same skeletal site. In addition, although a several QUS models are at present available on the market, especially for measurement at the calcaneus, only a small minority of these have had their scientific validity confirmed by clinical studies published in literature.

EXPERIENCE IN VITRO AND IN VIVO
Experimental Studies

The close correlation between SoS and density (r = 0.78–0.91) has been confirmed in several studies.[36,37] The SoS appears to be more greatly influenced by the mineral density and, to a lesser extent, by the elastic modulus of bone. The BUA, on the other hand, is influenced by trabecular porosity and other structural characteristics of trabecular bone.[36] Several studies have shown that neither SoS nor BUA can provide additional data on the characteristics of the mechanical resistance of the bone tissue different from those obtained with densitometry techniques.

The bone architecture of the phalanx influences in a different way some characteristics of the ultrasound wave that have propagated through it: the velocity (SoS), the shape (number of peaks), and the amplitude of the ultrasound signal (fast wave amplitude) (**Fig. 1**).[37,38] In a study performed on human phalanges of cadavers analyzed by bone ultrasound, dual-energy x-ray absorptiometry (DXA), and micro quantitative computed tomography, Wuster and colleagues[39] showed that the speed of the ultrasound and the amplitude of the signal are more closely connected with the mineralized spaces of the trabecular and cortical structure, whereas the frequency content of the signal, calculated by Fourier analysis, is linked with the inter trabecular spaces occupied by the marrow and the organic matrix.

Barkmann and colleagues[40] demonstrated in a clinical study on human phalanges that the duration (microseconds) of the fast ultrasound signal (bone transmission time, see **Fig. 1**) and the AD-SoS are able to reveal endosteal bone absorption, and are correlated with the dimensions of the cortical area and with the moment of inertia of the bone itself.

These observations are consistent with Biot's theory that foresee the propagation, in the two-phase heterogeneous media, of two types of ultrasound waves; one, faster, that moves within the mineralized materials, and the other, slower, that moves through the inter trabecular medullar structure.[41] **Table 1** lists the QUS parameters and the characteristics of bone tissue correlated according to the studies available in literature.

Recently, new methods of investigation by QUS technique at femur and spinal level have been developed. Studies in vitro have shown a high correlation between QUS measurement and bone mineral density (BMD) at femur level in samples of human bone (**Fig. 2**).[42,43] The accuracy achieved in vitro is undoubtedly good, and if a similar level of accuracy can also be maintained in vivo the new methodology will certainly be interesting and applicable because it will be possible to perform measurements in an axial, non-peripheral site, which is usually the site of fracture from fragility.

Several studies have attempted to obtain information on the modality of ultrasound propagation through the bone tissue by employing numerical modeling methods, with interesting results.[44] By analyzing different models of trabecular bone it has been observed that the SoS seems to be more greatly influenced by the bone volume rather than by other structural or elastic components, whereas the BUA appears to be influenced by scattering and viscoelastic mechanisms.[45]

CLINICAL EXPERIENCE
Clinical Validation in the Study of Osteoporosis

Clinical interest in quantitative bone ultrasound centers mainly on the problem of diagnosing

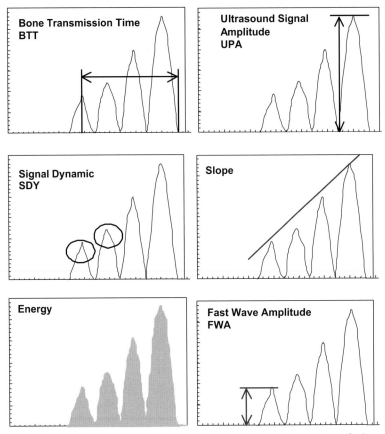

Fig. 1. Some QUS parameters that are computed by means of signal processing techniques applied to the ultrasound signal transmitted through the phalanx.

osteoporosis. Several studies have aimed at evaluating the performance of ultrasound devices in stability in time, precision, and ability to discriminate subjects with osteoporotic fractures.[4–7,46–48]

Numerous prospective studies of great importance have been performed to assess fracture risk by QUS at the calcaneus[4,5]; the latest of these, the EPIC-Norfolk prospective population study,[6] conducted on a British male and female population, has proved the effectiveness of QUS at calcaneus in predicting fracture risk. The study involved 14,824 subjects between 42 and 82 years of age, with a mean follow-up of 1.9(0.7) years, and found significant values of fracture risk for men and women, as reported in **Table 2**.

The European multicenter study (phalangeal osteoporosis study [PhOS]),[46] performed on more than 10,000 women provided important confirmation and clinical validation of the QUS method at phalanx. It was demonstrated that the QUS method has high precision (below 1% at short and long term), and excellent ability to detect osteoporotic subjects with vertebral or hip fractures. Comparisons with x-ray methods and morphometric

analysis of hand radiographs, made by Guglielmi and colleagues,[7] found no significant differences among the methods analyzed, with regard to receiver operating characteristic (ROC) analysis (**Table 3**).

Three European studies have recently reported similar findings using QUS whether at phalanx or at calcaneus. Hartl and colleagues,[48] in the basel osteoporosis study for detecting spinal fractures, have shown that the performances of the instruments at calcaneus and at phalanx are comparable with the results obtained with axial DXA. Krieg and colleagues performed an investigation on an elderly (70–80 years of age) Swiss population, to assess the ability of QUS methods at calcaneus and phalanx in discriminating subjects with hip fracture. Though both methods showed positive results in discriminating fractured subjects, QUS at calcaneus proved more effective in the elderly population.[49] The OPUS study has shown that the QUS method at phalanx and calcaneus is effective in discriminating subjects with spinal fracture in a population recruited in France, the United Kingdom, and Germany (**Table 4**).[35]

Table 1
Main QUS parameters and relationships with bone tissue properties evidenced in experimental studies

QUS Parameter	Bone Tissue Properties
SOS	Density, Glüer et al[36]
BUA	Trabecular structure, Glüer et al [36] Sasso et al[45]
Number of peaks	Connectivity of mineralized matrix structure, Cadossi & Canè[38]
Energy	Elasticity, de Terlizzi et al[37]
Fast wave amplitude	Elasticity; density, de Terlizzi et al[37]; medullary canal size, Barkmann et al[40]
Ultrasound peak amplitude	Trabeculae dimensions, Wuster et al[39]
Bone transmission time	Cortical area; moment of inertia, Barkmann et al[40]
AD-SoS	Cortical area; moment of inertia;density, Barkmann et al[40]
Fourier analysis	Medullary volume, Wuster et al[39]

An Italian study has outlined how QUS at phalanx is more sensitive in discriminating subjects with spinal fracture immediately post-menopause, before 70 years of age, whereas QUS at calcaneus is more sensitive in the subsequent period, at more than 70 years of age.[50]

In the numerous clinical studies in the literature, it has been demonstrated how the linear correlation between ultrasound and densitometry values is positive and statistically significant; however,

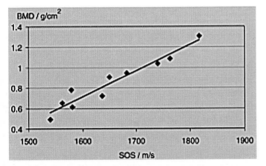

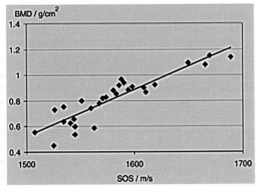

Fig. 2. Estimation of DXA BMD from SOS in Kiel (*upper graph*) and Paris (*lower graph*). (*From* Barkmann R, Laugier P, Moser U, et al. A method for the estimation of femoral bone mineral density from variables of ultrasound transmission through the human femur. Bone 2007;40(1):37–44; with permission.)

this is not sufficient to make it possible, through ultrasound measurement, to determine the value of axial BMD (rachis or femur).[46,47,51,52]

These observations show how QUS cannot be claimed to replace densitometry, but rather combines with it; pathologic ultrasound values must be considered a factor of fracture risk independent of BMD, and therefore their clinical validity cannot be neglected.

Recently, Kanis and colleagues[53] have also published the tables for calculating fracture risk at 10 years by means of QUS at phalanx, thus identifying the criteria for risk assessment based on QUS measurement at phalanx and in regard to age.

Ultrasound for the study of postmenopausal osteoporosis is by now completely validated, and this is supported by ample scientific documentation. The International Society for Clinical Densitometry (ISCD) recently published the new position of the society regarding QUS. As reported by Hans and Krieg[54] in their last review article, there are several QUS devices in the market with different level of evidence reached in the assessment of osteoporotic fracture risk (**Table 5**).

Scientific societies of several European countries have included bone ultrasound in their national guidelines for the management of osteoporosis problems, especially for the evaluation of risk for osteoporotic fracture in women who are menopausal, in the perspective of treatment.[55,56] In Italy, "note 79" regarding the prescription of anti-osteoporosis drugs has been updated to include QUS, on par with DXA, in the model for estimating fracture risk at 10 years, using the combination of clinical risk factors and T-score values.[57]

Further Clinical Applications of Quantitative Bone Ultrasound Technique

New interest in the field of male osteoporosis has led to the development of new research in this

Table 2
Relative risk for fracture by calcaneus QUS

	BUA		SoS	
	RR (95% CI)	P value	RR (95% CI)	P value
By sex				
Men	1.87 (1.23–2.86)	0.003	1.65 (1.17–2.33)	.003
Women	1.90 (1.36–2.66)	<0.0001	1.62 (1.26–2.08)	<.0001

Results from the EPIC-Norfolk study.
Abbreviation: RR, relative risk.
Data from Khaw KT, Reeve J, Luben R, et al. Prediction of total and hip fracture risk in men and women by quantitative ultrasound of the calcaneus: EPIC-Norfolk prospective population study. Lancet 2004;363:197–202.

field. Reference curves for male population have been built recently for phalangeal QUS technique in the Italian and Polish populations.[58,59] Important results have been found in the discrimination of subjects with spine and hip fractures from non-fractured subjects[15,16,60] for calcaneus and phalangeal QUS.

The QUS parameters (bone transmission time [BTT] and pure speed of sound [pSoS]) have shown characteristics of precision, stability in time and independence of the presence of soft tissue, enabling effective follow-up of osteo-trophic therapies to be performed. In a longitudinal study on subjects on hormone replacement therapy, Mauloni and colleagues,[61] taking into consideration the precision of the method and the expected variations in time, calculated that an interval of 18 months between one measurement and the next is required. Also treatment with alendronate,[62] raloxifene,[63] and teriparatide[64] can be monitored by bone ultrasound at the phalanx. Similar studies by ultrasound at the calcaneus have shown that the technique is able to reveal the effects of calcitonin therapy or hormone replacement therapy after 2 years.[65,66]

The versatility of ultrasound technique has suggested that its potential might be evaluated in fields of bone investigation other than those concerning osteoporosis. In the pediatric field, the possibilities of technique for studying skeletal maturation, given its absence of ionizing radiation, have been considered appealing. Reference growth charts have been produced, at the level of phalanx, radius, tibia and calcaneus, in subjects ranging from 3 to 18 years of age in seven countries.[18–20,67–71]

The effectiveness of the QUS technique in the study of pediatric pathologies regarding the skeleton has been assessed by several researchers. Baroncelli and colleagues[21] performed an important study in which they compared QUS at phalanx, lumbar DXA, and metacarpal X ray in a population of children and adolescents with pathologies of mineral and bone metabolism, also evaluating the discrimination between pathologic subjects with low-energy fractures and pathologic subjects without fracture.

The QUS technique in longitudinal transmission at radius and tibia has been applied to populations of obese children,[72] several handicapped institutionalized children[73] and adolescents, and children and adolescents with type 1 diabetes.[74] In all cases, recorded T scores have been significantly below the normal values.

Table 3
Relative risk for vertebral fractures by phalangeal QUS, axial DXA, axial QCT, and morphologic variables measured at the phalanges of the hand by x-ray imaging

Variables	AUC	Odds Ratio (95% CI)	P value
AD-SoS	0.70 ± 0.05	2.51 (1.48–4.26)	<.001
UBPI	0.74 ± 0.05	3.21 (1.56–6.60)	<.0001
QCT BMD (mg/cm³)	0.75 ± 0.05	4.28 (2.12–8.65)	<.0001
PA-DXA (g/cm²)	0.75 ± 0.05	4.06 (2.07–7.96)	<.0001
Cortical thickness (mm)	0.75 ± 0.05	4.10 (2.06–8.21)	<.0001
Medullary canal thickness (mm)	ns	ns	ns
Cortical ratio (%)	0.72 ± 0.05	0346 (0.19–0.63)	<.001

Abbreviations: AUC, area under the curve; DXA, dual energy X-ray absorptiometry; ns, non significant; PA, posterior-anterior; QCT, quantitative computed tomography; QUS, quantitative ultrasound; UBPI, ultrasound bone profile index.

Table 4
Results from the main three comparison studies between calcaneus and phalanges QUS relative risks and areas under the ROC curve

Parameter	Vertebral Fx Age Range 55–65 y Female Population (Hartl et al[48]) Odds Ratio (CI 95%)	Vertebral Fx Age Range 55–79 y Female Population (Glüer et al[35]) Odds Ratio (CI 95%)	Hip Fx Age Range 70–80 y Female Population (Krieg et al[49]) Odds Ratio (CI 95%)
DXA lumbar spine	2.1 (1.2–3.9)	1.46 (1.24–1.72)	—
DXA neck	1.9 (1.0–3.3)	1.38 (1.17–1.63)	—
DBM sonic AD-SoS	2.1 (1.3–3.4)	1.28 (1.09–1.50)	1.4 (1.1–1.7)
DBM sonic UBPI	2.2 (1.1–4.4)	—	—
Achilles BUA	2.7 (1.5–4.8)	1.26 (1.07–1.47)	2.3 (1.8–3.0)
Achilles SoS	2.8 (1.5–5.2)	1.52 (1.28–1.80)	2.5 (2.0–3.3)
Achilles stiffness	3.0 (1.6–5.6)	1.44 (1.22–1.69)	2.7 (2.1–3.5)
Sahara BUA	3.6 (1.8–7.0)	—	2.1 (1.6–2.7)
Sahara SoS	3.5 (1.7–7.5)	—	2.4 (1.8–3.1)
Sahara QUI	3.8 [1.8–8.2]	—	2.4 (1.8–3.2)
DTU-1 BUA	—	1.23 (1.06–1.43)	—
DTU-1 SOS	—	1.45 (1.23–1.71)	—
UBIS 5000 BUA	—	1.29 (1.11–1.51)	—
UBIS 5000 SOS	—	1.47 (1.24–1.74)	—
QUS-2 BUA	—	1.31 (1.12–1.53)	—

Abbreviation: AD-SoS, amplitude dependent speed of sound.

In neonatology, QUS is employed in the study and treatment of newborns and preterm infants. Humerus and tibia are the sites currently measured.[22–25] Significant links have been found with the gestational age, the axiometric parameters, and the postnatal age in preterm newborns at the humerus and tibia (**Table 6**). Longitudinal studies have also evaluated the variations in SoS in preterm subjects stimulated with early physical activity intervention, and it has been remarked that this kind of intervention prevents the diminution of the SoS observed after birth in preterm infants.[75]

Table 5
Level of evidence in fracture risk assessment for current available QUS devices

Manufacturer	Model	Ability to Assess Hip Fracture Risk	Ability to Assess Spine Fracture Risk
General Electric-medical	Achilles	Proven in most populations	Proven in most populations
DMS	UBIS 3000/5000	Some evidence	Some evidence
Hologic	Sahara	Proven in Caucasian	Proven in Caucasian
Norland	Cuba Clinical	Proven in Caucasian	Some evidence
IGEA	DBM Sonic BP	Proven in Caucasian	Proven in Caucasian
BeamMed	Omnisense	Some evidence	Some evidence
Meditech	DTU-One	No evidence	Some evidence
Aloka	AOS-100	Some evidence	No evidence
Elk Co	CM-100/200	—	No evidence

Table 6
Correlations among QUS parameters and auxometric and gestational variables in preterm and term neonates

Author	Skeletal Site	Variable	Number	GA	Weight	Length	Postnatal Age	Post-Conception Age
Nemet et al[24]	Tibia	SoS	44 term and preterm	R = 0.78 $P<.0005$	R = 0.74 $P<.0005$	—	R = −0.78 $P<.0005$	—
Littner et al[25]	Tibia	SoS	73 term and preterm	R = 0.61 $P<.001$	R = 0.48 $P<.001$	—	—	—
Rubinacci et al[23]	Humerus	SoS	51 preterm	R = 0.50 $P<.0001$	R = 0.58 $P<.0001$	R = 0.64 $P<.0001$	—	R = −0.32 $P<.05$
Rubinacci et al[23]	Humerus	BTT	51 preterm	R = 0.48 $P<.0001$	R = 0.56 $P<.0001$	R = 0.59 $P<.0001$	—	R = −0.20 ns
Ritschl et al[26]	Metacarpus	SoS	132 term and preterm	R = 0.55 $P<.0001$	R = 0.52 $P<.0001$	R = 0.47 $P<.0001$	R = −0.39 $P<.0001$	—
Ritschl et al[26]	Metacarpus	BTT	132 term and preterm	R = 0.84 $P<.0001$	R = 0.80 $P<.0001$	R = 0.76 $P<.0001$	R = −0.08 ns	—

Abbreviations: GA, gestational age; ns, non significant.

The technique has also been introduced in nephrology; several studies have applied it in populations of subjects who are uremic and on chronic dialysis. QUS at the phalanx can be used in combination with biochemical markers of bone turnover in the follow-up of patients who are on dialysis who present pathologies or alterations affecting bone.[11,76–85]

QUS studies have yielded very promising results in survivors of malignant bone tumors or acute lymphoblastic leukemia[86,87]: Down's syndrome; Martin Bell syndrome; Marfan Mass phenotype and genetic,[88–90] osteoporosis induced by corticosteroids,[12] rheumatoid arthritis,[8,9] osteomalacia,[13] thalassemia,[91] osteogenesis imperfecta,[92] hyperparathyroidism,[93] arthritic psoriasis,[94] epilepsy[10] and cystic fibrosis.[95]

SUMMARY

Quantitative bone ultrasound provides a valid support for clinical study of all pathologies involving the bone tissue, where determination of bone mass alone does not appear sufficient to complete the patients' clinical/history picture, nor to completely determine how the bone is affected in relation to its fragility and its risk for fracturing. The versatility of the method makes it applicable to the whole population: women, men, children, newborns, and preterm infants.

The ultrasound technique for the study of bone tissue also meets the requirements of the European Directive 97/43/Euratom of June 30, 1997, recently ratified in Italy by the Decree Law "Implementation of EURATOM/97/43 directive regarding the health protection of persons against the dangers of ionizing radiation connected with medical exposure" of May 26, 2005, number 187, article 3.1, which prescribes use of "…available alternative techniques, having the same objective but not involving exposure to ionizing radiation…"

REFERENCES

1. Nieh CF, Hans D, Fuerst, et al. Quantitative ultrasound: assessment of osteoporosis and bone status. London: Martin Dunitz Ltd; 1999. p. 1–20.
2. Hans D, Njeh CF, Genant HK, et al. Quantitative ultrasound in bone status assessment. Rev Rhum Engl Ed 1998;65(7–9):489–98.
3. Gluer CC. The International Quantitative Ultrasound Consensus Group. Quantitative ultrasound techniques for the assessment of osteoporosis: expert agreement on current status. J Bone Miner Res 1997;12:1280–8.
4. Hans D, Dargent-Molina P, Schott AM, et al. Ultrasonographic heel measurements to predict hip fracture in elderly women: the EPIDOS prospective study. Lancet 1996;348:511–4.

5. Bauer DC, Gluer CC, Cauley JA, et al. Broadband ultrasound attenuation predict fractures strongly and independently of densitometry in older women. A prospective study. Arch Intern Med 1997;157: 629–34.

6. Khaw KT, Reeve J, Luben R, et al. Prediction of total and hip fracture risk in men and women by quantitative ultrasound of the calcaneus: EPIC-Norfolk prospective population study. Lancet 2004;363: 197–202.

7. Guglielmi G, Njeh CF, de Terlizzi F, et al. Phalangeal quantitative ultrasound, phalangeal morphometric variables, and vertebral fracture discrimination. Calcif Tissue Int 2003;72(4):469–77.

8. Roben P, Barkmann R, Ullrich S, et al. Assessment of phalangeal bone loss and erosions in patients with rheumatoid arthritis by quantitative ultrasound. Ann Rheum Dis 2001;60:670–7.

9. Birkett V, Ring EF, Elvins DM, et al. A comparison of bone loss in early and late rheumatoid arthritis using quantitative phalangeal ultrasound. Clin Rheumatol 2003;22:203–7.

10. Pluskiewicz W, Nowakowska J. Bone status after long-term anticonvulsant therapy in epileptic patients: evaluation using quantitative ultrasound of calcaneus and phalanxes. Ultrasound Med Biol 1997;23:553–8.

11. Montagnani A, Gonnelli S, Cepollaro C, et al. Quantitative ultrasound in the assessment of skeletal status in uremic patients. J Clin Densitom 1999;2:389–95.

12. Tauchmanova L, Rossi R, Nuzzo V, et al. Bone loss determined by quantitative ultrasonometry correlates inversely with disease activity in patients with endogenous glucocorticoid excess due to adrenal mass. Eur J Endocrinol 2001;145:241–7.

13. Luisetto G, Camozzi V, de Terlizzi F. Use of quantitative ultrasonography in differentiating osteomalacia from osteoporosis: preliminary study. J Ultrasound Med 2000;19:251–6.

14. Camozzi V, Lumachi F, Mantero F, et al. Phalangeal quantitative ultrasound technology and dual energy X-ray densitometry in patients with primary hyperparathyroidism: influence of sex and menopausal status. Osteoporos Int 2003;14:602–8.

15. Montagnani A, Gonnelli S, Cepollaro C, et al. Usefulness of bone quantitative ultrasound in management of osteoporosis in men. J Clin Densitom 2001;4(3): 231–7.

16. Zitzmann M, Brune M, Vieth V, et al. Monitoring bone density in hypogonadal men by quantitative phalangeal ultrasound. Bone 2002;31:422–9.

17. Passeri G, Pini G, Troiano L, et al. Low vitamin D status, high bone turnover, and bone fractures in centenarians. J Clin Endocrinol Metab 2003;88(11): 5109–15.

18. Baroncelli GI, Federico G, Bertelloni S, et al. Bone quality assessment by quantitative ultrasound of proximal phalanxes of the hand in healthy subjects aged 3 – 21 years. Pediatr Res 2001;49:713–8.

19. Baroncelli GI, Federico G, Vignolo M, et al. The Phalangeal Quantitative Ultrasound Group. Cross-sectional reference data for phalangeal quantitative ultrasound from early childhood to young-adulthood according to gender, age, skeletal growth, and pubertal development. Bone 2006;39:159–73.

20. Barkmann R, Rohrschenider W, Vierling M, et al. German pediatric reference data for quantitative transverse transmission ultrasound of finger phalanges. Osteoporos Int 2002;13:55–61.

21. Baroncelli GI, Federico G, Bertelloni S, et al. Assessment of bone quality by quantitative ultrasound of proximal phalanges of the hand and fracture rate in children and adolescents with bone and mineral disorders. Pediatr Res 2003;54:125–36.

22. Gonnelli S, Montagnani A, Gennari L, et al. Feasibility of quantitative ultrasound measurements on the humerus of newborn infants for the assessment of the skeletal status. Osteoporos Int 2004;15(7): 541–6.

23. Rubinacci A, Moro GE, Moehm G, et al. Quantitative ultrasound (QUS) for the assessment of osteopenia in preterm infants. Eur J Endocrinol 2003;149(4): 307–15.

24. Nemet D, Dolfin T, Wolach B, et al. Quantitative ultrasound measurements of bone speed of sound in premature infants. Eur J Pediatr 2001;160:736–40.

25. Littner Y, Mandel D, Mimouni FB, et al. Bone ultrasound velocity curves of newly born term and preterm infants. J Pediatr Endocrinol 2003;16:43–7.

26. Ritschl E, Wehmeijer K, de Terlizzi F, et al. Assessment of skeletal development in preterm and term infants by quantitative ultrasound. Pediatr Res 2005;58(2):341–6.

27. Montagnani A, Gonnelli S, Cepollaro C, et al. Graphic trace analysis of ultrasound at the phalanges may differentiate between subjects with primary hyperparathyroidism and with osteoporosis: a pilot study. Osteoporos Int 2002;13:222–7.

28. Kleerekoper M, Nelson DA, Flynn MJ, et al. Comparison of radiologic absorptiometry with dual energy X-ray absorptiometry and quantitative computed tomography in normal older white and black women. J Bone Miner Res 1994;9:1745–50.

29. Barkmann R, Kantorovich E, Singal C, et al. A new method for quantitative ultrasound measurements at multiple skeletal sites. J Clin Densitom 2000;3:1–7.

30. Thijssen JM, Weijers G, de Korte CL. Objective performance testing and quality assurance of medical ultrasound equipment. Ultrasound Med Biol 2007;33(3):460–71.

31. Paggiosi MA, Blumsohn A, Barkmann R, et al. Effect of temperature on the longitudinal variability of quantitative ultrasound variables. J Clin Densitom 2005; 8(4):436–44.

32. Krieg MA, Cornuz J, Hartl F, et al. Quality controls for two heel bone ultrasounds used in the Swiss Evaluation of the Methods of Measurement of Osteoporotic Fracture Risk Study. J Clin Densitom 2002; 5(4):335–41.

33. Hans D, Wacker W, Genton L, et al. Longitudinal quality control methodology for the quantitative ultrasound Achilles+ in clinical trial settings. Osteoporos Int 2002;13(10):788–95.

34. Hans D, Alekxandrova I, Njeh C, et al. Appropriateness of internal digital phantoms for monitoring the stability of the UBIS 5000 quantitative ultrasound device in clinical trials. Osteoporos Int 2005;16(4):435–45.

35. Glüer CC, Eastell R, Reid DM, et al. Association of five quantitative ultrasound devices and bone densitometry with osteoporotic vertebral fractures in a population-based sample: the OPUS Study. J Bone Miner Res 2004;19(5):782–93.

36. Glüer CC, Wu CY, Jergas M, et al. Three quantitative ultrasound parameters reflect bone structure. Calcif Tissue Int 1994;55:46–52.

37. de Terlizzi F, Battista S, Cavani F, et al. Influence of bone tissue density and elasticity on ultrasound propagation: an in vitro study. J Bone Miner Res 2000;15:2458–66.

38. Cadossi R, Canè V. Pathways of transmission of ultrasound energy through the distal metaphysis of the second phalanx of pigs: an in vitro study. Osteoporos Int 1996;6:196–206.

39. Wuster C, de Terlizzi F, Becker S, et al. Usefulness of quantitative ultrasound in evaluating structural and mechanical properties of bone: comparison of ultrasound, dual-energy X-ray absorptiometry, microcomputed tomography, and mechanical testing of human phalanges in vitro. Technol Health Care 2005;13:1–14.

40. Barkmann R, Lüsse S, Stampa B, et al. Assessment of the geometry of human finger phalanges using quantitative ultrasound in vivo. Osteoporos Int 2000;11:745–55.

41. McKelvie ML, Palmer SB. The interaction of ultrasound with cancellous bone. Phys Med Biol 1991; 36:1331–40.

42. Barkmann R, Laugier P, Moser U, et al. A method for the estimation of femoral bone mineral density from variables of ultrasound transmission through the human femur. Bone 2007;40(1):37–44.

43. Dencks S, Barkmann R, Padilla F, et al. Wavelet-based signal processing of in vitro ultrasonic measurements at the proximal femur. Ultrasound Med Biol 2007;33(6):970–80.

44. Haïat G, Padilla F, Peyrin F, et al. Variation of ultrasonic parameters with microstructure and material properties of trabecular bone: a 3D model simulation. J Bone Miner Res 2007;22:665–74.

45. Sasso M, Haïat G, Yamato Y, et al. Dependence of ultrasonic attenuation on bone mass and microstructure in bovine cortical bone. J Biomech 2008;41(2):347–55.

46. Wüster C, Albanese C, de Aloysio D, et al. Phalangeal osteosonogrammetry study (PhOS): age related changes, diagnostic sensitivity and discrimination power. J Bone Miner Res 2000; 15(8):1603–14.

47. Guglielmi G, Cammisa M, De Serio A, et al. Phalangeal US velocity discriminates between normal and vertebrally fractured subjects. Eur Radiol 1999;9: 1632–7.

48. Hartl F, Tyndall A, Kraenzlin M, et al. Discriminatory ability of quantitative ultrasound parameters and bone mineral density in a population-based sample of postmenopausal women with vertebral fractures: result of the Basel Osteoporosis Study. J Bone Miner Res 2002;17:321–30.

49. Krieg MA, Cornuz J, Ruffieux C, et al. Burckhardt. Comparison of three bone ultrasounds for the discrimination of subjects with and without osteoporotic fractures among 7562 elderly women. J Bone Miner Res 2003;18:1261–6.

50. Camozzi V, De Terlizzi F, Zangari M, et al. Quantitative bone ultrasound at phalanges and calcanues in osteoporotic postmenopausal women: influence of age and measurement site. Ultrasound Med Biol 2007;33(7):1039–45.

51. Rosenthall L, Tenehouse A, Camijnis J. A correlative study of ultrasound calcaneal and dual-energy X-ray absorptiometry bone measurements of the lumbar spine and femur in 1000 women. Eur J Nucl Med 1995;22:402–6.

52. Schott AM, Weill-Engerer S, Hans D, et al. Ultrasound discriminates patients with hip fracture equally well as dual energy X-ray absorptiometry and independently of bone mineral density. J Bone Miner Res 1995;10(2):243–9.

53. Kanis JA, Johnell O, Oden A, et al. Ten-year probabilities of clinical vertebral fractures according to phalangeal quantitative ultrasonography. Osteoporos Int 2005;16:1065–70.

54. Hans D, Krieg MA. Quantitative ultrasound for the detection and management of osteoporosis. Salud Publica Mex 2009;51(Suppl 1):S25–37.

55. National Osteoporosis Society. The use of quantitative ultrasound in the management of osteoporosis. Position statement of 31st January 2002.

56. Schattauer GmbH. Evidence-Based DVO Guidelines Osteoporosis in Germany; prophylaxis, diagnosis and therapy in postmenopausal women and men over 60 years. Verlag fur medizin und naturwissenschaften, 70174 Stuttgart 2006.

57. Agenzia Italiana Del Farmaco. Note AIFA 2006-2007 per l'uso appropriato dei farmaci. Supplemento ordinario alla "Gazzetta Ufficiale" n. 7 del 10 gennaio 20-Serie generale, Nota 79. 4 Gennaio 2007.

58. Montagnani A, Gonnelli S, Cepollaro C, et al. Quantitative ultrasound at the phalanges in healthy Italian men. Osteoporos Int 2000;11:499–504.

59. Drozdzowska B, Pluskiewicz W. Skeletal status in males aged 7–80 years assessed by quantitative ultrasound at the hand phalanges. Osteoporos Int 2003;14:295–300.

60. Ekman A, Michaelsson K, Petrén-Mallmin M, et al. Dual X-ray absorptiometry of hip, heel ultrasound, and densitometry of fingers can discriminate male patients with hip fractures from controls subjects: a comparison of four different methods. J Clin Densitom 2002;5(1):79–85.

61. Mauloni M, Rovati LC, Cadossi R, et al. Monitoring bone effect of transdermal hormone replacement therapy by ultrasound investigation at the phalanx. A four year follow up study. Menopause 2000;7:402–12.

62. Ingle BM, Machado ABC, Pereda CA, et al. Monitoring alendronate and oestradiol therapy with quantitative ultrasound and bone mineral density. J Clin Densitom 2005;8:278–86.

63. Agostinelli D, de Terlizzi F. QUS in monitoring raloxifene and estrogen-progestogens: a 4-year longitudinal study. Ultrasound Med Biol 2007;33(8):1184–90.

64. Gonnelli S, Martini G, Caffarelli C, et al. Teriparatide's effects on quantitative ultrasound parameters and bone density in women with established osteoporosis. Osteoporos Int 2006;17(10):1524–31.

65. Gonnelli S, Cepollaro C, Pondrelli C. Ultrasound parameters in osteoporotic patients treated with salmon calcitonin: a longitudinal study. Osteoporos Int 1996;6:303–7.

66. Giorgino R, Lorusso D, Paparella P. Ultrasound bone densitometry and 2-year hormonal replacement therapy efficacy in the prevention of early postmenopausal bone loss. Osteoporos Int 1996;6(Suppl 1):S341.

67. Halaba Z, Pluskiewicz W. The assessment of development of bone mass in children by quantitative ultrasound through the proximal phalanxes of the hand. Ultrasound Med Biol 1997;23:1331–5.

68. Gimeno Ballester J, Azcona San Julián C, Sierrasesúmaga Ariznabarreta L. Bone mineral density determination by osteosonography in healthy children and adolescents: normal values. An Esp Pediatr 2001;54(6):540–6.

69. Sawyer A, Moore S, Fielding KT, et al. Calcaneus ultrasound measurements in a convenience sample of healthy youth. J Clin Densitom 2001;4(2):111–20.

70. Sundberg M, Gardsell P, Johnell O, et al. Comparison of quantitative ultrasound measurements in calcaneus with DXA and SXA at other skeletal sites: a population-based study on 280 children aged 11–16 years. Osteoporos Int 1998;8:410–27.

71. Zadik Z, Price D, Diamond G. Pediatric reference curves for multi-site quantitative ultrasound and its modulators. Osteoporos Int 2003;14:857–62.

72. Eliakim A, Nemet D, Wolach B. Quantitative ultrasound measurements of bone strength in obese children and adolescents. J Pediatr Endocrinol Metab 2001;14:159–64.

73. Hartman C, Brik R, Tamir A, et al. Bone quantitative ultrasound and nutritional status in severely handicapped institutionalized children and adolescents. Clin Nutr 2004;23:89–98.

74. Damilakis J, Galanakis E, Mamoulakis D, et al. Quantitative ultrasound measurements in children and adolescents with type 1 diabetes. Calcif Tissue Int 2004;74(5):424–8.

75. Litmanovitz I, Dolfin T, Friedland O, et al. Early physical activity intervention prevents decrease of bone strength in very low birth weight infants. Pediatrics 2003;112:15–9.

76. Pluskiewicz W, Adamczyk P, Drozdzowska B, et al. Skeletal status in children, adolescents and young adults with end-stage renal failure treated with hemo- or peritoneal dialysis. Osteoporos Int 2002;13:353–7.

77. Pluskiewicz W, Adamczyk P, Drozdzowska B. Skeletal status in children and adolescents with chronic renal failure before onset of dialysis or on dialysis. Osteoporos Int 2003;14:283–8.

78. Pluskiewicz W, Adamczyk P, Drozdzowska B, et al. Skeletal status in adolescents with end-stage renal failure: a longitudinal study. Osteoporos Int 2005;16:289–95.

79. Rico H, Aguado F, Revilla M, et al. Ultrasound bone velocity and metacarpal radiogrammetry in hemodialyzed patients. Miner Electrolyte Metab 1994;20:103–6.

80. Przedlacki J, Pluskiewicz W, Wieliczko M, et al. Quantitative ultrasound of phalanxes and dual-energy X-ray absorptiometry of forearm and hand in patients with end-stage renal failure treated with dialysis. Osteoporos Int 1999;10:1–6.

81. Taal MW, Cassidy MJ, Pearson D, et al. Usefulness of quantitative heel ultrasound compared with dual-energy X-ray absorptiometry in determining bone mineral density in chronic haemodialysis patients. Nephrol Dial Transplant 1999;14:1917–21.

82. Arici M, Ertuk H, Altun B. Bone mineral density in haemodialysis patients: a comparative study of dual-energy X-ray absorptiometry and quantitative ultrasound. Nephrol Dial Transplant 2000;15:1847–51.

83. Peretz A, Penaloza A, Mesquita M, et al. Quantitative ultrasound and dual X-ray absorptiometry measurements of the calcaneus in patients on maintenance hemodialysis. Bone 2000;27:287–92.

84. Pluskiewicz W, Przedlacki J, Drozdzowska B, et al. Quantitative ultrasound at hand phalanges in adults

with end-stage renal failure. Ultrasound Med Biol 2004;30(4):455–9.

85. Guglielmi G, de Terlizzi F, Aucella F, et al. Quantitative ultrasound technique at the phalanges in discriminating between uremic and osteoporotic patients. Eur J Radiol 2006;60(1):108–14.

86. Azcona C, Burghard E, Ruza E, et al. Reduced bone mineralization in adolescent survivors of malignant bone tumors: comparison of quantitative ultrasound and dual-energy x-ray absorptiometry. J Pediatr Hematol Oncol 2003;25(4):297–302.

87. Pluskiewicz W, Luszczynska A, Halaba Z, et al. Skeletal status in survivors of childhood acute lymphoblastic leukemia assessed by quantitative ultrasound: a pilot cross-sectional study. Ultrasound Med Biol 2002;28:1279–84.

88. Pluskiewicz W, Pyrkosz A, Drozdzowska B, et al. Quantitative ultrasound of the hand phalanges in patients with genetic disorders: a pilot case-control study. Osteoporos Int 2003;14:787–92.

89. Guglielmi G, de Terlizzi F, Torrente I, et al. Quantitative ultrasound of the hand phalanges in a cohort of monozygotic twins: influence of genetic and environmental factors. Skeletal Radiol 2005;34(11):727–35.

90. Halaba Z, Pyrkosz A, Adamczyk P, et al. Longitudinal changes in ultrasound measurements: a parallel study in subjects with genetic disorders and healthy controls. Ultrasound Med Biol 2006;32:409–13.

91. Filosa A, de Terlizzi F. Quantitative ultrasound (QUS): a new approach to evacuate bone status in thalassemic patients. Ital J Pediatr 2002;28:310–8.

92. Cepollaro C, Gonnelli S, Pondrelli C, et al. Osteogenesis Imperfecta: bone turnover, bone density, and ultrasound parameters. Calcif Tissue Int 1999;65:129–32.

93. Gonnelli S, Montagnani A, Cepollaro C, et al. Quantitative ultrasound and bone mineral density in patients with primary hyperparathyroidism before and after surgical treatment. Osteoporos Int 2000;11:255–60.

94. Taccari E, Sensi F, Spadaro A, et al. Ultrasound measurements at the proximal phalanges in male patients with psoriatic arthritis. Osteoporos Int 2001;12:412–6.

95. Rossini M, Viapiana O, Del Marco A, et al. Quantitative ultrasound in adults with cystic fibrosis: correlation with bone mineral density and risk of vertebral fractures. Calcif Tissue Int 2007;80(1):44–9.

Quantitative Computed Tomography

Thomas F. Lang, PhD

KEYWORDS
- Computed tomography • Osteoporosis • Bone density
- Bone geometry • Bone strength

Osteoporosis is one of the major public health problems facing the elderly population,[1] and hip fractures are the most serious manifestation of osteoporosis, affecting over 250,000 elderly in the United States annually and resulting in a 20% mortality rate and substantial loss of quality of life.[2] The number of osteoporotic fractures is expected to increase as the population ages, resulting both from age-related changes in skeletal material properties and geometry that adversely affect bone strength, and from age-related increases in the risk of falling. Thus, with increasing age, decreased skeletal strength is combined with an increased probability of falls and other events that increase the risk of pathologic loads on bone.

Bone strength is a function of skeletal geometry and of material properties, elastic modulus, and material strength, at each point, as they vary throughout the structure.[3] Image-based methods operate in the clinical setting as surrogate measures for bone strength. Image-based methods range from dual x-ray absorptiometry (DXA), which measures the mass and areal bone mineral density (BMD) of large volumes of bone tissue, to DXA-based hip structure analysis, which derives simple geometric measurements from DXA images.[4] Quantitative computed tomography (QCT) methods range from compartmental measures of trabecular and cortical bone mineral density, to simple measures of bone geometry and structure, and ultimately to QCT-based finite element modeling,[3,5–12] which uses voxel-based estimates of material properties across the bone structure to directly calculate whole bone strength and stiffness.

Until relatively recently, x-ray-based imaging has been principally employed for density measurement. Areal BMDs by DXA is the most widely employed clinical surrogate for bone strength. In DXA studies, a one SD reduction in femoral BMD compared with age-matched normal BMD resulted in an approximately threefold increase in fracture risk, depending on the femoral subregion assessed.[7,8] Additionally, geometric measurements, such as hip axis length or increased trochanteric width,[9,10] have also been related to hip fracture risk. QCT, on the other hand, provides measurements of cortical and trabecular volumetric BMD (vBMD).[11] Epidemiologic studies have documented that individual subregions based on trabecular and cortical compartments are independent predictors of hip fracture,[12] and clinical trials have shown that the cortical and trabecular compartments demonstrate differential responses to pharmacologic interventions in osteoporosis.[13] Although BMD measures, whether by DXA or QCT, have strong associations with incident and prevalent fracture, they are poor fracture predictors on an individual basis. Many individuals with high BMD sustain fractures, and many with low BMD do not. Further, changes in BMD do not appear to account for the large changes in fracture risk associated with pharmacologic interventions. Over time, these findings and others have led to the investigation of other skeletal factors not captured in BMD measurements, including measures of bone macroarchitecture, such as bone shape and size, and microarchitecture related to the microstructure of trabecular and cortical bone.

Joint Bioengineering Graduate Group, and Department of Radiology and Biomedical Imaging, University of California, San Francisco, San Francisco, CA 94143-0946, USA
E-mail address: Thomas.Lang@Radiology.ucsf.edu

Radiol Clin N Am 48 (2010) 589–600
doi:10.1016/j.rcl.2010.03.001
0033-8389/10/$ – see front matter © 2010 Elsevier Inc. All rights reserved.

This article focuses on volumetric QCT (vQCT) imaging, both for measures of BMD and for more novel measures that take into account the ability of QCT to quantify the distribution of BMD within skeletal envelopes as it relates to bone strength. In addition to bone strength estimates, vQCT has also been shown to provide measures of muscle size and composition that also relate to risk of fracture through their ability to take into account nonskeletal risk factors such as muscle weakness and falls. Whereas other techniques have evolved, such as MR imaging, or high-resolution peripheral QCT and micro-CT, which can examine the detailed trabecular and cortical microarchitecture of peripheral skeletal sites, these topics will not be discussed here.

QCT: IMAGE ACQUISITION

CT is a three-dimensional (3D) radiographic absorptiometric measurement that provides the distribution of linear attenuation coefficient in a thin cross section of tissue. **Fig. 1** depicts the geometry of a CT measurement. The cross section of the object being scanned is contained within a fan of x-rays defined between the edges of the detector array and a x-ray point source. The x-ray attenuation of the patient is measured along ray-paths corresponding to the lines defined between individual detector elements and the x-ray source. Along the length of the scanning system, the x-ray beam is shaped to radiate a relatively thin "slice" of tissue, ranging from 0.5mm to 10 mm in the case of clinical scanners. The fan of x-rays circumscribes a circular field of view, which is itself contained within a square image matrix that typically consists of two-dimensional arrays of square pixel elements, or "pixels." Because the image represents a cross section of tissue, the picture elements are effectively volume elements, or "voxels." The voxel dimensions depend on the number of elements in the matrix and the size of the field of view. They may thus be adjusted depending on the size of the organ being imaged. Depending on the type of scanner, the voxel dimensions range from the hundreds of microns to roughly 1 mm "in plane" and up to several millimeters in slice thickness. The CT image is acquired when the x-ray source and detector rotate around the patient, and the absorption is continuously measured for each detector element. Through a full acquisition, in which the detector may rotate from 180° to 360°, each voxel is intersected by several ray-paths. The x-ray absorption measurements taken at the different angles are recorded in a computer and combined in a process known as filtered back-projection to calculate the linear attenuation coefficient at each voxel. In the resulting CT image, the voxel values are based on the linear attenuation coefficients. Because these linear attenuation coefficients depend on the effective x-ray energy (which varies between CT scanner models and different peak kilovoltage [kVp] settings of the same scanner), a simple scale, known as the Hounsfield scale, is used to standardize them. The gray-scale value of each voxel is represented as a Hounsfield unit (HU), which is defined as the difference of the linear attenuation coefficient of a given voxel from that of water, divided by the linear attenuation coefficient of water. The HU scale is a linear scale in which air has a value of −1000, water 0, muscle 30, with bone typically ranging from 300 to 3000 units.

The value of the HU for a given voxel depends on several technical factors related primarily to the size of the voxel and the spatial resolution of the imaging system, but also on the linearity of the attenuation coefficient measurements. First, if the sizes of the structures in the tissue are

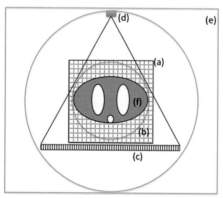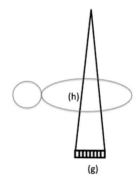

Fig. 1. Simplified A multidetector CT system. Frontal view: (a) image matrix, (b) reconstruction circle, (c) detector array, (d) x-ray source (vertex of fan encompassing edges of detector array and reconstruction circle), (e) CT gantry, (f) transverse view of patient including lung and spine, (g) side view of detector array showing multiple detector rows, and (h) side view of patient.

smaller than the dimensions of the voxel, the HU value is subject to partial volume averaging, in which the HU value is the average HU of the constituent tissues of the voxel, weighted by their volume fractions. For example, a 0.78mm × 0.78mm × 10mm voxel of trabecular bone is a mixture of bone, collagen, cellular marrow, and fatty marrow, and HU is the volume-weighted average of these four constituents. Beam hardening is a second source of variation in HU. In a CT image, the result of this is that for the same tissue, attenuation coefficients at the outside of the patient are systematically higher than those in the interior. Although manufacturers of CT equipment have implemented beam-hardening corrections, the efficacy of these corrections varies between manufacturers and between technical settings on different machines.

Image data for multiple cross sections are acquired with motion of the patient table through the CT gantry. Currently, modern CT scanners are of the multidetector design, with a detector system formed from a rectangular array of detector elements. Typically, this array might consist of 700 to 1000 detector elements along the transverse dimension of the array, with 16 to 256 elements along the direction of the imaging table. Initial multidetector systems ranged from 4 to 16 elements with the most modern systems having 64 to 256 arrays of detectors. Imaging involves helical acquisitions in which the x-ray tube and detector array rotate continuously while the imaging table translates continuously through the CT gantry. The x-ray spot thus describes a spiral trajectory, with use of interpolation to fill in data between the arms of the spiral. Introduction of this technology resulted in significant reductions in image acquisition time[14,15] and combined with the advent of powerful, inexpensive computer workstations, has enabled the clinical development of vQCT analyses of the spine and hip as will be discussed below. Modern scanners allow for acquisition of CT cross sections of submillimeter thickness, resulting in the ability to acquire high-quality volumetric scans with the resolution along the table axis comparable to the in-plane spatial resolution. As will be described, this technology allows for improved analyses of skeletal sites such as the proximal femur, which must be resampled through oblique reformations of the scan data.

QCT: CALIBRATION OF HU VALUES TO BMD

CT BMD assessment is based on quantitative analysis of the HU in volumes of bone tissue. Most calibration approaches involve a solid calcium hydroxyapatite-based bone mineral reference phantom that is scanned simultaneously with the patient. Depending on the acquisition, the phantom may be placed underneath the lumbar spine or between the hips of the patient, with the goal of minimizing differences in the local beam-hardening environment between the phantom and the bone tissue being quantified. Several manufacturers have provided calibration standards along with special software to define regions of interest and quantify BMD. The Image Analysis (Columbia, KY, USA) standard consists of rods with varying concentrations (200 mg/cm^3, 100 mg/cm^3, and 50 mg/cm^3) of calcium hydroxyapatite mixed in a water-equivalent solid resin matrix.[16] Two other manufacturers, Mindways and Siemens, offer similar calibration standards. Another approach, phantomless calibration, uses histograms of HU values placed in regions of subcutaneous fat and skeletal muscle, assuming fixed properties for each tissue types to determine a HU calibration. After calibration, during the analysis of the QCT image, regions of interest are placed in each of the calibration objects, and linear regression analysis is used to determine a relationship between the mean HU measured in each region and the known concentrations of bone-equivalent material. This calibration relationship is then used to convert the mean HU in the patient region of interest (ROI) (for example, vertebra or proximal femur) into a concentration (reported in mg/cm^3, ie, the mass of bone per unit tissue volume) of bone-equivalent material in the ROI. Unlike areal BMD, the QCT density measurement is independent of bone size, and thus is more robust measure for comparisons of bone density between populations and potentially for growing children.

The principal source of error in QCT bone-density assessment is the partial volume effect, which has an important influence on measurements of both trabecular and cortical BMD. Because the voxel dimensions in QCT measurements (0.8–1.0 mm in the imaging plane; 3–10 mm slice thicknesses) are larger than the dimensions and spacing of trabeculae, a QCT voxel includes both bone and marrow constituents. Thus, a QCT measurement is the mass of bone in a volume containing bone, red marrow, and marrow fat. A single-energy QCT measurement is capable of determining the mass of bone in a volume consisting of two components (eg, bone and red marrow), but not in a three-component system. Resolving the mass fractions of bone, red marrow, and marrow fat in the QCT voxel requires a dual-energy QCT measurement. Because fat has a HU value of

−200, compared with 30 HU for red marrow and 300 to 3000 HU for bone, the presence of fat in the QCT volume depresses the HU measurement. Thus, the presence of marrow fat causes single-energy QCT to underestimate the mass of bone per unit tissue volume, an error which can be corrected using dual-energy acquisitions in which two images are acquired serially at two kVp values, typically 80 kVp and 140 kVp. The effect of marrow fat on QCT measurements is larger at the spine than at the hip or peripheral skeletal sites. Whereas the conversion from red to fatty marrow tends to finish by the mid-20s in the hip and peripheral skeleton, the vertebrae show a gradual age-related increase in the proportion of fat in the bone marrow, which starts in youth and continues through old age.[17] The inclusion of fatty marrow in the vertebral BMD measurement results in accuracy errors ranging from 5% to 15% depending on the age group. However, because the increase in marrow fat is age related, single-energy CT data can be corrected using age-related reference databases, and the residual error is not considered to be clinically relevant. Provided that the QCT scan is acquired at low effective energies (ie, 80–90 kVp), the population SD in marrow fat accounts for roughly 5 mg/cm3 of the 25 to 30 mg/cm3 population SD in spinal trabecular BMD. This residual error is not considered large enough to merit clinical use of dual-energy techniques, which are more accurate but which have larger radiation doses and precision errors. Interest in dual-energy QCT has recently increased due to increased scientific attention on age-, disease-, and drug-related effects on bone marrow adipocytes. The field would benefit from improved methodology to assess the adipose content of bone marrow. The resurgent interest in this topic has been fueled by the advent of CT scanners with dual-source technology. The initial variant of this CT scanner type, features two x-ray tubes placed 90% apart in the gantry, operated at two kVp values, and allowing for simultaneous dual-energy acquisitions.

MEASUREMENT OF STRUCTURE AND BMD USING VOLUMETRIC CT IMAGES OF THE SPINE AND HIP

The advent of multidetector CT systems and inexpensive high-performance computer workstations has made possible the rapid acquisition and processing of 3D scans from large volumes of bone tissue such as the proximal femora and spinal column. For assessment of the central skeleton, analytic methods have been developed that quantify structural and density measurements from 3D reconstructions of these skeletal sites. One of the most powerful applications of helical CT scanning and 3D-image analysis is for assessment of BMD, geometry, and strength of the proximal femur. Analysis approaches range from assessment of density, geometry, and macrostructural features based on reconstruction of cross sections and volumes of femoral neck tissue to finite element modeling approaches to model the strength of the hip based on bone geometry and material properties mapped from CT image values.

Densitometric and structural assessments based on 3D reconstructions of the proximal femur based on CT scans have been developed at the University of California, San Francisco (UCSF),[18,19] the University of Erlangen,[20,21] the Mindways Company,[22] Image Analysis,[23] and the Mayo Clinic.[24] The approaches developed at UCSF, Mindways, and Erlangen involve reformatting of the QCT scans along the femoral neck axis and segmentation of the entire proximal femoral envelope, with combinations of mathematical morphology and thresholding, and edge detection approaches to derive the cortical envelope for volume and thickness assessments. The computer algorithm described by Kang and colleagues[20,21] performs volumetric analyses of the femoral neck and the approach described by Lang and colleagues[18,19] at UCSF (**Fig. 2**) processes 3D CT images of the proximal femur to measure BMD in the femoral neck, the total femur, and in a region that combines the trochanteric and intertrochanteric subregions similar to those of DXA systems. Within each anatomic subregion, the density, mass, and volume are computed for the cortical and trabecular components as well as for the integral bone envelope. For trabecular BMD measurements, the precision of this method in vivo was found to range from 0.6% to 1.1% depending on the volume of interest assessed.[18] Both the Erlangen and UCSF approaches carry out geometric and structural analyses of the minimum femoral neck cross section, computing cross-sectional area, estimates of cortical volume and thickness, and moments of inertia for strength estimation. The approach for proximal femoral analysis developed at the Mayo clinic[24,25] does not reconstruct the whole proximal femoral volume, a single cross section of the femoral neck is reconstructed, and measures of integral, cortical and medullary density, and cross-sectional area (CSA) are

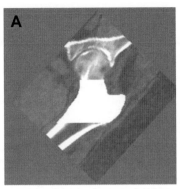 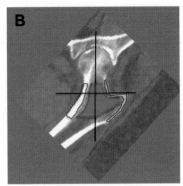

Fig. 2. QCT hip density analysis: coronal midsection through hip. (*A*) Segmentation of total proximal femur region with white pixels signifying bone tissue within periosteal boundaries. (*B*) Separation into cortical and trabecular compartments. Black vertical line is femoral neck axis and black horizontal line is division between femoral neck and trochanteric subvolumes.

computed in addition to bending and axial compressive strength indices.

QCT AND DISCRIMINATION OF HIP FRACTURE

Whereas earlier studies using QCT have documented that density and structural measures are associated with proximal femoral strength in vitro,[18] recent data have confirmed that measures of density and structure are associated with hip fracture in vivo. Cheng and colleagues[26] compared postmenopausal Chinese women imaged within 48 hours of a hip fracture to age- and body-size–matched controls, showing that hip fracture was significantly associated with reduced vBMD in the cortical, integral, and trabecular compartments, as well as reduced measures of cortical volume and thickness. Two interesting findings of the study were that fracture status was associated with increased femoral neck cross-sectional area, consistent with an earlier finding of increased proximal femoral intertrochanteric width from pelvic x-rays in the Study of Osteoporotic Fractures.[27] The study also reported an independent association with hip fracture of femoral neck trabecular bone density and cortical tissue volume. In a subsequently published prospective study in men, Black and colleagues[12] reported that the percentage of proximal femoral tissue volume occupied by cortical tissue, a measure of cortical thickness, and the CSA of the femoral neck, were both associated with incident hip fracture in men aged 69 to 90 years, independently of BMD measured either volumetrically by QCT or areally by DXA. The percentage cortical volume in the femoral neck was a particularly powerful predictor. A reduction of one SD of percentage cortical volume increased the relative

risk of fracture nearly threefold.[12] Interestingly, however, the predictive power for incident hip fracture of QCT BMD and the independently associated geometric parameters in a multivariate model were not better than that of hip DXA. This may be because, as described earlier, areal BMD by hip DXA comprises information regarding bone density and bone size, both of which are hip fracture risk factors.

VOXEL-BASED MORPHOMETRY OF THE PROXIMAL FEMUR: ASSOCIATION WITH HIP FRACTURE

Li and colleagues[28–30] have proposed a novel approach to using CT scans to quantify the spatial distribution of BMD within the proximal femur as it relates to fracture and other endpoints. This method involves using intersubject registration to register CT scans from an entire cohort (for example, containing subjects with and without hip fractures, or a set of subjects before and after drug treatment) onto a common proximal femoral anatomic template, which is typically a representative normal image from the cohort. The resulting composite image is a voxel-based atlas of the entire population, with each voxel mapped to the corresponding voxels from the individual images that were registered onto the template. Thus, each voxel of the composite image corresponds to the spectrum of BMD values from the individual scans mapped to that location. This representation of the cohort CT data allows for statistical tests to be performed within each voxel, allowing visualization of the spatial distribution of BMD associated with a particular endpoint, such as fracture or drug treatment. Using the CT scans from the cross-sectional study in Chinese women described above, first employed an intersubject image registration approach to register all of the scans onto a common hip coordinate system, creating a voxelized 3D model of the entire cohort. Li and colleagues[29] then divided the cohort into training and test subgroups, with each subgroup containing half of the fracture and control subjects, and with a voxel-based model for each subgroup. Within the training subgroup, they performed an analysis of variance to determine which voxels in the training 3D model were most highly correlated with hip fracture status. This resulted in a ROI, called the biomechanical ROI (B-ROI), corresponding to voxels with highest association with hip fracture (**Fig. 3**). They then mapped this region into the scans of the test subject, and compared BMD measured in that region between the fracture subjects and control, observing that it tended to be more strongly associated with hip fracture status than standard regions of BMD assessment, such as femoral neck or total femur.[29] In addition to this approach, which computed mean BMD in a set of voxels associated with fracture, the same group has also proposed use of the anatomic atlas to use the distribution of BMD values rather than the mean value of a B-ROI to assess the degree of fracture risk. With this newer method, the image of a given subject could be mapped to images of subjects known to be healthy or to have fractures of the contralateral hip. Fracture risk was assessed as the degree of similarity of the subject image to the images of subjects with fractures, as assessed by metrics of image similarity such as normalized mutual

information, In a receiver operating characteristic analysis of area under the curve (AUC), Li and colleagues[30] found that image similarity measures, when combined with QCT-derived femoral neck integral vBMD, had superior ability to discriminate fracture compared with femoral neck BMD alone (AUC=0.92 for combined model vs AUC=0.835, $P = .0046$).

CORRELATION OF QCT BMD AND STRUCTURE MEASURES TO AGE, DRUG TREATMENT, AND DISUSE

In addition to fracture status, recent studies have delineated the correlation of QCT measures to age,[25,31] drug treatment,[13,32] and changes in mechanical loading.[33] Using vQCT in a seminal cross-sectional study of aging, Riggs and colleagues[25] compared measures of proximal femoral volumetric density, cortical geometry, and femoral neck CSA between young normal and aging subjects of the Rochester Study. In addition to powerful age-related declines across multiple indices of volumetric cortical and trabecular BMD and cortical thickness, they observed higher femoral neck cross-sectional areas in the older subjects, supporting the idea of periosteal apposition as a compensation for age-related bone loss.[25,34,35] Consistent findings of age-related increases in measures of femoral neck, femoral shaft, and vertebral CSA were supported by other cross-sectional studies reported by Sigurdsson and colleagues,[34] who studied a cohort of Icelandic men and women aged 66 to 90 years, by Marshall and colleagues,[35,36] who studied aging American men and by Meta and colleagues,[31] who compared young and elderly American women. Currently, several studies have documented the response of bone density and structure variables measured by QCT to pharmacologic interventions. There have been several studies in which QCT has been employed to characterize the differential effects of parathyroid hormone (PTH) treatment of cortical and trabecular bone. In the proximal femur, studies of PTH (1–84) and teriparatide (12 and 18 months, respectively) have shown concurrent increases in trabecular vBMD and decreases in cortical vBMD.[13,32] Black and colleagues[13] have reported that 1 year of PTH (1–84) therapy resulted in an increased of cortical tissue volume consistent with increased amount of cortical tissue having low mineralization. Studies of antiresorptive medications have reported smaller increases in proximal femoral trabecular and cortical BMD by QCT. However, in these cases, positive changes have been associated with increases in both compartments.

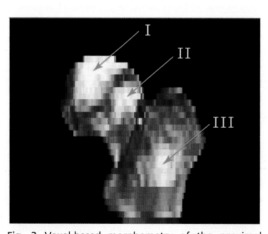

Fig. 3. Voxel-based morphometry of the proximal femur. Hip atlas compiled from 37 subjects with fractures of the contralateral hip and 44 controls. Brightness of voxels represent t-values, with clusters I, II, and III representing clusters of voxels with most statistically significant differences between fractures and controls. Regions II and III correspond to femoral neck and trochanteric fracture sites.

QCT-based studies regarding the response of proximal femoral density and structure variables to changes in mechanical loading has been provided by two longitudinal studies of astronauts undergoing and recovering from spaceflights of roughly 6-month duration on the International Space Station. Lang and colleagues[19] reported that crews on long-duration spaceflight lose on average of 1% to 2.7% of their proximal femoral bone mass per month of spaceflight, depending on anatomic subregion and compartment. A study following the same subjects 1 year after their return from their mission observed that, although indices of bone mass recovered nearly completely, indices of vBMD only recovered to a small extent, and that this discrepancy could be explained by an increase in the bone size during the year after flight, supporting the idea that periosteal apposition could be a response to resumed weight bearing after the loss of large amounts of bone during the flight.[33]

QCT ASSESSMENT OF HIP AND THIGH MUSCULATURE: RELATION TO HIP FRACTURE RISK

In addition to the skeletal anatomy, QCT images of the hip also depict the muscle and adipose tissue surrounding the proximal femur. These images provide information about the total pelvic adipose and lean content as well information on the cross-sectional areas and HU values (a measure of tissue x-ray attenuation) of the functional muscle groups in the field of view. CT measurements of the CSA and mean HU of the abdomen and midthigh

muscle bundle are well established measurements in epidemiologic studies of physical function in the elderly.[37–39] The CSA is a measure of overall muscle size and is strongly correlated to muscle strength and fall-related measures of physical function.[40] The HU value is a measure of the inter- and intracellular adipose content of the muscles, with decreasing HU proportional to increasing fattiness.[40,41] In the thigh, the CSA and HU are independently correlated to knee extensor strength,[42] and low mean HU is associated with reduced current physical function, lower strength, and onset of disability.[38,39] Lang and colleagues[43] recently developed a computer program that computes the CSA and mean HU of the hip extensor, adductor, abductor, and flexor muscle groups (**Fig. 4**). Using images from the cross-sectional study of hip fracture described by Cheng and colleagues,[26] they tested the hypothesis that the measures of size and HU of the hip muscles, by providing independent information on fall-related aspects on physical function, would improve the ability of QCT hip images to estimate fracture risk compared with proximal femoral BMD alone. Compared to controls fracture subjects had higher muscle adiposity as indicated by lower attenuation in the adductor, abductor, and flexor groups ($0.00001 < P < .02$). Fracture subjects also had lower extensor and adductor CSA values ($P < .0001$). After adjusting for differences in age and body mass index, the extensor and adductor CSA values, and the adductor attenuation values remained significantly lower in the fracture subjects ($0.001 < P < .05$). In receiver operating characteristic analyses, models combining QCT-

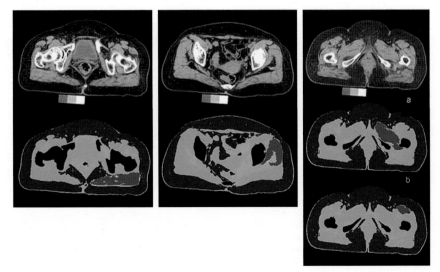

Fig. 4. Proximal femoral muscle regions of interest (*red*) superimposed on reconstructed cross-sections through a hip QCT scan. (*Left*) Hip extensors. (*Middle*) Hip adductors. (*Right*) (*A*) Hip adductors and (*B*) hip flexors.

derived areal BMD with soft tissue measures had higher AUC than models containing only BMD (0.001<P<.05) supporting the idea that combining measures of muscle size and HU with bone density may improve fracture prediction compared with bone measures alone. In a subsequently published report, Lang and colleagues[44] observed that measures of muscle CSA and HU obtained in the midthigh, were associated with incident hip fracture in a population of American men and women enrolled in the prospective Health Aging and Body Composition Study. In prediction models corrected for age, gender, race, height, body mass index, and total percentage fat by DXA, decrements of one SD in thigh muscle bundle CSA and lean tissue attenuation respectively conferred 65% and 58% increases in hip fracture risk. When the model was adjusted by DXA total femur BMD, thigh muscle lean HU, but not CSA, continued to be associated with incident hip fracture, with a one SD decrement conferring an increased risk of 46%.

3D QCT OF THE VERTEBRAE

In the spine, the use of vQCT measurements affects precision more than discriminatory capability. The ability to improve the precision of spinal measurements relates to the use of 3D anatomic landmarks to guide the placement of volumes of interest and to correct for differences of patient positioning, which affects single slice scans. Currently, single-slice QCT techniques are highly operator dependent, requiring careful slice positioning and angulation as well as careful ROI placement. Lang and colleagues[45] developed a volumetric spinal QCT approach in which an image of the entire vertebral body is acquired

and anatomic landmarks such as the vertebral endplates and the spinous process are used to fix the 3D orientation of the vertebral body, allowing for definition of new trabecular and integral regions that contain most of the bone in the vertebral centrum, as shown in **Fig. 5**. Although measuring a larger volume of tissue may enhance precision, these new regions are highly correlated with the midvertebral subregions assessed with standard QCT techniques and may not contain significant new information about vertebral strength. Consequently, volumetric studies of regional BMD, which examine specific subregions of the centrum that may vary in their contribution to vertebral strength, and studies of the cortical shell, the condition of which may be important for vertebral strength in osteoporotic individuals, are of interest for future investigation.

FINITE ELEMENT MODELING

Finite element modeling (FEM) is a mathematical technique used by engineers to evaluate the strength of complex structures such as engine parts, bridges, and, more recently, bones. The structure is divided into "finite elements" (FEs) (discrete pieces of the structure) to form an "FE mesh" so that it can be analyzed. The advantage of using FEM in this study is that this method can account for the material heterogeneity and irregular geometry of the femur, factors that cannot be considered using other approaches. Until recently, it has not been possible to analyze individual bones owing to the extraordinary amount of labor involved in generating the FE mesh. The complex 3-D geometry must be defined and the material properties, which vary dramatically within the bone, must be specified. As a result, researchers have often spent

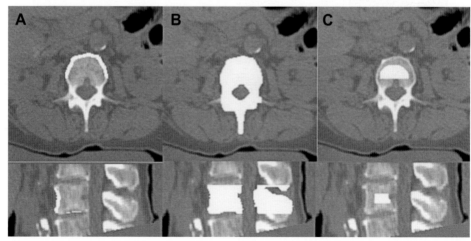

Fig. 5. Regions of interest (white pixels) superimposed on axial (top row) and sagittal (bottom row) mid-vertebral views. (*A*) Cortical. (*B*) Total vertebral body integral. (*C*) Trabecular.

months, or even years, to create just one FE model, and even then, the model often lacked adequate refinement. To address this problem, researchers have developed methods to derive FEMs from CT scans of the hip and spine. These methods involve vQCT whole hip[3,46–49] or whole vertebra images[5,6,50] obtained with 1-mm or 3-mm slice thickness (**Fig. 6**). The finite element modeling application involves three steps. First, the bone geometry information is obtained by determining the outer boundaries of the proximal femora or vertebra on each imaged cross section on the stack of cross-sections that encompass the bone. Next, material properties, such as elastic modulus and strength are computed for each voxel within the bone boundaries. These are computed using parametric relationships between BMD and material properties obtained by scanning and then mechanically testing samples of trabecular and cortical bone. Once the material properties and bone geometry have been defined, load vectors are applied, which simulate the forces applied to bone in normal loading, or in traumatic events such as falls. Keyak and colleagues[3,49,50] have developed an automated, CT scan-based method of generating patient specific FE models of the hip. This method takes advantage of the voxel-based nature of quantitative CT scan data to achieve fully automated mesh generation and,

more significantly, to allow heterogeneous material properties to be specified. The FE models can be analyzed using a loading condition simulating a load on the femur in a single-legged gait or a fall backward and to the side with an impact on the greater trochanter. For each voxel, elastic modulus and strength are estimated as material properties and the factor of safety (FOS) is determined as the strength at each element divided by the stress, with FOS less than 1 representing mechanical failure. A fracture is considered to occur if 15 contiguous elements fail. The outcome variable produced by the modeling technique is failure load, which is defined as the load magnitude required to produce a fracture. This procedure has been extensively tested in vitro, with high correlations to measured failure load for both loading conditions ($r = 0.95$ and 0.96 for fall and stance loading conditions respectively).[3] In addition to their close correlation with fracture load, the FE models depict areas of high strain that occur at the sites where the bones fracture in vitro, and where fractures occur in vivo. The application of FEM to clinical studies has been limited in the past, but is now growing with the wide employment of CT scanning in clinical osteoporosis research. Black and colleagues[12] recently reported that proximal femoral strength and the ratio of applied load to proximal femoral strength were strongly

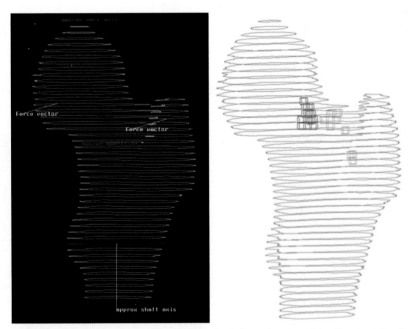

Fig. 6. Proximal femoral FEM (fall to the side) using methodology developed by Keyak and colleagues.[53] (*Left*) Contour map of hip geometry showing approximate femoral neck and shaft axes, and directions of forces vectors for sideways impact onto femoral head and trochanter. (*Right*) Predicted site of fracture in fall loading. Dark cluster of voxels signifies 15 contiguous voxels in which applied stress has exceeded the estimated strength (taken as a material property).

associated with incident hip fracture in elderly men. In particular, load to strength ratio remained strongly and significantly associated with incident hip fracture even after areal BMD was taken into account. Keaveny and colleagues[51] reported on the use of FEM to estimate changes of proximal femoral strength associated with 1 year's administration of PTH (1–84), alendronate, and a combination of these two therapies. In the second year of the study, the PTH group was split into alendronate and placebo treated subgroup, and the combination and alendronate groups were followed up with alendronate. For the first year of treatment, both the PTH and alendronate group showed small but significant increases of femoral strength from baseline and, in the second year, femoral strength continued to increase for all groups but the placebo group, with the group initially treated by PTH showing the largest overall change in strength. It seems that the relatively modest increases in strength reported for the PTH group are consistent with the idea that PTH treatment has an initially negative effect on cortical bone, which counteracts the large increases in trabecular bone mineral density. Keaveny and colleagues[6] recently applied FEM to compare the effects of teriparatide and alendronate on estimated vertebral strength and vertebral bone density, and Lian and colleagues[52] employed FEM to compare estimated proximal femoral strength between subjects with glucocorticoid-induced osteoporosis and age-matched controls. In addition to studies of fracture risk and drug treatment, FEM of the hip has also been used to study the effect of mechanical unloading of the proximal femur in long-duration spaceflight. Keyak and colleagues[53] reported that crewmembers undergoing International Space Station missions of 6 months average length showed loss of proximal femoral strength on the order of 2% to 2.6% per month of flight, which is roughly double the rate of bone loss reported for studies of integral bone density by DXA and QCT. **Fig. 6** shows an example of the application of single-legged stance and posterolateral fall loading conditions to a FE model of the proximal femur, as computed by Keyak.[53]

SUMMARY

Recent advances in CT scanning and computer workstations have made it possible to extend QCT beyond its original function of assessing trabecular BMD in the spine into 3D assessment of cortical and trabecular BMD, cortical thickness, and sectional and whole bone strength in the proximal femur. The ability of QCT images to depict the bone macroarchitecture in 3D, coupled to advanced processing techniques such as FEM, voxel-based morphometry and assessment of muscle size and HU, make QCT a promising technique for assessment of bone quality and fracture risk in the clinical research and clinical settings.

REFERENCES

1. Sasser AC, Rousculp MD, Birnbaum HG, et al. Economic burden of osteoporosis, breast cancer, and cardiovascular disease among postmenopausal women in an employed population. Womens Health Issues 2005;15(3):97–108.
2. Cummings SR, Nevitt MC, Browner WS, et al. Risk factors for hip fracture in white women. Study of Osteoporotic Fractures Research Group [comments]. N Engl J Med 1995;332(12):767–73.
3. Keyak JH, Kaneko TS, Tehranzadeh J, et al. Predicting proximal femoral strength using structural engineering models. Clin Orthop Relat Res 2005;437: 219–28.
4. Beck TJ, Ruff CB, Warden KE, et al. Predicting femoral neck strength from bone mineral data. A structural approach. Invest Radiol 1990;25(1):6–18.
5. Crawford RP, Rosenberg WS, Keaveny TM. Quantitative computed tomography-based finite element models of the human lumbar vertebral body: effect of element size on stiffness, damage, and fracture strength predictions. J Biomech Eng 2003;125(4): 434–8.
6. Keaveny TM, Donley DW, Hoffmann PF, et al. Effects of teriparatide and alendronate on vertebral strength as assessed by finite element modeling of QCT scans in women with osteoporosis. J Bone Miner Res 2007;22(1):149–57.
7. Cummings SR, Black DM, Nevitt MC, et al. Bone density at various sites for prediction of hip fractures: the study of osteoporotic fractures. Lancet 1993;341:72–5.
8. Schott AM, Cormier C, Hans D, et al. How hip and whole-body bone mineral density predict hip fracture in elderly women: the EPIDOS Prospective Study. Osteoporos Int 1998;8(3):247–54.
9. Glüer CC, Cummings SR, Pressman A, et al. Prediction of hip fractures from pelvic radiographs: the study of osteoporotic fractures. J Bone Miner Res 1994;9:671–7.
10. Faulkner KG, Cummings SR, Glüer CC, et al. Simple measurement of femoral geometry predicts hip fracture: the study of osteopotic fractures. J Bone Miner Res 1993;8:1211–7.
11. Genant HK, Cann CE, Ettinger B, et al. Quantitative computed tomography of vertebral spongiosa: a sensitive method for detecting early bone loss after oophorectomy. Ann Intern Med 1982;97(5): 699–705.

2. Black DM, Bouxsein ML, Marshall LM, et al. Proximal femoral structure and the prediction of hip fracture in men: a large prospective study using QCT. J Bone Miner Res 2008;23(8):1326–33.

3. Black DM, Greenspan SL, Ensrud KE, et al. The effects of parathyroid hormone and alendronate alone or in combination in postmenopausal osteoporosis. N Engl J Med 2003;349(13):1207–15.

4. Kalender WA, Polacin A. Physical performance of spiral CT scanning. Med Phys 1991;18(5):910–5.

5. Kalender WA, Seissler W, Klotz E, et al. Spiral volumetric CT with single-breath-hold technique, continuous transport and continuous scanner rotation. Radiology 1990;176:181–3.

6. Faulkner KG, Glüer CC, Grampp S, et al. Cross calibration of liquid and solid QCT calibration standards: corrections to the UCSF normative data. Osteoporos Int 1993;3:36–42.

7. Dunnill M, Anderson J, Whitehead R. Quantitative histological studies on age changes in bone. J Pathol Bacteriol 1967;94:275–91.

8. Lang TF, Keyak JH, Heitz MW, et al. Volumetric quantitative computed tomography of the proximal femur: precision and relation to bone strength. Bone 1997;21(1):101–8.

9. Lang T, LeBlanc A, Evans H, et al. Cortical and trabecular bone mineral loss from the spine and hip in long-duration spaceflight. J Bone Miner Res 2004;19(6):1006–12.

10. Kang Y, Engelke K, Kalender WA. A new accurate and precise 3-D segmentation method for skeletal structures in volumetric CT data. IEEE Trans Med Imaging 2003;22(5):586–98.

11. Kang Y, Engelke K, Fuchs C, et al. An anatomic coordinate system of the femoral neck for highly reproducible BMD measurements using 3D QCT. Comput Med Imaging Graph 2005;29(7):533–41.

12. MindWays. Available at: http://www.qct.com. Accessed March 31, 2010.

13. Image analysis. Available at: http://www.image-analysis.com. 2009. Accessed March 31, 2010.

14. Camp JJ, Karwoski RA, Stacy MC, et al. A system for the analysis of whole-bone strength from helical CT images. Proc SPIE 2004;5369:74–88.

15. Riggs BL, Melton Iii LJ 3rd, Robb RA, et al. Population-based study of age and sex differences in bone volumetric density, size, geometry, and structure at different skeletal sites. J Bone Miner Res 2004;19(12):1945–54.

16. Cheng X, Li J, Lu Y, et al. Proximal femoral density and geometry measurements by quantitative computed tomography: association with hip fracture. Bone 2007;40(1):169–74.

17. Gluer CC, Cummings SR, Pressman A, et al. Prediction of hip fractures from pelvic radiographs: the study of osteoporotic fractures. The Study of Osteoporotic Fractures Research Group. J Bone Miner Res 1994;9(5):671–7.

28. Li W, Kezele I, Collins DL, et al. Voxel-based modeling and quantification of the proximal femur using inter-subject registration of quantitative CT images. Bone 2007;41(5):888–95.

29. Li W, Kornak J, Harris T, et al. Identify fracture-critical regions inside the proximal femur using statistical parametric mapping. Bone 2009;44(4):596–602.

30. Li W, Kornak J, Harris TB, et al. Bone fracture risk estimation based on image similarity. Bone 2009;45(3):560–7.

31. Meta M, Lu Y, Keyak JH, et al. Young-elderly differences in bone density, geometry and strength indices depend on proximal femur sub-region: a cross sectional study in Caucasian-American women. Bone 2006;39(1):152–8.

32. McClung MR, San Martin J, Miller PD, et al. Opposite bone remodeling effects of teriparatide and alendronate in increasing bone mass. Arch Intern Med 2005;165(15):1762–8.

33. Lang TF, Leblanc AD, Evans HJ, et al. Adaptation of the proximal femur to skeletal reloading after long-duration spaceflight. J Bone Miner Res 2006;21(8):1224–30.

34. Sigurdsson G, Aspelund T, Chang M, et al. Increasing sex difference in bone strength in old age: the age, gene/environment susceptibility-Reykjavik Study (AGES-REYKJAVIK). Bone 2006;39(3):644–51.

35. Marshall LM, Lang TF, Lambert LC, et al. Dimensions and volumetric BMD of the proximal femur and their relation to age among older U.S. men. J Bone Miner Res 2006;21(8):1197–206.

36. Marshall LM, Zmuda JM, Chan BK, et al. Race and ethnic variation in Proximal femur structure and BMD among older men. J Bone Miner Res 2008;23(1):121–30.

37. Goodpaster BH, Park SW, Harris TB, et al. The loss of skeletal muscle strength, mass, and quality in older adults: the health, aging and body composition study. J Gerontol A Biol Sci Med Sci 2006;61(10):1059–64.

38. Visser M, Goodpaster BH, Kritchevsky SB, et al. Muscle mass, muscle strength, and muscle fat infiltration as predictors of incident mobility limitations in well-functioning older persons. J Gerontol A Biol Sci Med Sci 2005;60(3):324–33.

39. Visser M, Kritchevsky S, Goodpaster B, et al. Leg muscle mass and composition in relation to lower extremity performance in men and women aged 70–79: The Health Aging and Body Composition Study. J Am Geriatr Soc 2002;50(5):897–905.

40. Goodpaster BH, Kelley DE, Thaete FL, et al. Skeletal muscle attenuation determined by computed tomography is associated with skeletal muscle lipid content. J Appl Physiol 2000;89(1):104–10.

41. Larson-Meyer DE, Smith SR, Heilbronn LK, et al. Muscle-associated triglyceride measured by computed tomography and magnetic resonance spectroscopy. Obesity (Silver Spring) 2006;14(1): 73–87.

42. Goodpaster BH, Carlson CL, Visser M, et al. Attenuation of skeletal muscle and strength in the elderly: The Health ABC Study. J Appl Physiol 2001;90(6):2157–65.

43. Lang T, Koyama A, Li C, et al. Pelvic body composition measurements by quantitative computed tomography: association with recent hip fracture. Bone 2008;42(4):798–805.

44. Lang TF, Cauley JA, Tylavsky F, et al. Computed tomography measurements of thigh muscle cross-sectional area and attenuation coefficient predict hip fracture: the Health, Aging and Body Composition Study. J Bone Miner Res 2009. [Epub ahead of print].

45. Lang TF, Li J, Harris ST, et al. Assessment of vertebral bone mineral density using volumetric quantitative CT. J Comput Assist Tomogr 1999;23(1):130–7.

46. Keyak JH. Improved prediction of proximal femoral fracture load using nonlinear finite element models. Med Eng Phys 2001;23(3):165–73.

47. Keyak JH, Rossi SA, Jones KA, et al. Prediction of fracture location in the proximal femur using finite element models. Med Eng Phys 2001;23(9):657–64.

48. Cody DD, Gross GJ, Hou FJ, et al. Femoral strength is better predicted by finite element models than QCT and DXA. J Biomech 1999 32(10):1013–20.

49. Cody DD, Hou FJ, Divine GW, et al. Short term in vivo precision of proximal femoral finite element modeling. Ann Biomed Eng 2000;28(4):408–14.

50. Faulkner KG, Cann CE, Hasegawa BH. Effect of bone distribution on vertebral strength: assessment with patient-specific nonlinear finite element analysis. Radiology 1991;179(3):669–74.

51. Keaveny TM, Hoffmann PF, Singh M, et al. Femoral bone strength and its relation to cortical and trabecular changes after treatment with PTH, alendronate and their combination as assessed by finite element analysis of quantitative CT scans. J Bone Miner Res 2008;23(12):1974–82.

52. Lian KC, Lang TF, Keyak JH, et al. Differences in hip quantitative computed tomography (QCT) measurements of bone mineral density and bone strength between glucocorticoid-treated and glucocorticoid-naive postmenopausal women. Osteoporos Int 2005;16(6):642–50.

53. Keyak JH, Koyama AK, LeBlanc A, et al. Reduction in proximal femoral strength due to long-duration spaceflight. Bone 2009;44(3):449–53.

High-Resolution Imaging Techniques for the Assessment of Osteoporosis

Roland Krug, PhD[a],*, Andrew J. Burghardt, BS[a],
Sharmila Majumdar, PhD[a,b], Thomas M. Link, MD[a]

KEYWORDS

- Magnetic resonance imaging
- High-resolution peripheral quantitative computed tomography (HR-pQCT)
- Micro computed tomography • Trabecular bone imaging
- Cortical bone imaging

Osteoporosis is a metabolic disease characterized by low bone mass and structural deterioration with an increased fracture risk. Atraumatic fragility fractures mainly affect the proximal femur, the spine, and distal radius. Osteoporosis is a major public health problem, with a high impact on quality of life and high rates of morbidity. At present the established modality to diagnose and monitor osteoporosis in a clinical setting is dual-energy X-ray absorptiometry (DXA), which provides areal bone mineral density (BMD). DXA is a projectional imaging technique and hence measures integral BMD of both cortical and trabecular bone. In addition to DXA, volumetric quantitative computed tomography (vQCT) has been used to assess BMD. This 3-dimensional (3D) technique measures volumetric BMD (vBMD) and thus permits separate characterization of bone geometry and bone density as elements of fracture risk. Furthermore, vQCT can examine cortical and trabecular bone separately. The aforementioned modalities only measure BMD and macroscopic geometry. However, there is a disparity between bone density and bone microarchitecture

in the assessment of bone strength and fracture risk. It has been found that BMD only explains about 70% to 75% of the variance in strength, while the remaining variance is due to the cumulative and synergistic effect of other factors such as bone architecture, tissue composition, and micro damage. Also in the context of therapeutic changes, it has been shown that density alone has limitations in predicting the outcome. Furthermore, in a multicenter fracture intervention trial, the antifracture effects of all drugs tested in trials was only partially explained by their effects on BMD. In fact, BMD explained less than half the effect.[1] In a meta-analysis of 38 studies investigating measures of bone strength, it was concluded that BMD is a limited predictor of fracture risk and that the bone's architectural make-up significantly contributes to bone strength.[2] Besides trabecular thinning, changes in topology, notably a conversion from trabecular plates to rods, and eventually disconnection of trabeculae all contribute to architectural deterioration and loss of bone strength.[3] Furthermore, cortical thinning and cortical porosity contribute to increased

This work was supported by NIH R01 AR057336 (R.K.), NIH 1P30AR058899 (S.M.), NIH AG017762 (S.M.), 1RC1AR058405-01 (T.M.L.), and UC Discovery Grants (7Tesla) LSIT01-10107 and ITL-BIO04-10148.
[a] MQIR, Department of Radiology and Biomedical Imaging, University of California, San Francisco, CA, USA
[b] University of California San Francisco-University of California Berkeley Joint Graduate Group in Bioengineering, CA, USA
* Corresponding author. Department of Radiology and Biomedical Imaging, UCSF, China Basin Landing, 185 Berry Street, Suite 350, Box 0946, San Francisco, CA 94107, USA.
E-mail address: Roland.Krug@radiology.ucsf.edu

0033-8389/10/$ – see front matter © 2010 Elsevier Inc. All rights reserved.

bone fragility.[4] Accordingly, there is a demand for high-resolution imaging techniques to evaluated bone microstructure.

GENERAL CONSIDERATIONS FOR BONE IMAGING

For the assessment of bone structure, both trabecular and cortical bone play important roles. Sites containing predominantly trabecular bone such as the hip, spine, and wrist are also sites of increased fracture risk. Furthermore, trabecular bone remodels up to an order of magnitude faster than cortical bone and is thus the main target of therapeutic approaches. Cancellous bone is prevalent near the joints of long bone (wrist, ankle) and in the axial skeleton (hip, spine), and is surrounded by a cortical bone shell. Cortical bone is usually very compact (cortical thickness varies between 1 and 5 mm) and is primarily found in the shafts of long bones such as the femur, tibia, and radius. Cortical bone constitutes about 80% of the skeleton. In previous studies, it has been emphasized that cortical thinning[5,6] as well as increased cortical porosity,[4,7] are important factors in the assessment of osteoporosis and bone strength. Especially in the context of the proximal femur, a site with high fracture rates and morbidity, the importance of cortical bone structure has been established in previous publications.[8,9] The cortical bone ratio is more than a magnitude higher in the femur than, for instance, in the shaft or diaphysis of the radius. Considering the ratio of trabecular versus cortical bone, the vertebral body is primarily trabecular (up to 90%), the intertrochanteric region of the proximal femur is approximately 50% trabecular and the femoral neck is only 25% trabecular. The structure of cortical bone is related to its mechanical strength and thus plays an important role in bone strength.[10] Furthermore, age, gender, and osteoporotic status all affect the cortical bone structure. There has recently been an increased focus on porosity of the cortical bone that can be attributed to resorption spaces, merging of haversional canals, and clustering of osteons. Because cortical porosity has a significant impact on mechanical properties of cortical bone,[11] characterizing cortical porosity is also important in the context of bone strength and prediction of fracture risk.

The trabecular network has traditionally been assessed from bone biopsies by 2-dimensional (2D) histomorphometry. More recently, these techniques were replaced by 3D imaging techniques, which depict the bone architecture more accurately. Using microcomputed tomography, bone biopsies from the iliac crest can be analyzed with an isotropic voxel size less than 8 µm. The disadvantage of this method is its invasiveness and the restriction to small local regions fo bone assessment, which are not critical fracture sites. Multidetector computed tomography (MDCT) has been used to image bone structure in the axial skeleton in vivo, but is associated with high radiation exposure and limited spatial resolution. Another CT-based method to assess bone structure at peripheral sites, albeit with much lower radiation dose, is high-resolution peripheral quantitative computed tomography (HR-pQCT), with isotropic voxel size as small as 41 µm in a clinical setting. An additional modality that is increasingly being used for high-resolution assessment of bone is magnetic resonance imaging (MRI). The absence of ionizing radiation and its excellent soft tissue contrast render MRI a prime modality for in vivo assessment of bone structure. This article focuses mainly on the two latter techniques (HR-pQCT and MRI), which are presently the most promising for the assessment of bone structure in vivo. Multidetector CT is also briefly discussed.

MAGNETIC RESONANCE IMAGING

MRI is an emerging technology for acquiring high-resolution images of cortical and trabecular bone in vivo. MRI is a noninvasive modality and does not require ionizing radiation. Therefore, it is well suited for assessing bone structure in a clinical setting. In conventional MRI, bone yields a low signal and appears dark due to the relatively low abundance of protons and an extremely short T2 relaxation time (<1 ms) similar to most solid-state tissues. The MR signal stems largely from bone marrow, and depends on the pulse sequence used and the fat content of the marrow (fatty vs hematopoietic bone marrow). As a result, in MRI bone is usually depicted with a negative contrast relative to the high background signal from bone marrow. Information regarding structure, topology, and orientation of the trabecular bone network as well as cortical thickness and area can be extracted from the images by applying digital postprocessing techniques. A large number of analysis parameters have been investigated in the past and have been related to osteoporotic fracture risk and response to treatment, as outlined below. Because there are different requirements for the measurement and analysis of trabecular versus cortical bone, this article discusses each in separate sections.

Trabecular Bone Assessment Using MRI

MR image acquisition

Signal to noise and spatial resolution In MRI, spatial resolution and signal to noise (SNR) are trade-off parameters, and it is not yet clear whether enhancing resolution at the expense of SNR increases or decreases detection sensitivity and what errors are incurred by imaging at aniso-tropic resolution. Li and colleagues[12] investigated the impact of limited spatial resolution and noise on structural parameters. These investigators noted systematic changes in the derived structural parameters with decreasing SNR below a certain threshold; they also showed that these errors at smaller SNR levels are correctable using simple linear transformations, thereby allowing the data to be normalized. Rajapakse and colleagues[13] investigated the implications of noise and resolution on mechanical properties of trabecular bone as estimated by image-based finite element analysis (FEA), and found that the elastic moduli computed from simulated MR images were highly correlated with those obtained from micro-CT (μCT) ($R^2 = 0.99$). The elastic moduli became increasingly underestimated with decreasing SNR. However, the high correlation between elastic parameters derived from μCT and simulated MR data suggested that there is potential for estimating mechanical moduli on the basis of in vivo MR images.

Although there has been a lot of effort to develop trabecular bone imaging of peripheral sites such as the radius, tibia, and calcaneus, very little work has been done on the proximal femur, a site of high fracture incidence. This lack of research is primarily due to SNR limitations for deep body locations, and is related to the fact that the radiofrequency (RF) signal is attenuated by surrounding tissues such as fat and muscle. Only recently, through pulse sequence and coil optimization, the femur was made accessible for trabecular bone analysis.[14] Further optimization in the authors' laboratory led to enhanced SNR efficiency and improved MR images of the proximal femur (**Fig. 1**). The depicted in vivo images are acquired in 12 minutes with a high spatial resolution of $234 \times 234 \times 500$ μm³.

Pulse sequences A pulse sequence is a preselected set of defined RF and gradient pulses, usually repeated many times during a scan. The signal reception and thus the contrast of the image depend on the exact sequence executed. Pulse sequences are computer programs that control all hardware aspects of the MR measurement process. In principle, two main types of pulse sequences can be defined and are both used for

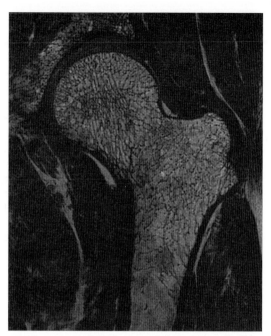

Fig. 1. In vivo MR image of the proximal femur acquired in 12 minutes using a balanced steady-state gradient-echo pulse sequence along with an 8-channel phased array RF coil. The images have a spatial resolution of $234 \times 234 \times 500$ μm³.

bone imaging: spin-echo–based pulse sequences and gradient-echo–based pulse sequences. A gradient-echo is usually always required to read out the necessary wave numbers of the Fourier transformation. A second RF pulse can additionally create a spin-echo. This method ensures that all spins are in phase at the time of the gradient-echo no matter what field inhomogeneities they experience. Deviations from the main magnetic field are particularly strong near trabecular bone and bone marrow transitions. As bone is more diamagnetic than bone marrow, off-resonance frequencies of 100 Hz and more are expected[15] at 3 Tesla (T) and more than 200 Hz at ultra-high field strength of 7 T.[16] The result is an intravoxel spin dephasing, which can lead to significant signal attenuation or even complete signal cancellation. To choose a suitable pulse sequence for bone MRI, a few guidelines have to be considered. First, a 3D excitation usually provides higher SNR than a 2D sequence. However, 2D acquisition techniques have also been used previously to image the trabecular structure of the calcaneus[17–19] albeit with lower spatial resolution. Second, the gradient-echo has to be acquired immediately after the excitation pulse to avoid signal loss due to T2 relaxation. Finally, the imaging time has to be in a clinically feasible range.

The simplest sequence that fulfills the afore-mentioned requirements is a basic gradient-echo sequence. By adjusting the flip angle, the steady state of gradient-echo pulse sequences can be maximized in terms of signal efficiency (signal per unit time) if the scan time (and repetition time TR) is short.[20] Further improvements of SNR efficiency can be made by fully balancing all magnetic gradients during one repetition. The so-called balanced steady-state gradient-echo pulse sequence (bSSFP) maximizes SNR efficiency but is also very prone to magnetic field inhomogeneities. Krug and colleagues[21] pointed out some advantages of this signal attenuation. Smaller trabeculae that would normally disappear due to partial volume effects were enhanced and thus visible because of increased signal cancellation using bSSFP[22] compared with a spin-echo approach. Bauer and colleagues[23] found a similar advantage when imaging 43 calcaneus specimens at 3 T and 1.5 T. Because these susceptibility effects scale with field strength, the trabecular structure is usually enhanced at higher field strength. Bauer and colleagues showed that previously demonstrated advances at the higher field strength for visualization and quantification of trabecular structure are only partially dependent on SNR and that the susceptibility induced accentuation of small structures was most beneficial at higher noise levels, which yielded a superior image quality at 3 T regarding the trabecular bone network. Therefore, due to its very high SNR efficiency, SSFP has become the sequence of choice among gradient-echo–based pulse sequences for trabecular bone imaging.[14–16,24–27]

Spin-echo–based pulse sequences avoid these susceptibility induced off-resonance effects entirely at the time of the gradient-echo.[21,28] However, spin-echo pulse sequences usually demand relatively long scan times due to larger TRs (TR >60 ms). One advantage of the longer TR is the possibility to implement motion correction for the relatively long scans.[29] Song and Wehrli[30] presented a retrospective 2D correction of translational motion for spin-echo imaging using navigator echoes albeit without correcting for rotational patient movements. In the authors' laboratory, careful patient positioning has been proved to largely prevent motion artifacts. Furthermore, imaging time was considerably reduced by employing accelerated image acquisition techniques (parallel imaging). For trabecular bone imaging, this was first introduced by Banerjee and colleagues[31] for gradient-echo imaging followed by Krug and colleagues[21] for spin-echo–based pulse sequences. Both implementations were done using generalized autocalibrating partially parallel acquisitions (GRAPPA).[32]

Image analysis and postprocessing

Image analysis of trabecular bone images in MR involves several postprocessing steps; mainly the outlining of the trabecular bone region of interest (ROI), the correction of the coil sensitivity, bone-marrow segmentation, structural calculations and, if needed, serial image registration.[33] Before analysis, the ROI containing the trabecular bone structure has to be defined; this can be done manually by an operator or in a semiautomatic fashion as suggested by Newitt and colleagues.[33] The next steps in the processing chain are described here.

Coil correction To accurately analyze the MR images, the spatial variations due to the coil's sensitivity profile have to be corrected. For quadrature or birdcage coils with satisfactory in-plane homogeneity, a simple phantom-based correction can be applied, as demonstrated by Newitt and colleagues.[33] However, this method strongly depends on the accurate placement of the scanner landmark at the center of the coil. Another approach previously used for images acquired with surface coils[33] is based on a low-pass filter (LPF) correction scheme described by Wald and colleagues,[34] whereby the image is low-pass filtered by convolution with a Gaussian kernel. Vasilic and Wehrli[35] estimated the local bias field by finding the intensity for which the discrete Laplacian is zero as a part of a local thresholding algorithm. More recently, Folkesson and colleagues[36] compared the performance of LPF with a fully automatic coil correction scheme based on a nonparametric nonuniform intensity normalization N3 approach[37] for coil-induced intensity inhomogeneities in trabecular bone MR imaging. The investigators concluded that N3 coil correction preserves image information while accurately correcting for coil-induced intensity inhomogeneities, which makes it very suitable for quantitative analysis of trabecular bone.

Image postprocessing There are many different approaches for extracting structural information from 3D images of the trabecular bone. The most fundamental parameter in MRI is related to bone volume fraction (BVF) and is also denoted BV/TV (bone volume to total volume fraction). This number can be easily extracted from high-resolution images in which the intensity histogram is bimodal by setting a single threshold and counting the number of bone pixels and total pixels within an ROI. In the presence of partial volume effects, this becomes much more difficult, and the 2 peaks of the intensity histogram blur into a single peak. Different approaches have been used to solve this problem. One approach is to binarize the image into bone and bone marrow phases. This technique requires a threshold, which can be found empirically.[38] The drawback of this method is a significant loss of image information through binarization due to partial volume effects. Other methods seek to circumvent the binarization step and instead investigate the original gray-scale image. Hwang and Wehrli[39] introduced a method for noise removal by deconvolution. From the resulting noiseless image, a BVF map can be generated and from the voxel intensities the marrow volume fraction can be determined. Vasilic and Wehrli[35] presented an alternative method based on local thresholding, which estimates the local marrow intensities within a nearest-neighbor framework.

Trabecular bone analysis Structural parameters are commonly divided into 3 classes including scale, topology, and orientation.[40,41] Scale is primarily described by the volume of bone in a ROI and the thickness of the trabeculae or the spacing between the trabeculae. Topology can be assessed by investigating the plate- or rodlike structure of the network. Finally, orientation methods characterize the degree of anisotropy of the structure. Early assessment of trabecular bone by applying the principles of stereology are based on scale. In MRI, trabecular thickness can be obtained from the mean intercept length (MIL) of parallel test lines across the ROI averaged over multiple angles. From MIL and BV/TV measurements, trabecular thickness (Tb.Th), trabecular spacing (Tb.Sp), and trabecular number (Tb.N) are obtained as described by Majumdar and colleagues.[38] 3D approaches have also been proposed. Krug and colleagues[42] used 3D wavelets to compute a trabecular bone thickness map without the need for image binarization. The investigators calculated BV/TV from these maps by counting the number of pixels with thickness values different from zero, and by dividing this number by the total number of pixels in the corresponding ROI.

Saha and Wehrli[43] introduced a fuzzy distance transform for trabecular bone analysis whereby the Tb.Th is obtained by computing the fuzzy distance along the medial axis of the trabeculae. The method obviated the need of image binarization and is very robust to noise. Carballido-Gamio and colleagues[44] used fuzzy clustering for trabecular bone segmentation and to evaluate BV/TV measurements. More recently, Folkesson and colleagues[45] extended this approach by incorporating a local bone enhancement feature at multiple scales (BE-FMC). This method allows noise suppression while enhancing local relative intensity anisotropy, thus accounting for partial volume effects, noise, and signal intensity inhomogeneities. The new method proved to perform better than both the fuzzy clustering and the dual thresholding approach. BE-FCM could also significantly differentiate between control and fracture groups of 30 calcaneus specimens (from 17 subjects with and 13 without vertebral fracture).

In the literature it has been emphasized that osteoporotic bone loss is strongly associated with changes in bone topology, which results in a fenestration of trabecular plates and ultimately loss of connectivity. Saha and colleagues[46] introduced digital topological analysis (DTA) and applied it to trabecular bone topology.[47] With this method, each voxel is classified into 3 categories it belongs to: curve, surface, or junction. The disadvantage of this approach is the requirement for binarized images because the trabecular network has to be skeletonized before DTA analysis. As previously discussed, the determination of an appropriate threshold is challenging and alters the result. Gomberg and colleagues[47] used a fixed threshold at BVF = 0.25. Pothuaud and colleagues[48] presented a 3D skeletonization technique based on topological invariant and implemented it with a sequential thinning algorithm. A 3D skeleton graph analysis was then implemented to count and to isolate all the vertices and branches of the skeleton graph. Carballido-Gamio and colleagues[49] introduced a new technique to provide a complete assessment of scale, topology, and anisotropy using geodesic topological analysis (GTA). GTA quantifies the trabecular bone network in terms of its junctions, which play a central role in connectivity, and geodesic distances, defined as the shortest path between two points as demonstrated in **Fig. 2**. The investigators found that fracture discrimination was improved by combining GTA parameters as shown by logistic regression analysis. It was further demonstrated that GTA combined with BMD allowed for better discrimination than BMD alone (area under the curve = 0.95; $P<.001$).

It is intuitively clear that to maximize bone strength, the trabecular orientation has to follow major stress lines. Very early, this concept was applied to trabecular bone structure using MIL[50] and was used to investigate its relation to bone strength and bone loss. More recent approaches include topology-based orientation analysis of trabecular bone networks,[47] and 3D spatial autocorrelation function (ACF).[51,52] Wald and colleagues[52] compared the structural anisotropy

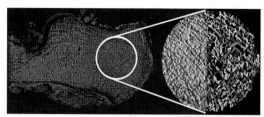

Fig. 2. High-resolution MR image of the calcaneus acquired at 3 T and a selected region of interest (ROI). The left side of the zoomed region is the original ROI and the right part is the color-coded map that illustrates the different assignments of bone voxel to their closest junction based on minimum geodesic distances. (*Courtesy of* Dr Julio Carballido-Gamio.)

and principal direction of the computed fabric tensor for ACF with MIL in 10 healthy postmenopausal women, and found that ACF is faster and considerably more robust to noise. Good agreement was found between the 2 methods, but ACF analysis yielded greater anisotropy than MIL for both trabecular bone thickness and spacing.

Image registration For treatment monitoring it is important to analyze the same trabecular sections at baseline and follow these up to detect small changes in the fine trabecular structure. Two basic registration approaches have been proposed. The images can be aligned after acquisition (retrospective registration) or the acquisition process of the follow-up scan is adapted with respect to field of view (FOV) to exactly match the baseline scan. The latter technique is termed prospective registration, and has only recently been applied to trabecular bone imaging.[53–55] Newitt and colleagues[33] used the coronal scout image on which the high-resolution scan was prescribed to provide a longitudinal anatomic reference point for comparing results in similar regions between subjects. For follow-up scans on the same subject, retrospective registration was done using only rigid body translations and rotations, and the

aligned image was generated using nearest-neighbor interpolation. Magland and colleagues[56] developed an algorithm that uses local pattern of the trabecular structure near 100 randomly selected points to enable true 3D registration. Prospective registration for trabecular bone MR was first implemented by Blumenfeld and colleagues.[53] This method does not require image interpolation because the images are aligned at the acquisition stage; this is a significant advantage for high-resolution MRI, where the slice thickness is usually larger than the in-plane resolution and partial volume effects may be substantial. Thus, some image information and structure is lost during the interpolation process. Furthermore, the technique ensures that the ROI is placed on the same slice for both the baseline and follow-up, and thus simplifies the subsequent postprocessing. The method presented by Blumenfeld and colleagues works as follows. First, the baseline images of the subject are acquired including a 3D low-resolution scan and a high-resolution bSSFP scan. For the follow-up scan, one low spatial resolution scan is obtained for registration purposes (about 4 minutes scan time). The low-resolution axial baseline and follow-up scans are then registered using mutual information[57] based on a rigid registration scheme and the new FOV is adapted to the previous baseline scan. This registration is performed while the patient remains in the scanner and usually takes less than one minute, including the time to upload the baseline and follow-up volumes. **Fig. 3** visualizes the difference between prospective registered follow-up images of the proximal femur and nonregistered follow-up images. As seen in **Fig. 4**, there is a substantial difference between the slices in the calculated BV/TV comparing baseline and follow-up scans of nonregistered images, which could lead to substantial errors when monitoring treatment over a longer time interval. The method was validated in 5 healthy subjects. The registration error found was approximately 0.2° for

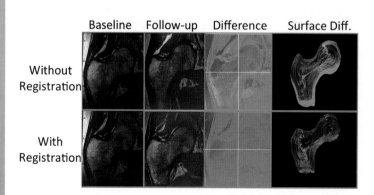

Baseline   Follow-up   Difference   Surface Diff.

Without Registration

With Registration

Fig. 3. Comparison of follow-up MR scans with image registration versus follow-up scans without image registration. The difference image is a subtraction of baseline and follow-up, and the surface difference image is a 3D rendering of registered and nonregistered proximal femur surfaces (*green* = baseline, *red* = follow-up). (*Courtesy of* Dr Janet Goldenstein.)

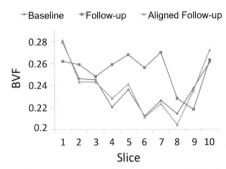

Fig. 4. Change in bone volume fraction (BVF), slice by slice, moving from anterior to posterior. The difference between the red line, the BVF without image registration and the green line, the BVF with image registration, represents the error removed due to an aligned VOI. (*Courtesy of* Dr Janet Goldenstein.)

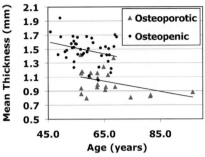

Fig. 5. Mean cortical thickness is depicted for each subject in 2 populations. The regression lines for the osteoporotic and osteopenic populations show a similar age trend. The osteoporotic subjects have significantly decreased cortical thickness.

rotations and approximately 1.1 mm for translations. The coefficient of variance was within a 2% to 4.5% range.

Cortical Bone Assessment Using MRI

MR image acquisition
The advantage of using MRI for cortical bone measures is the ability to align the FOV perpendicular to the femoral neck and thus to depict its 3D cortical architecture more accurately.[58] In contrast, HR-pQCT can image the cortical shell in much shorter scan time and isotropic voxel size,[27] but is restricted to peripheral sites like the distal radius and the distal tibia. As previously mentioned, in conventional MRI bone appears with background signal intensity. Thus, the cortex is usually nicely distinguished from the bone marrow, which provides high signal intensity. However, the outer cortical shell yields less contrast with the surrounding dark muscle (long T1) and dark connective tissues like tendons and ligaments (short T2). Another issue for segmentation is partial volume averaging, which demands high spatial resolution. Furthermore, the chemical shift of fatty bone marrow requires relatively high readout bandwidths. Investigating the cortical thickness of 41 postmenopausal osteopenic women (age 58.6 ± 6.4 years) and 22 postmenopausal osteoporotic women with spine fractures (65.7 ± 9.95 years), Hyun and colleagues[59] found similar age trends but also significant changes in the cortical thickness between the 2 groups (**Fig. 5**), underlining the importance of geometric measurements of the cortical bone.

More recently, Goldenstein and colleagues[60] looked at intracortical porosity using MRI. These investigators compared HR-pQCT with MRI (**Fig. 6**), which allows the visualization of soft tissues such as bone marrow and thus a quantification of the amount of cortical porosity that contains bone marrow. In this work, images of the distal radius and distal tibia of 49 postmenopausal osteopenic women (age 56 ± 3.7 years) were acquired at an image resolution of 156 × 156 × 500 μm^3. After aligning the images from both modalities using a normalized mutual information registration algorithm, the percentage, the number, and the size of each cortical pore containing marrow as seen in the MR images were determined. Although the amount of cortical porosity did not vary greatly between subjects, the type of cortical pore, containing marrow versus not containing marrow, varied highly between subjects. In addition, the number of cortical pores containing marrow did not depend on the amount of porosity and there was no relationship between cortical pore size and the presence of bone marrow. The data suggested that cortical pore spaces contain different components, and that there may be more than one mechanism for the development of cortical porosity and more than one type of bone fluid present in cortical pores. It must be noted, however, that this approach only captures relatively large cortical pores, which can be visualized within the resolution limits of the modality.

Another method of more recent interest is the quantification of bone water in the microscopic pores of the haversian and the lacunocanalicular systems of cortical bone containing approximately 20% water by volume. A smaller water fraction is also bound to collagen and the matrix substrate, and imbedded in the crystal structure of the mineral. These micropores are in general too small (a few micrometers) to be captured within one voxel, but the quantification of bone water using MRI could potentially provide a surrogate measure of bone porosity without resolving the individual

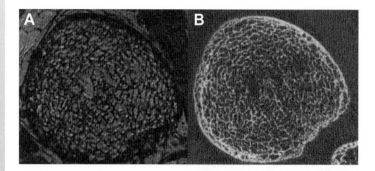

Fig. 6. (*A*) MR image of the distal tibia acquired at 3 T. The thin cortical bone shell with some marrow infiltration can be appreciated from this image. (*B*) The same subject scanned by HR-pQCT. Due to the smaller voxel size, the porosity within the cortical bone is more pronounced. (*Courtesy of* Dr Galateia Kazakia.)

pores. Because the pore water protons possess a very short T2 (T2 <500 μs), ultrashort echo times (UTE) have to be employed to capture the decaying signal immediately after RF excitation. The hydrated state of bone is essential in conferring bone material its unique viscoelastic properties. Techawiboonwong and colleagues[61] implemented a UTE pulse sequence and validated bone water quantification measurements in sheep and human cadaveric specimens. These investigators also performed a pilot study to evaluate the method's sensitivity to distinguish subjects of different age and disease state. The data were compared with areal and volumetric BMD from DXA and peripheral quantitative CT, respectively. The bone water content was calibrated with the aid of an external reference (10% H_2O in D_2O doped with 27 mmol/L $MnCl_2$), which was attached anteriorly to the subject's tibial midshaft. Excellent agreement ($R^2 = 0.99$) was found in the specimen between the water displaced by using D_2O exchange and water measured with respect to the reference sample. In vivo, the bone water content was increased 65% in the postmenopausal group compared with the premenopausal group. Issever and colleagues[62] further improved the spatial resolution of 3D-UTE MRI to an

isotropic voxel size of 0.4 × 0.4 × 0.4 mm³, allowing instant image reformation. Their imaging was performed on a human cadaver proximal femur (**Fig. 7**). Bone marrow was largely removed before imaging. For reference purposes, two 27 mmol/L $MnCl_2$ doped phantoms consisting of 10% H_2O and 20% D_2O concentrations were used as shown in **Fig. 7**, similar to Techawiboonwong and colleagues.[61]

Pulse sequences Hyun and colleagues[59] acquired MR images of the distal radius (**Fig. 8A**) at 1.5 T using a 3D fast gradient recalled echo (FGRE) pulse sequence featuring an in-plane resolution of 0.16 × 0.16 mm² and 2-mm slice thickness. The same protocol was employed by Kazakia and colleagues,[27] who measured the distal radius and the distal tibia at 3 T field strength. Gomberg and colleagues[58] imaged the tibial cortex using a 2D fast spin-echo (FSE) sequence with a voxel size of 0.47 × 0.47 × 2 mm³. The authors also acquire images of the proximal femur with an in-plane resolution of 0.625 μm and 2-mm slice thickness. The hip joint is a very important site for cortical bone measurements, and might be responsible for intracapsular hip fractures.[9] Cortical analysis of the hip is complicated by its

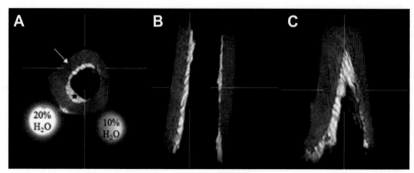

Fig. 7. 3D UTE images of a human femoral shaft are depicted in axial (*A*), sagittal (*B*), and coronal (*C*) plane with isotropic voxel size (0.4 × 0.4 × 0.4 mm³). The green cross locates the reconstructed slice position in each of the 3 planes. The white arrow indicates the cortical bone. Residual bone marrow is marked with a black star. (*Courtesy of* Dr Ahi Issever).

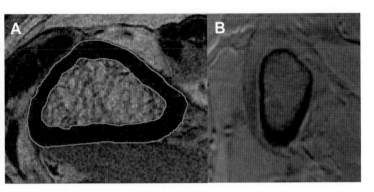

Fig. 8. (A) MR in vivo image of the distal radius acquired by Hyun and colleagues with a 3D FGRE pulse sequence at 1.5 T. (B) Double-oblique MR image of the femoral neck acquired by R. Krug at 3 T using a 2D FGRE pulse sequence.

deep location within the pelvis and the double-oblique angle between the neck and the body's orthogonal axes. Thus, the measurements by Gomberg and colleagues were performed on oblique slices perpendicular to the femoral axes using a 2D spoiled gradient recalled echo (2D-SPGR) pulse sequence (TR = 150 ms, echo time TE = 4.8 ms). More recently, one of the authors (R. Krug) further maximized the contrast between the dark cortical bone and the relatively dark muscle signal (Fig. 8B), using a 2D FGRE sequence with long TR (TR = 300 ms) and shorter TE (TE = 2.29 ms). Because muscle has a relatively long T1 relaxation time of more than 1 ms,[63] a very long TR is preferred to increase SNR. Although 3D pulse sequences deliver higher SNR, the advantage of a 2D pulse sequence is the possibility of multiple interleaved acquisitions allowing for much longer TR without compromising the clinically feasible scan time. For measurements of cortical porosity, Goldenstein and colleagues[60] chose a bSSFP sequence with parameters similar to Banerjee and colleagues[15] to maximize spatial image resolution in order to resolve the small cortical pores. For UTE MRI, both 2D and 3D pulse sequences with radial readout have been used in the past. Issever and colleagues[62] applied a 3D UTE pulse sequence with an echo time as short as TE = 64 μs. Similar values can also be achieved with 2D UTE pulse sequences for cortical bone measurements [61,64] on clinical MR scanners.

Image analysis and postprocessing

Hyun and colleagues[59] designed a semiautomatic segmentation algorithm to segment both the endosteal and periosteal cortical boundary from their surroundings. The algorithm featured a deformable contour to conform to the strongest gradient edges in the neighborhood of the user-placed model. The accuracy of the method was tested by comparing MR images 0.16 × 0.16 × 2 mm^3 at 1.5 T to CT images (voxel size 0.07 × 0.07 × 0.8 mm^3) of ex vivo porcine femora specimens, as depicted in Fig. 9. The in vivo feasibility was also tested in the distal radius of a cohort of human subjects. The cortical area was calculated as the area enclosed by the concentric contours. The mean thickness was calculated as area divided by mean contour length. Using this method, Hyun and colleagues found very good in vivo reproducibility for cortical volume (coefficient of variation CV = 2.19%) and

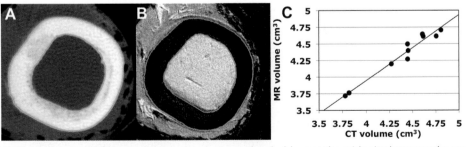

Fig. 9. (A) CT images. Cortical bone was segmented using a threshold set at the midpoint between the peaks representing the high-intensity bone and low-intensity soft tissue. (B) MR images: Inner and outer cortical boundary contours were generated with a semiautomatic segmentation program using a deformable contour and then adjusted by a trained operator. (C) Scatter plot of cortical volume for each specimen for a 16-mm long section centered on the minimum cross-sectional area. A good agreement between CT- and MR-derived measures was found (R^2 = 0.96).

for cortical thickness (CV = 1.96%). Kazakia and colleagues[27] used the distance transform method[65] to further improve the measurements of cortical thickness by fitting a sphere into the segmented cortical shell; they also compared thickness measurements from MR data with HR-pQCT and found significant correlations. Gomberg and colleagues[58] presented a semiautomatic segmentation approach whereby after a rough manual outline of the cortical contour, radial profiles perpendicular to the cortex were normalized to the marrow signal and further processed by morphologic operators before computing the cross-sectional area and thickness. Gomberg and colleagues found a similar CV of around 2% for the reproducibility of their technique.

Clinical Applications

Over the past few years, the technological developments have made quantitative MRI of bone structure more clinically practical. The substantial improvement in fracture discrimination by including structural information in addition to BMD has been well established. Wehrli and colleagues[66] showed that topological bone parameters investigated in 79 women (29 with vertebral fracture) could much better discriminate the fracture group from the non-fracture group than BMD. Benito and colleagues[67] investigated the effect of testosterone replacement on trabecular architecture in hypogonadal men in the distal tibial metaphysis of 10 severely testosterone-deficient hypogonadal men. These investigators found dramatic topological changes in the bone, suggesting that antiresorptive treatment results in improved structural integrity. Chesnut and colleagues[68] looked at the effect of salmon calcitonin on bone structure at the distal radius and calcaneus of 91 postmenopausal women during a period of 2 years. The treatment group showed improved trabecular structure compared with the placebo group, but no significant change in BMD was detected. More recently, Wehrli and colleagues[69] reported on topological changes of the trabecular bone network after menopause and the protective effect of estradiol. Short-term temporal changes in trabecular architecture were observed after menopause, and a protective effect of estradiol in maintaining the platelike trabecular architecture was observed. Wehrli and colleagues concluded that MRI-based in vivo assessment of trabecular bone has great promise as a tool for monitoring osteoporosis treatment. Zhang and colleagues[70] tested the hypothesis that testosterone replacement in hypogonadal men would improve the mechanical properties of their bone.

The results of their study suggested that 24 months of testosterone treatment of hypogonadal men improves estimated elastic moduli of tibial trabecular bone by increased trabecular plate thickness.

Most of the previous studies were done at 1.5 T field strength. However, as high field (3 T) and ultra-high field (7 T and higher) modalities become more widely available at clinical sites, there is an increasing trend to use these scanners for bone imaging. Sell and colleagues[71] found high correlations between trabecular bone structure measured in vitro at 3 T using 15 femoral head specimens, compared with μCT, as the standard of reference. Phan and colleagues[72] compared 1.5-T with 3-T MRI in differentiating donors with spinal fractures from those without spinal fractures. The investigators concluded that MR imaging at 3 T provided a better depiction of the trabecular bone structure than did MR imaging at 1.5 T. Banerjee and colleagues[15] compared and optimized different gradient-echo pulse sequences for trabecular bone imaging in vivo at 1.5 T and 3 T field strength. These investigators scanned eight healthy subjects at the proximal femur, calcaneus, and the distal tibia, and found a significant increase in SNR at the higher field strength but also increased susceptibility-induced effects between the more diamagnetic bone and the bone marrow. Krug and colleagues[16,25,26] investigated the impact on bone imaging using field strengths as high as 7 T, imaging 6 healthy subjects at 3 T and 7 T and additionally with HR-pQCT. Krug and colleagues found a substantial increase in SNR at 7 T and also an alteration in structural bone parameters, as expected from susceptibility induced off-resonances.[25]

COMPUTED TOMOGRAPHY IMAGING

CT is a 3D x-ray imaging technique. Unlike most MRI musculoskeletal applications, CT provides positive contrast of mineralized tissues. The image formation process begins with the acquisition of serial radiographic projections over a range of angular positions around the object of interest. The cross-sectional FOV is then reconstructed using established computational techniques based on Radon projection theory. Similar to simple radiography, the reconstructed image intensity values represent the local x-ray attenuation—a material property related to the electron density. Contrast between soft and mineralized tissues in CT is high due to the relative electron-dense inorganic component (calcium hydroxyapatite) of the bone matrix.[73] Quantitative calibration of x-ray attenuation to BMD is accomplished by imaging reference phantoms containing objects of known hydroxyapatite concentrations.

Several classes of CT devices are presently used for high-resolution imaging of trabecular and cortical bone microarchitecture. Application of standard whole-body MDCT to imaging trabecular bone in the axial and peripheral skeleton has been investigated at several research institutes.[74–78] A standard MDCT gantry recently has been combined with 2D flat panel detector technology to provide rapid continuous acquisitions at high isotropic spatial resolution.[79,80] In the last 5 years a high-resolution, limited FOV CT device has become commercially available for dedicated imaging of bone structure in the peripheral skeleton (high-resolution peripheral QCT, HR-pQCT).[27,81–83]

Multidetector Computed Tomography

MDCT is a clinical CT technique, which is available in most diagnostic imaging departments and thus a dedicated scanner is not required. The spatial resolution of this technique is limited; minimum slice thickness in clinical studies is on the order of 0.6 mm while minimum pixel sizes range around 0.25 to 0.3 mm. These spatial resolutions are above trabecular dimensions and imaging of individual trabeculae is subjected to significant partial volume effects; however, it has been shown that trabecular bone parameters obtained with this technique correlate with those determined in contact radiographs from histologic bone sections and μCT.[84,85] In one of these studies, corresponding sections of contact radiographs and MDCT images of the distal radius were analyzed and structure parameters analogous to bone histomorphometry were determined. Significant correlations between MDCT-derived structure parameters and those derived from the contact radiographs were found ($P<.01$) with R values of up to 0.70.[85]

The advantage of the MDCT technique is that more central regions of the skeleton such as the spine and proximal femur can be visualized; these are sites were osteoporotic fractures are found and which would be important to monitor therapy. However, to achieve adequate spatial resolution and image quality the required radiation exposure is substantial, which offsets the technique's applicability in clinical routine and scientific studies. High-resolution CT scanning is associated with a considerably higher radiation dose compared with standard techniques for measuring BMD. Compared with the 0.01 to 0.05 mSv effective dose associated with DXA in adult patients and 0.06 to 0.3 mSv delivered through 2D QCT of the lumbar spine, studies show that protocols used to examine vertebral microstructure using high-

resolution MDCT provide an effective dose of about 3 mSv (1.5 years of natural background radiation).[74,76]

MDCT has been used in vivo to study the trabecular bone at the lumbar spine, and results have been promising in differentiating subjects with and without osteoporotic spine fractures and in monitoring therapy-induced changes of trabecular microarchitecture.[74,76] Ito and colleagues[74] demonstrated that MDCT-derived trabecular bone structure parameters of the L3 vertebral body better separated patients with and without vertebral fractures than did BMD of the spine, obtained by DXA. Graeff and colleagues[76] showed that teriparatide treatment effects were better monitored by architectural parameters of the spine obtained through MDCT than by BMD.

Using clinical imaging in more central regions of the skeleton such as spine and femur, however, it is still noted that the trabecular bone architecture visualized with MDCT is more a texture of the trabecular bone than a true visualization of the individual trabecular structure (**Fig. 10**).

High-Resolution Peripheral Quantitative Computed Tomography

A dedicated extremity imaging system designed for trabecular-scale imaging is currently available from a single manufacturer (XtremeCT, Scanco Medical AG, Brüttisellen, Swizterland). The development of HR-pQCT represents the convergence of clinical CT with many of the technological features of desktop μCT used widely for basic research in specimen and small animal models of skeletal disorders.[86,87] This device has the advantage of significantly higher SNR and spatial

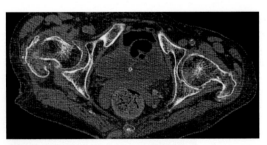

Fig. 10. MDCT of the proximal femur obtained using 120 kVp, automatic current modulation between 70 and 500 mA, noise index of 50, 0.625-mm slice thickness, and reconstructed at 1.25 mm. A standard bone kernel algorithm was used to reconstruct the axial images. Note osteoporotic right intertrochanteric fracture. The left proximal femur was used for trabecular bone structure analysis; however, due to the significant noise level in this section, the resulting image shows more of a texture instead of individual bone trabeculae.

resolution compared with MDCT and MRI (nominal isotropic voxel dimension of 82 μm). Furthermore, the radiation dose is several orders of magnitude lower compared with whole-body CT, and primarily does not involve critical, radiosensitive organs. There are also several disadvantages to this technology. Most notably, it is limited to peripheral skeletal sites and therefore can provide no direct insight into bone quality in the lumbar spine or proximal femur—common sites for osteoporotic fragility fractures, which are associated with the most significant financial and quality of life burden for patients. In addition, there are presently a limited number of devices installed across the world and they are primarily located in major research institutions.

Image acquisition

Hardware The HR-pQCT imaging system consists of a microfocus x-ray source with a 70-μm focal spot size. The scanner operates at a fixed voltage of 60 kVp and current of 900 μA. Filters of 0.3 mm Cu and 1 mm Al are positioned at the aperture to filter soft x-rays to reduce patient dose and limit beam-hardening effects. The cone beam x-ray field is incident on a structured cesium iodide (40 mg/cm^2) scintillator coupled by a fiberoptic taper to a 2D 3072 × 256 element CCD detector with a 41-μm pitch. The x-ray source and detector ensemble interface a high-resolution motorized gantry that allows translation along the z-axis of the scanner and axial rotation across 180° for tomographic acquisitions. The readout electronics of the detector interface a computer workstation and associated data storage resources through a small computer system interface connection.

Scan setup A standard, manufacturer-recommended scan protocol has been used in most of the published literature to date. The techniques involved were primarily adapted from a previous generation pQCT device.[88] The subject's forearm or ankle is immobilized in a carbon fiber cast that is fixed within the gantry of the scanner. A single dorsal-palmar projection image of the distal radius or tibia is acquired to define the tomographic scan region. This region spans 9.02 mm in length (110 slices) and is localized to a fixed offset proximal from the mid-jointline and extending proximally. In the radius the offset is 9.5 mm while in the tibia it is 22.5 mm (**Fig. 11**). It is important to note that this method does not account for differences in bone length and therefore may be a confounding source of variability in cross-sectional studies.[89] In the radius, the default axial scan location has been found to partially overlap with the most common site for fracture and region of the most significant biomechanical consequence.[90]

There are several different protocol modifications that have been employed for developmental studies in children and adolescents to account for patient size, and designed to avoid radiation exposure to the epiphyseal growth plate. In a cross-sectional study of age- and gender-related differences in the microstructure of the distal forearm of adolescent boys and girls, Kirmani and colleagues[91] used a fixed offset (1 mm) with respect to the proximal extent of the distal epiphyseal growth plate of the radius. This protocol ensured no direct irradiation of the growth plate and is consistent with the most common site of forearm fractures during adolescence.[92] In a similar population participating in a longitudinal

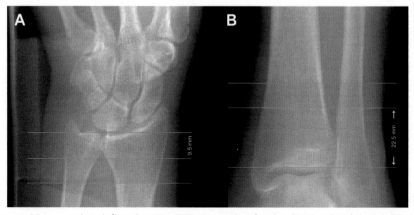

Fig. 11. Scout acquisition used to define the HR-pQCT scan region for the distal radius (A) and distal tibia (B). The solid green region corresponds to the imaging location and consists of 110 slices spanning 9.02 mm longitudinally. In the radius the scan region is fixed 9.5 mm proximal from the mid-jointline, while in the tibia the scan region is 22.5 mm proximal from the tibial plafond.

study of bone development, Burrows and colleagues[93] selected a region offset 8% of the total tibial length proximal to the tibial plafond. In their cohort this approach resulted in no overlap with the growth plate, allowed comparable localization for longitudinal measurements during growth, and did not require operator identification of the proximal extent of the growth plate, which can be highly variable and is therefore a potential source of operator-related error. While there are several studies underway investigating other scan locations in adults, including more proximal sites dominated by cortical bone, hardware constraints for this device preclude imaging true diaphyseal sites in the radius or tibia.

Tomography Before each tomographic acquisition, a precalibration procedure is performed to measure the dark bias signal in the detector (x-ray shutter closed) and the reference intensity of the x-ray source with an empty FOV (x-ray shutter open). For the actual tomographic acquisition, 750 projections are acquired over 180° with a 100-ms integration time at each angular position. The 12.6-cm FOV is reconstructed across a 1536 × 1536 matrix using a modified Feldkamp algorithm, yielding 82-μm isotropic voxels (**Fig. 12**).[94] The total scan time is 2.8 minutes and results in an effective dose to the subject of approximately 4.2 μSv, several orders of magnitude smaller than clinical CT and comparable to DXA and other planar radiographic modalities. In total, the raw projection data, reconstructed image data, and other derivative data require approximately 1 GB (1024 MB) of digital storage space per scan.

Image analysis and postprocessing

The reconstructed images are analyzed using a standard protocol provided by the manufacturer. The operator initiates the segmentation process by drawing an approximate contour around the periosteal perimeter of the radius or tibia in the first slice of the dataset. This contour is then automatically adjusted using an edge detection process to precisely identify the periosteal boundary. The software iteratively proceeds through the remaining slices in the dataset while the operator visually verifies the accurate contouring of the periosteal surface, adjusting where necessary. The cortical bone compartment is segmented using a 3D Gaussian smoothing filter followed by a simple

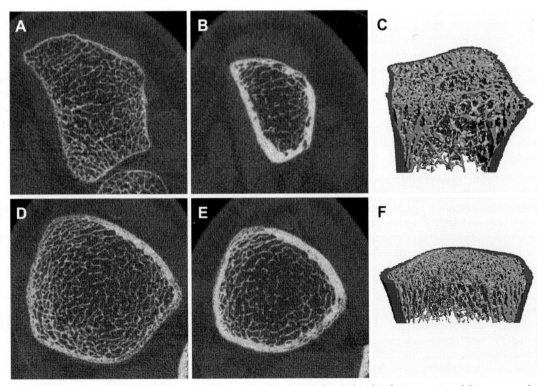

Fig. 12. Typical HR-pQCT images from the distal radius (*A–C*) and distal tibia (*D–F*). Images *A* and *D* correspond to the distalmost slices of the scan, while images *B* and *E* correspond to the proximalmost slices. Images *C* and *F* are 3D reconstructions of the extracted mineralized structure, with the segmented cortical compartment highlighted in dark gray.

fixed threshold. The trabecular compartment is identified by digital subtraction of the cortical bone from the region enclosed by the periosteal contours. The trabecular bone structure is extracted using a Laplace-hamming edge-enhancement process followed by a second fixed threshold.[95] Based on this semiautomated contouring and segmentation process, the trabecular and cortical compartments are segmented automatically for subsequent densitometric, morphometric, and biomechanical analyses. For some scenarios, this segmentation procedure may be unsatisfactory,[27,96] and more sophisticated techniques are an active area of research.[97,98] In general, reproducibility of densitometric measures is very high (CV <1%), while biomechanical and morphometric measures typically have a CV of 4% to 5%.[27,81,82,99,100]

Densitometric analysis The linear attenuation values of the tomographic images are converted to hydroxyapatite (HA) mineral densities using a beam-hardening correction and phantom calibration procedure previously described for an ex vivo μCT system.[101] The calibration phantom (Scanco Medical AG, Brüttisellen, Switzerland) is composed of 5 cylinders of HA-resin mixtures with a range of mineral concentrations (0, 100, 200, 400, 800 mg HA/cm^3) where 0 mg HA/cm^3 represents a soft tissue equivalent background devoid of mineral. Based on this calibration, volumetric BMD can be determined independently for cortical and trabecular bone compartments based on the segmentation process described above. HR-pQCT images have also been used to derive surrogate measures of areal BMD in the ultradistal radius.[102] This technique has shown a high level of agreement with multiple clinical DXA devices (R^2 >0.8).

Morphometric analysis Morphometric indices analogous to classic histomorphometry are calculated from the binary image of the trabecular bone. Unlike MRI and MDCT, which have a large slice thickness relative to the in-plane resolution, the high isotropic resolution of HR-pQCT (82 μm) permits direct, 3D assessment of intertrabecular distances. These measures have been well validated against μCT gold standards in several studies.[83,98,103] From the binary image of the extracted trabecular structure, 3D distance transformation techniques are used to calculated trabecular number (**Fig. 13**).[65] Whereas the intertrabecular distances are large compared with the voxel dimension, the average trabecular thickness (100–150 μm) is on average only 1 to 2 voxels wide. Accordingly, direct measures of thickness and bone volume are complicated by significant

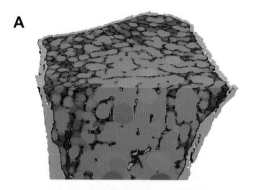

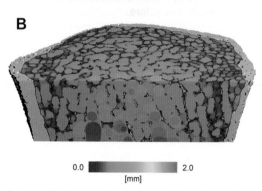

0.0 ▮▮▮▮▮▮ 2.0
[mm]

Fig. 13. 3D visualization in the distal radius (*A*) and distal tibia (*B*), with the color range indicating the magnitude of local intertrabecular distances calculated using a 3D distance transform. The mean value of this distance map is equivalent to the inverse of trabecular number (Tb.N).

partial volume effects. In the standard analysis protocol, BV/TV is derived from the trabecular volumetric BMD assuming a fixed mineralization of 1200 mg HA/cm^3 for compact bone (BV/TV = Tb.vBMD/1200). From the direct measure of Tb.N and the densitometrically derived BV/TV, trabecular thickness and separation (Tb.Th, Tb.Sp) are derived using standard stereological relations assuming a plate-model geometry.[88,104]

There are several potential concerns with this approach. First, phantom studies by Sekhon and colleagues[105] have documented significant errors in the measurement of trabecular vBMD related to biologically relevant variations in cortical thickness, as well as the magnitude of trabecular vBMD itself. This is most likely related to x-ray scatter effects—the HR-pQCT does not have a collimated detector to block Compton scattered x-rays—and residual beam-hardening artifacts. These errors are primarily a concern for cross-sectional studies when cortical thickness and trabecular vBMD may span a broad range. It is less of a concern, and indeed may not be significant, in longitudinal studies where percent-change s the primary end point as age, pathology, and therapy-related changes in cortical thickness and trabecular vBMD are comparatively small. Second, the assumption of a fixed matrix mineralization is not consistent with the established action of many common antifracture therapeutic agents.[106] Changes in bone tissue mineral density would be expected to cause an increase in vBMD irrespective of bone volume changes, and therefore result in an overestimation of BV/TV and propagate error to the derivative measures of trabecular thickness and separation, confounding any actual therapy-related effect on trabecular bone volume and structure.

Several studies have investigated other measures of bone microarchitecture and topology from HR-pQCT images including connectivity, structure model index (a measure of the rod or platelike appearance of the structure), and anisotropy. However, there is mixed evidence of their reliability at in vivo resolutions.[83,98,103,107] More sophisticated approaches to cortical bone segmentation have recently been proposed,[97] which allow direct 3D assessment of cortical thickness (Ct.Th) as well as quantification of cortical microarchitecture, including intracortical porosity (Fig. 14).[108,109]

Biomechanical analysis Although volumetric density and microarchitectural information provide improved fracture risk prediction and some explanation for treatment efficacy, more direct estimates of bone mechanical strength inherently accounting for geometry, microarchitecture, and even composition are the ultimate goals for improving fracture risk prediction and management of osteoporosis. To that end, computational modeling approaches have been introduced to take advantage of the detailed information in high-resolution images of bone. FEA is a common computational tool in classic engineering fields, critical to design and failure analysis. The basic concept is that the behavior of a complicated system under a simulated loading condition, in this case the biomechanical properties of bone, can be determined through subdivision into smaller constitutive elements for which the behavior is trivial to determine. Applied to high-resolution images of bone, the apparent biomechanical properties (eg, stiffness, elastic modulus) of a biologically complex microstructure are computed by decomposing the structure into small cubic elements (ie, the voxels) with assumed mechanical properties (Fig. 15).[110,111] For HR-pQCT this technique has been validated against both higher resolution models (μCT) as well as empirical measures of strength.[103,112] In addition to whole bone mechanics, micro-FEA (μFEA) can be used to determine the relative load distribution between cortical and trabecular compartments,[113] and estimate mechanical implications of specific structural features such as intracortical porosity.[108]

Longitudinal analysis For clinical investigations into longitudinal changes in HR-pQCT derived measures of bone quality, several important considerations must be addressed. First, because bone structure and geometry can change substantially along the axial direction,[89] it is critical that baseline and follow-up scans be matched. To this end the scout scan and reference line position for all baseline measurements are recorded automatically. When a follow-up measurement is performed, the operator is automatically presented with an image of the baseline scout denoted with the original reference position as a visual aid for positioning the reference line for the follow-up acquisition. Nevertheless, this is a subjective process subject to operator error. At the authors' imaging center, repeat measurements are typically associated with a margin of error in the axial positioning of approximately 1 mm. Accordingly, automated methods are needed to ensure that comparable regions of interest are used for the image analysis. To that end, the manufacturer provides software that automatically matches slices based on periosteal cross-sectional area and limits the analyzed region to the slices common

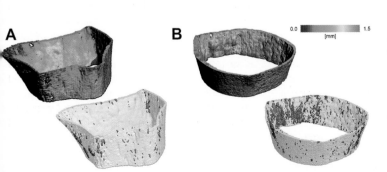

Fig. 14. 3D visualization from quantitative analyses of cortical bone geometry and microarchitecture in the distal radius (A) and distal tibia (B), showing direct 3D measures of cortical thickness (top) and the segmentation of intracortical pore volume (bottom).

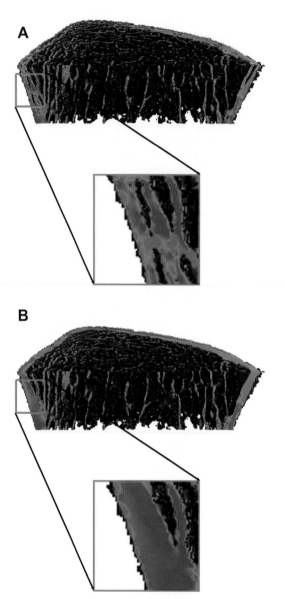

Fig. 15. 3D visualization from μFEA simulation of 1% axial compression in the distal tibia with (*A*) and without (*B*) intracortical porosity. The pseudocolor renderings show the distribution of strain energy density in each model.

to both baseline and follow-up.[88] Alternatively, MacNeil and Boyd[99] have demonstrated that 3D image registration techniques can provide improved short- and medium-term reproducibility compared with the default slice-matching approach. This approach may also be more appropriate in longitudinal studies where changes in cortical thickness would compromise registration, based strictly on cross-sectional area. As discussed earlier, meaningful longitudinal comparisons in children or adolescents experiencing rapid

growth is not trivial, and requires more careful consideration of standardization of scan positioning and analysis protocols.[93]

Clinical Applications

There is a growing body of clinical research literature featuring HR-pQCT assessment of bone quality. The first cross-sectional studies by Boutroy and colleagues[81] and Khosla and colleagues[82] demonstrated significant, gender-specific age-related differences in bone microarchitecture, while Dalzell and colleagues[114] and Burghardt and colleagues[108] have reported analogous findings for μFEA biomechanical measures. A microstructural basis for ethnicity-related differences in bone strength between East Asian and Caucasian women has been reported in two recent studies[115,116] Sornay-Rendu and colleagues[117] demonstrated cortical and trabecular morphology provided some additional fracture discrimination independent of areal BMD in osteopenic women. In the same OFELY cohort, Boutroy and colleagues[118] later showed that μFEA mechanical measures provided additional discriminatory power between osteopenic women with and without distal radius fractures. Although the initial focus has predominantly been investigations of postmenopausal osteopenia and osteoporosis, several more recent studies have used HR-pQCT to investigate developmental changes in bone quality and fracture risk[91,119,120] as well as secondary causes of bone loss.[121,122] While there are several single and multicenter longitudinal studies currently underway or recently completed, few results have yet to be published at the time of the preparation of this article.[123]

SUMMARY

High-resolution bone imaging has made tremendous progress in the recent past. Both imaging modalities, computed tomography as well as MR imaging, have improved image quality. New developments such as HR-pQCT now make it possible to acquire in vivo images at peripheral sites with isotropic voxel size in a very short time. Further enhancements in the MR field have made it possible to image more central body sites such as the proximal femur with very high spatial resolution. New analysis methods can obtain direct estimates of biomechanical properties and important information related to bone's topology, as well as parameters of scale and orientation. These accomplishments will be essential in the noninvasive assessment of osteoporosis and fracture risk, will provide insight into the mechanisms behind

bone loss, and will increasingly play a role as a tool
for assessing treatment efficacy.

REFERENCES

1. Black DM, Thompson DE, Bauer DC, et al. Fracture risk reduction with alendronate in women with osteoporosis: the Fracture Intervention Trial. FIT Research Group. J Clin Endocrinol Metab 2000; 85:4118.

2. Wehrli FW, Saha PK, Gomberg BR, et al. Role of magnetic resonance for assessing structure and function of trabecular bone. Top Magn Reson Imaging 2002;13:335.

3. Hildebrand T, Laib A, Muller R, et al. Direct three-dimensional morphometric analysis of human cancellous bone: microstructural data from spine, femur, iliac crest, and calcaneus. J Bone Miner Res 1999;14:1167.

4. Bousson V, Peyrin F, Bergot C, et al. Cortical bone in the human femoral neck: three-dimensional appearance and porosity using synchrotron radiation. J Bone Miner Res 2004;19:794.

5. Horikoshi T, Endo N, Uchiyama T, et al. Peripheral quantitative computed tomography of the femoral neck in 60 Japanese women. Calcif Tissue Int 1999;65:447.

6. Pistoia W, van Rietbergen B, Ruegsegger P. Mechanical consequences of different scenarios for simulated bone atrophy and recovery in the distal radius. Bone 2003;33:937.

7. Bousson V, Bergot C, Meunier A, et al. CT of the middiaphyseal femur: cortical bone mineral density and relation to porosity. Radiology 2000;217:179.

8. Alonso CG, Curiel MD, Carranza FH, et al. Femoral bone mineral density, neck-shaft angle and mean femoral neck width as predictors of hip fracture in men and women. Multicenter Project for Research in Osteoporosis. Osteoporos Int 2000;11:714.

9. Crabtree N, Loveridge N, Parker M, et al. Intracapsular hip fracture and the region-specific loss of cortical bone: analysis by peripheral quantitative computed tomography. J Bone Miner Res 2001; 16:1318.

10. Augat P, Reeb H, Claes LE. Prediction of fracture load at different skeletal sites by geometric properties of the cortical shell. J Bone Miner Res 1996;11: 1356.

11. Schneider P, Stauber M, Voide R, et al. Ultrastructural properties in cortical bone vary greatly in two inbred strains of mice as assessed by synchrotron light based micro- and nano-CT. J Bone Miner Res 2007;22:1557.

12. Li CQ, Magland JF, Rajapakse CS, et al. Implications of resolution and noise for in vivo micro-MRI of trabecular bone. Med Phys 2008;35:5584.

13. Rajapakse CS, Magland J, Zhang XH, et al. Implications of noise and resolution on mechanical properties of trabecular bone estimated by image-based finite-element analysis. J Orthop Res 2009;27:1263.

14. Krug R, Banerjee S, Han ET, et al. Feasibility of in vivo structural analysis of high-resolution magnetic resonance images of the proximal femur. Osteoporos Int 2005;16:1307.

15. Banerjee S, Han ET, Krug R, et al. Application of refocused steady-state free-precession methods at 1.5 and 3 T to in vivo high-resolution MRI of trabecular bone: simulations and experiments. J Magn Reson Imaging 2005;21:818.

16. Krug R, Carballido-Gamio J, Banerjee S, et al. In vivo bone and cartilage MRI using fully-balanced steady-state free-precession at 7 tesla. Magn Reson Med 2007;58:1294.

17. Link TM, Lotter A, Beyer F, et al. Changes in calcaneal trabecular bone structure after heart transplantation: an MR imaging study. Radiology 2000; 217:855.

18. Link TM, Saborowski, Kisters K, et al. Changes in calcaneal trabecular bone structure assessed with high-resolution MR imaging in patients with kidney transplantation. Osteoporos Int 2002;13:119.

19. Link TM, Vieth V, Matheis J, et al. Bone structure of the distal radius and the calcaneus vs BMD of the spine and proximal femur in the prediction of osteoporotic spine fractures. Eur Radiol 2002;12:401.

20. Ernst R, Bodenhausen G, Wokaun A. Principles of nuclear magnetic resonance in one and two dimensions, vol. 28. Oxford: Clarendon; 1987. p. 125.

21. Krug R, Han ET, Banerjee S, et al. Fully balanced steady-state 3D-spin-echo (bSSSE) imaging at 3 Tesla. Magn Reson Med 2006;56:1033.

22. Krug R, Carballido-Gamio J, Burghardt AJ, et al. Assessment of trabecular bone structure comparing magnetic resonance imaging at 3 Tesla with high-resolution peripheral quantitative computed tomography ex vivo and in vivo. Osteoporos Int 2008;19:653.

23. Bauer JS, Monetti R, Krug R, et al. Advances of 3T MR imaging in visualizing trabecular bone structure of the calcaneus are partially SNR-independent: analysis using simulated noise in relation to micro-CT, 1.5T MRI, and biomechanical strength. J Magn Reson Imaging 2009;29:132.

24. Bolbos RI, Zuo J, Banerjee S, et al. Relationship between trabecular bone structure and articular cartilage morphology and relaxation times in early OA of the knee joint using parallel MRI at 3T. Osteoarthritis Cartilage 2008;16:1150.

25. Krug R, Carballido-Gamio J, Banerjee S, et al. In vivo ultra-high-field magnetic resonance imaging

of trabecular bone microarchitecture at 7 T. J Magn Reson Imaging 2008;27:854.

26. Krug R, Stehling C, Kelley DA, et al. Imaging of the musculoskeletal system in vivo using ultra-high field magnetic resonance at 7 T. Invest Radiol 2009;44:613.

27. Kazakia GJ, Hyun B, Burghardt AJ, et al. In vivo determination of bone structure in postmenopausal women: a comparison of HR-pQCT and high-field MR imaging. J Bone Miner Res 2008;23:463.

28. Ma J, Wehrli FW, Song HK. Fast 3D large-angle spin-echo imaging (3D FLASE). Magn Reson Med 1996;35:903.

29. Gomberg BR, Wehrli FW, Vasilic B, et al. Reproducibility and error sources of micro-MRI-based trabecular bone structural parameters of the distal radius and tibia. Bone 2004;35:266.

30. Song HK, Wehrli FW. In vivo micro-imaging using alternating navigator echoes with applications to cancellous bone structural analysis. Magn Reson Med 1999;41:947.

31. Banerjee S, Choudhury S, Han ET, et al. Autocalibrating parallel imaging of in vivo trabecular bone microarchitecture at 3 Tesla. Magn Reson Med 2006;56:1075.

32. Griswold MA, Jakob PM, Heidemann RM, et al. Generalized autocalibrating partially parallel acquisitions (GRAPPA). Magn Reson Med 2002;47:1202.

33. Newitt DC, Van Rietbergen B, Majumdar S. Processing and analysis of in vivo high-resolution MR images of trabecular bone for longitudinal studies: reproducibility of structural measures and micro-finite element analysis derived mechanical properties. Osteoporos Int 2002;13:278.

34. Wald LL, Carvajal L, Moyher SE, et al. Phased array detectors and an automated intensity-correction algorithm for high-resolution MR imaging of the human brain. Magn Reson Med 1995;34:433.

35. Vasilic B, Wehrli FW. A novel local thresholding algorithm for trabecular bone volume fraction mapping in the limited spatial resolution regime of in vivo MRI. IEEE Trans Med Imaging 2005;24:1574.

36. Folkesson J, Krug R, Goldenstein J, et al. Evaluation of correction methods for coil-induced intensity inhomogeneities and their influence on trabecular bone structure parameters from MR images. Med Phys 2009;36:1267.

37. Sled JG, Zijdenbos AP, Evans AC. A nonparametric method for automatic correction of intensity nonuniformity in MRI data. IEEE Trans Med Imaging 1998; 17:87.

38. Majumdar S, Genant HK, Grampp S, et al. Correlation of trabecular bone structure with age, bone mineral density, and osteoporotic status: in vivo studies in the distal radius using high resolution magnetic resonance imaging. J Bone Miner Res 1997;12:111.

39. Hwang S, Wehrli F. Estimating voxel volume fractions of trabecular bone on the basis of magnetic resonance images acquired in vivo. Int J Imaging Syst Technol 1999;10:186.

40. Wehrli FW, Song HK, Saha PK, et al. Quantitative MRI for the assessment of bone structure and function. NMR Biomed 2006;19:731.

41. Wehrli FW. Structural and functional assessment of trabecular and cortical bone by micro magnetic resonance imaging. J Magn Reson Imaging 2007; 25:390.

42. Krug R, Carballido-Gamio J, Burghardt AJ, et al. Wavelet-based characterization of vertebral trabecular bone structure from magnetic resonance images at 3 T compared with micro computed tomographic measurements. Magn Reson Imaging 2007;25:392.

43. Saha PK, Wehrli FW. Measurement of trabecular bone thickness in the limited resolution regime of in vivo MRI by fuzzy distance transform. IEEE Trans Med Imaging 2004;23:53.

44. Carballido-Gamio J, Phan C, Link TM, et al. Characterization of trabecular bone structure from high-resolution magnetic resonance images using fuzzy logic. Magn Reson Imaging 2006; 24:1023.

45. Folkesson J, Carballido-Gamio J, Eckstein F, et al. Local bone enhancement fuzzy clustering for segmentation of MR trabecular bone images. Med Phys 2010;37:295.

46. Saha PK, Chaudhuri BB. 3D digital topology under binary transformation with applications. Comput Vis Image Underst 1996;63:418.

47. Gomberg BR, Saha PK, Song HK, et al. Topological analysis of trabecular bone MR images. IEEE Trans Med Imaging 2000;19:166.

48. Pothuaud L, Van Rietbergen B, Charlot C, et al. A new computational efficient approach for trabecular bone analysis using beam models generated with skeletonized graph technique. Comput Methods Biomech Biomed Engin 2004; 7:205.

49. Carballido-Gamio J, Krug R, Huber MB, et al. Geodesic topological analysis of trabecular bone microarchitecture from high-spatial resolution magnetic resonance images. Magn Reson Med 2009;61:448.

50. Whitehouse WJ. The quantitative morphology of anisotropic trabecular bone. J Microsc 1974;101:153.

51. Rotter M, Berg A, Langenberger H, et al. Autocorrelation analysis of bone structure. J Magn Reson Imaging 2001;14:87.

52. Wald MJ, Vasilic B, Saha PK, et al. Spatial autocorrelation and mean intercept length analysis of trabecular bone anisotropy applied to in vivo magnetic resonance imaging. Med Phys 2007; 34:1110.

53. Blumenfeld J, Carballido-Gamio J, Krug R, et al. Automatic prospective registration of high-resolution trabecular bone images of the tibia. Ann Biomed Eng 2007;35:1924.

54. Blumenfeld J, Studholme C, Carballido-Gamio J, et al. Three-dimensional image registration of MR proximal femur images for the analysis of trabecular bone parameters. Med Phys 2008;35:4630.

55. Rajapakse CS, Magland JF, Wehrli FW. Fast prospective registration of in vivo MR images of trabecular bone microstructure in longitudinal studies. Magn Reson Med 2008;59:1120.

56. Magland JF, Jones CE, Leonard MB, et al. Retrospective 3D registration of trabecular bone MR images for longitudinal studies. J Magn Reson Imaging 2009;29:118.

57. Hancu I, Blezek DJ, Dumoulin MC. Automatic repositioning of single voxels in longitudinal 1H MRS studies. NMR Biomed 2005;18:352.

58. Gomberg BR, Saha PK, Wehrli FW. Method for cortical bone structural analysis from magnetic resonance images. Acad Radiol 2005;12:1320.

59. Hyun B, Newitt DC, Majumdar S. Assessment of cortical bone structure using high-resolution magnetic resonance imaging. In: Proceedings 13th Scientific Meeting, International Society for Magnetic Resonance in Medicine, Miami, 7–13 May, 2005.

60. Goldenstein J, Kazakia G, Majumdar S. In vivo evaluation of the presence of bone marrow in cortical porosity in postmenopausal osteopenic women. Ann Biomed Eng 2009;38:235.

61. Techawiboonwong A, Song HK, Leonard MB, et al. Cortical bone water: in vivo quantification with ultrashort echo-time MR imaging. Radiology 2008;248:824.

62. Issever A, Larson P, Majumdar S, et al. High-resolution 3D UTE imaging of cortical bone. In: Proceedings 17th Scientific Meeting, International Society for Magnetic Resonance in Medicine, Honolulu, 18–24, April 2009, p. 3948.

63. Gold GE, Han E, Stainsby J, et al. Musculoskeletal MRI at 3.0 T: relaxation times and image contrast. AJR Am J Roentgenol 2004;183:343.

64. Techawiboonwong A, Song HK, Wehrli FW. In vivo MRI of submillisecond T(2) species with two-dimensional and three-dimensional radial sequences and applications to the measurement of cortical bone water. NMR Biomed 2008;21:59.

65. Hildebrand T, Ruegsegger P. A new method for the model-independent assessment of thickness in three-dimensional images. J Microsc 1997;185:67.

66. Wehrli FW, Gomberg BR, Saha PK, et al. Digital topological analysis of in vivo magnetic resonance microimages of trabecular bone reveals structural implications of osteoporosis. J Bone Miner Res 2001;16:1520.

67. Benito M, Vasilic B, Wehrli FW, et al. Effect of testosterone replacement on trabecular architecture in hypogonadal men. J Bone Miner Res 2005;20:1785.

68. Chesnut CH 3rd, Majumdar S, Newitt DC, et al. Effects of salmon calcitonin on trabecular microarchitecture as determined by magnetic resonance imaging: results from the QUEST study. J Bone Miner Res 2005;20:1548.

69. Wehrli FW, Ladinsky GA, Jones C, et al. In vivo magnetic resonance detects rapid remodeling changes in the topology of the trabecular bone network after menopause and the protective effect of estradiol. J Bone Miner Res 2008;23:730.

70. Zhang XH, Liu XS, Vasilic B, et al. In vivo microMRI-based finite element and morphological analyses of tibial trabecular bone in eugonadal and hypogonadal men before and after testosterone treatment. J Bone Miner Res 2008; 23:1426.

71. Sell CA, Masi JN, Burghardt A, et al. Quantification of trabecular bone structure using magnetic resonance imaging at 3 Tesla—calibration studies using microcomputed tomography as a standard of reference. Calcif Tissue Int 2005;76:355.

72. Phan CM, Matsuura M, Bauer JS, et al. Trabecular bone structure of the calcaneus: comparison of MR imaging at 3.0 and 1.5 T with micro-CT on the standard of reference. Radiology 2006;239:488.

73. Berger MJ, Hubbell JH, Seltzer SM, et al. XCOM: Photon cross sections database version 1.3. National Institute of Standards and Technology. Gaithersburg (MD): 2005. Available at: http://physics.nist.gov/xcom.

74. Ito M, Ikeda K, Nishiguchi M, et al. Multi-detector row CT imaging of vertebral microstructure for evaluation of fracture risk. J Bone Miner Res 2005;20:1828.

75. Bauer JS, Link TM, Burghardt A, et al. Analysis of trabecular bone structure with multidetector spiral computed tomography in a simulated soft-tissue environment. Calcif Tissue Int 2007;80:366.

76. Graeff C, Timm W, Nickelsen TN, et al. Monitoring teriparatide-associated changes in vertebral microstructure by high-resolution CT in vivo: results from the EUROFORS study. J Bone Miner Res 2007;22:1426.

77. Diederichs G, Link T, Marie K, et al. Feasibility of measuring trabecular bone structure of the proximal femur using 64-slice multidetector computed tomography in a clinical setting. Calcif Tissue Int 2008;83:332.

78. Issever AS, Link TM, Kentenich M, et al. Trabecular bone structure analysis in osteoporotic spine using a clinical in-vivo set-up for 64-slice MDCT imaging: Comparison to muCT imaging and muFE modeling. J Bone Miner Res 2009;24:1628.

79. Reichardt B, Sarwar A, Bartling SH, et al. Musculo-skeletal applications of flat-panel volume CT. Skeletal Radiol 2008;37:1069.

80. Gupta R, Grasruck M, Suess C, et al. Ultra-high resolution flat-panel volume CT: fundamental principles, design architecture, and system characterization. Eur Radiol 2006;16:1191.

81. Boutroy S, Bouxsein ML, Munoz F, et al. In vivo assessment of trabecular bone microarchitecture by high-resolution peripheral quantitative computed tomography. J Clin Endocrinol Metab 2005; 90:6508.

82. Khosla S, Riggs BL, Atkinson EJ, et al. Effects of sex and age on bone microstructure at the ultradistal radius: a population-based noninvasive in vivo assessment. J Bone Miner Res 2006;21:124.

83. Macneil JA, Boyd SK. Accuracy of high-resolution peripheral quantitative computed tomography for measurement of bone quality. Med Eng Phys 2007;29:1096.

84. Issever AS, Vieth V, Lotter A, et al. Local differences in the trabecular bone structure of the proximal femur depicted with high-spatial-resolution MR imaging and multisection CT. Acad Radiol 2002;9:1395.

85. Link T, Vieth V, Stehling C, et al. High resolution MRI versus Multislice spiral CT—which technique depicts the trabecular bone structure best? Eur Radiol 2003;13:663.

86. Kohlbrenner A, Koller B, Hammerle S, et al. In vivo micro tomography. Adv Exp Med Biol 2001;496:213.

87. Muller R, Ruegsegger P. Micro-tomographic imaging for the nondestructive evaluation of trabecular bone architecture. Stud Health Technol Inform 1997;40:61.

88. Laib A, Hauselmann HJ, Ruegsegger P. In vivo high resolution 3D-QCT of the human forearm. Technol Health Care 1998;6:329.

89. Boyd SK. Site-specific variation of bone micro-architecture in the distal radius and tibia. J Clin Densitom 2008;11:424.

90. Mueller TL, van Lenthe GH, Stauber M, et al. Regional, age and gender differences in architectural measures of bone quality and their correlation to bone mechanical competence in the human radius of an elderly population. Bone 2009;45:882.

91. Kirmani S, Christen D, van Lenthe GH, et al. Bone structure at the distal radius during adolescent growth. J Bone Miner Res 2008;24:1033.

92. Bailey DA, Wedge JH, McCulloch RG, et al. Epidemiology of fractures of the distal end of the radius in children as associated with growth. J Bone Joint Surg Am 1989;71:1225.

93. Burrows M, Liu D, McKay H. High-resolution peripheral QCT imaging of bone micro-structure in adolescents. Osteoporos Int 2009;21:515.

94. Feldkamp LA, Davis LC, Kress JW. Practical cone-beam algorithm. J Opt Soc Am A 1984;1:612.

95. Laib A, Ruegsegger P. Comparison of structure extraction methods for in vivo trabecular bone measurements. Comput Med Imaging Graph 1999;23:69.

96. Davis KA, Burghardt AJ, Link TM, et al. The effects of geometric and threshold definitions on cortical bone metrics assessed by in vivo high-resolution peripheral quantitative computed tomography. Calcif Tissue Int 2007;81:364.

97. Buie HR, Campbell GM, Klinck RJ, et al. Automatic segmentation of cortical and trabecular compartments based on a dual threshold technique for in vivo micro-CT bone analysis. Bone 2007;41:505.

98. Burghardt AJ, Kazakia GJ, Majumdar S. A local adaptive threshold strategy for high resolution peripheral quantitative computed tomography of trabecular bone. Ann Biomed Eng 2007;35:1678.

99. MacNeil JA, Boyd SK. Improved reproducibility of high-resolution peripheral quantitative computed tomography for measurement of bone quality. Med Eng Phys 2008;30:792.

100. Mueller TL, Stauber M, Kohler T, et al. Non-invasive bone competence analysis by high-resolution pQCT: An in vitro reproducibility study on structural and mechanical properties at the human radius. Bone 2009;44:364.

101. Burghardt AJ, Kazakia GJ, Laib A, et al. Quantitative assessment of bone tissue mineralization with polychromatic micro-computed tomography. Calcif Tissue Int 2008;83:129.

102. Burghardt AJ, Kazakia GJ, Link TM, et al. Automated simulation of areal bone mineral density assessment in the distal radius from high-resolution peripheral quantitative computed tomography. Osteoporos Int 2009;20:2017.

103. Liu XS, Zhang XH, Sekhon KK, et al. High-resolution peripheral quantitative computed tomography can assess microstructural and mechanical properties of human distal tibial bone. J Bone Miner Res 2009. [Epub ahead of print].

104. Parfitt AM, Drezner MK, Glorieux FH, et al. Bone histomorphometry: standardization of nomenclature, symbols, and units. Report of the ASBMR Histomorphometry Nomenclature Committee. J Bone Miner Res 1987;2:595.

105. Sekhon K, Kazakia GJ, Burghardt AJ, et al. Accuracy of volumetric bone mineral density measurement in high-resolution peripheral quantitative computed tomography. Bone 2009;45:473.

106. Boivin GY, Chavassieux PM, Santora AC, et al. Alendronate increases bone strength by increasing the mean degree of mineralization of bone tissue in osteoporotic women. Bone 2000; 27:687.

107. Sode M, Burghardt AJ, Nissenson RA, et al. Resolution dependence of the non-metric trabecular structure indices. Bone 2008;42:728.

108. Burghardt AJ, Kazakia GJ, Ramachandran S, et al. Age and gender related differences in the geometric properties and biomechanical significance of intra-cortical porosity in the distal radius and tibia. J Bone Miner Res 2009. [Epub ahead of print].

109. Nishiyama KK, Macdonald HM, Buie HR, et al. Postmenopausal women with osteopenia have higher cortical porosity and thinner cortices at the distal radius and tibia than women with normal aBMD: an in vivo HR-pQCT study. J Bone Miner Res 2009. [Epub ahead of print].

110. van Rietbergen B, Weinans H, Huiskes R, et al. A new method to determine trabecular bone elastic properties and loading using micromechanical finite-element models. J Biomech 1995;28:69.

111. Muller R, Ruegsegger P. Three-dimensional finite element modelling of non-invasively assessed trabecular bone structures. Med Eng Phys 1995;17:126.

112. Macneil JA, Boyd SK. Bone strength at the distal radius can be estimated from high-resolution peripheral quantitative computed tomography and the finite element method. Bone 2008;42:1203.

113. MacNeil JA, Boyd SK. Load distribution and the predictive power of morphological indices in the distal radius and tibia by high resolution peripheral quantitative computed tomography. Bone 2007;41:129.

114. Dalzell N, Kaptoge S, Morris N, et al. Bone micro-architecture and determinants of strength in the radius and tibia: age-related changes in a population-based study of normal adults measured with high-resolution pQCT. Osteoporos Int 2009;20:1683.

115. Wang XF, Wang Q, Ghasem-Zadeh A, et al. Differences in macro- and micro-architecture of the appendicular skeleton in young Chinese and Caucasian women. J Bone Miner Res 2009;24:1946.

116. Walker MD, McMahon DJ, Udesky J, et al. Application of high-resolution skeletal imaging to measurements of volumetric BMD and skeletal microarchitecture in Chinese-American and white women: explanation of a paradox. J Bone Miner Res 2009;24:1953.

117. Sornay-Rendu E, Boutroy S, Munoz F, et al. Alterations of cortical and trabecular architecture are associated with fractures in postmenopausal women, partially independent of decreased BMD measured by DXA: the OFELY study. J Bone Miner Res 2007;22:425.

118. Boutroy S, Van Rietbergen B, Sornay-Rendu E, et al. Finite element analysis based on in vivo HR-pQCT images of the distal radius is associated with wrist fracture in postmenopausal women. J Bone Miner Res 2008;23:392.

119. Burrows M, Liu D, Moore S, et al. Bone microstructure at the distal tibia provides a strength advantage to males in late puberty: a HR-pQCT study. J Bone Miner Res 2009. [Epub ahead of print].

120. Chevalley T, Bonjour JP, Ferrari S, et al. Deleterious effect of late menarche on distal tibia microstructure in healthy 20-year-old and premenopausal middle-aged women. J Bone Miner Res 2009;24:144.

121. Bacchetta J, Boutroy S, Guebre-Egziabher F, et al. The relationship between adipokines, osteocalcin and bone quality in chronic kidney disease. Nephrol Dial Transplant 2009;24:3120.

122. Bacchetta J, Boutroy S, Vilayphiou N, et al. Early impairment of trabecular microarchitecture assessed with HR-pQCT in patients with stage II-IV chronic kidney disease. J Bone Miner Res 2009;. [Epub ahead of print].

123. Chavassieux P, Asser Karsdal M, Segovia-Silvestre T, et al. Mechanisms of the anabolic effects of teriparatide on bone: insight from the treatment of a patient with pycnodysostosis. J Bone Miner Res 2008;23:1076.

Pediatric Bone Densitometry

Cornelis van Kuijk, MD, PhD

KEYWORDS

- Bone densitometry • Osteoporosis • Bone fracture
- Dual x-ray absorptiometry

Bone densitometry is an established diagnostic tool in adults to assess bone quantity and to stratify patients and healthy individuals for the prevention of bone fracture. It has become a powerful tool in monitoring diseases and treatments that have an impact on bone metabolism, such as primary osteoporosis or drug-induced secondary osteoporosis. Although there are several techniques to assess bone density (eg, radiogrammetry, dual x-ray absorptiometry [DXA], quantitative CT [QCT], and quantitative ultrasound [QUS]), the most widely used technique is DXA.

Diseases of bone metabolism in childhood and treatment strategies in children for several diseases, such as cancer treatment, that influence bone metabolism, require a diagnostic follow-up of bone status. Skeletal maturation and bone density development are monitored over time and, when possible, treatments are started to ensure that children have appropriate bone status to prevent bone weakness and fractures.

Next to specific endocrinopathic diseases, such as hypogonadism and Cushing syndrome, there is a vast number of chronic medical conditions, such as chronic kidney disease, immunologic disorders, malabsorption syndromes, and malignancies, that have a negative effect on bone maturation and development. In addition, many medications are known to influence bone status and maturation, of which glucocorticoids and chemotherapeutic agents are the most well known, having a negative effect. As the medical community gets better at treating these children with a variety of disorders, it is recognized that there is a need to optimize bone status for these children. Bone densitometry (especially DXA) is the tool for monitoring these children and has become popular over the past 10 years (**Figs. 1** and **2**). There are some pitfalls

and problems, however. Clinicians, including radiologists, should be aware of these problems before requesting or interpreting bone densitometry studies in children.[1–5]

THE DXA PROBLEM

DXA is a 2-D measurement of a 3-D object. Using x-ray technology, the attenuation of the x-ray spectrum caused by tissue (eg, bone and soft tissue) is measured using 2 different scan energies. The measurement is converted into grams of bone-equivalent tissue and divided by the scan area; the outcome parameter is, therefore, in grams per square centimeter (g/cm^2). This is not a real and true bone density that should have a unit of grams per cubic centimeter (g/cm^3). In adults, this is a relative problem, because bone size does not change over time. On the contrary, bone size changes in growing children in 3 dimensions. When measuring children with DXA and following them over time, growth is measured more than actual changes in bone density. The differences in bone density (growth) curves between DXA and QCT are illustrative. QCT is the only bone densitometry measurement technique that directly relates to actual bone density (in g/cm^3). Several articles have investigated normal values in pediatric bone densitometry. When measured with QCT, there is a more or less stable bone density until puberty kicks in. At that time, there is an increase in bone density that levels off when growth has stopped.[6] Clear differences are seen between girls and boys. The true increase of bone density starts at an earlier age in girls (around the age of 10 in girls and around age 12 in boys). By the age of 17, boys

Department of Radiology, VU University Medical Center, PO Box 7057, 1007 MB Amsterdam, The Netherlands
E-mail address: C.vanKuijk@vumc.nl

Radiol Clin N Am 48 (2010) 623–627
doi:10.1016/j.rcl.2010.02.017
0033-8389/10/$ – see front matter © 2010 Elsevier Inc. All rights reserved.

radiologic.theclinics.com

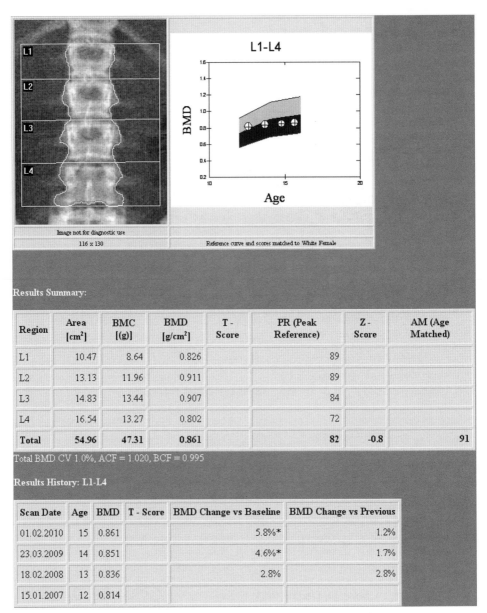

Fig. 1. Follow-up spinal pediatric DXA in child with treatment influencing bone density.

Results Summary:

Region	Area [cm²]	BMC [(g)]	BMD [g/cm²]	T - Score	PR (Peak Reference)	Z - Score	AM (Age Matched)
L1	10.47	8.64	0.826		89		
L2	13.13	11.96	0.911		89		
L3	14.83	13.44	0.907		84		
L4	16.54	13.27	0.802		72		
Total	54.96	47.31	0.861		82	-0.8	91

Total BMD CV 1.0%, ACF = 1.020, BCF = 0.995

Results History: L1-L4

Scan Date	Age	BMD	T - Score	BMD Change vs Baseline	BMD Change vs Previous
01.02.2010	15	0.861		5.8%*	1.2%
23.03.2009	14	0.851		4.6%*	1.7%
18.02.2008	13	0.836		2.8%	2.8%
15.01.2007	12	0.814			

have caught up and have more or less the same range of normal values.

In DXA, however, there is a continuous increase of so-called bone density (in g/cm²) over time with acceleration during puberty.[7] The prepubertal increase, however, is largely caused by bone growth and not by real bone density. The pubertal (accelerated) increase is caused by actual increase of bone density and by bone growth. As such, pediatric DXA can be misleading. Because it measures largely bone growth, the interpretation becomes cumbersome in children who have problems with bone maturation and have a discrepant skeletal age. These children (often with chronic disorders or medication) should never be compared with age-matched reference (normal) values. They should be compared with children with the same maturation status (skeletal age).

Correction for this growth problem has been tried by several investigators. By assuming a cylindrical shape of the vertebral body in spinal DXA, the volume of the vertebral body is estimated from the width of the vertebral body. Then, the outcome parameter becomes apparent bone density in g/cm³. This mathematical best guess correction, however, is not more than an

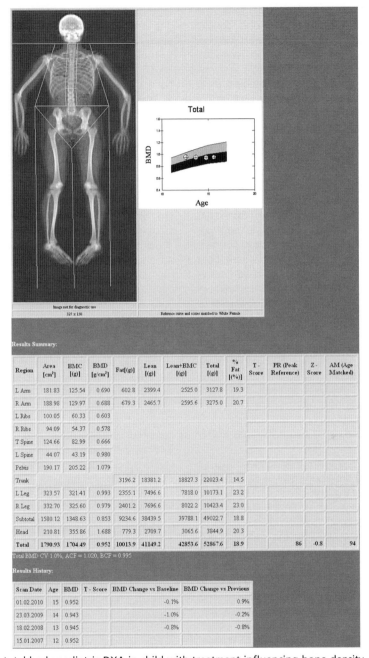

Results Summary:

Region	Area [cm²]	BMC [(g)]	BMD [g/cm²]	Fat[(g)]	Lean [(g)]	Lean+BMC [(g)]	Total [(g)]	% Fat [(%)]	T-Score	PR (Peak Reference)	Z-Score	AM (Age Matched)
L Arm	181.83	125.54	0.690	602.8	2399.4	2525.0	3127.8	19.3				
R Arm	188.98	129.97	0.688	679.3	2465.7	2595.6	3275.0	20.7				
L Ribs	100.05	60.33	0.603									
R Ribs	94.09	54.37	0.578									
T Spine	124.66	82.99	0.666									
L Spine	44.07	43.19	0.980									
Pelvis	190.17	205.22	1.079									
Trunk				3196.2	18381.2	18827.3	22023.4	14.5				
L Leg	323.57	321.41	0.993	2355.4	7496.6	7818.0	10173.1	23.2				
R Leg	332.70	325.60	0.979	2401.2	7696.6	8022.2	10423.4	23.0				
Subtotal	1580.12	1348.63	0.853	9234.6	38439.5	39788.1	49022.7	18.8				
Head	210.81	355.86	1.688	779.3	2709.7	3065.6	3844.9	20.3				
Total	1790.93	1704.49	0.952	10013.9	41149.2	42853.6	52867.6	18.9		86	-0.8	94

Total BMD CV 1.0%, ACF = 1.020, BCF = 0.995

Results History:

Scan Date	Age	BMD	T - Score	BMD Change vs Baseline	BMD Change vs Previous
01.02.2010	15	0.952		-0.1%	0.9%
23.03.2009	14	0.943		-1.0%	-0.2%
18.02.2008	13	0.945		-0.8%	-0.8%
15.01.2007	12	0.952			

Fig. 2. Follow-up total body pediatric DXA in child with treatment influencing bone density.

approximation. When done, the normal reference values show a trend to be comparable with QCT: stable bone density before puberty and a sharp increase during puberty.[7]

Other problems when interpreting pediatric DXA studies exist. A significant change in (extraosseous) body composition can cause erroneous data. Furthermore, vast changes in bone marrow composition can influence the data.[2] Last but not least, there is considerable variation between DXA machines and between different versions of analysis software.[8]

TO DO OR NOT TO DO?

After the previous introduction to the pitfalls, readers would probably wonder if it makes any sense to do bone densitometry in children. Ideally true bone density is needed to have a reliable estimate of the pediatric bone status. QCT of the vertebral bodies in the lumbar spine is the preferred method. It provides a bone density measurement in g/cm^3 and can separate cortical from trabecular bone. Because the vertebral trabecular network has a high metabolic activity, changes in bone density can be detected early (high sensitivity to change) and the reproducibility of the measurement using the correct protocol and the correct analysis algorithm is approximately 1% to 2% coefficient of variation, comparable with DXA. It seems to be the ideal method; so, why is it not used more often? One of the reasons is the radiation burden. It is estimated that the effective dose equivalent when using a low-dose technique is approximately 30 to 300 µSv for QCT whereas that for DXA is approximately 3 µSv. Because children are more susceptible to radiation-induced cancer, this is a concern because these children are usually already medically challenged and have different types of imaging studies for their underlying diseases.[5,9] Furthermore, it is easier to make a DXA scan than a QCT scan. CT scanners are used for a variety of reasons, indications, and anatomic areas. In busy CT machines, QCT is not more then a special option or add-on possibility, whereas DXA-scanners are dedicated to bone densitometry. Furthermore, reimbursement issues exist in certain countries. Last but not least, CT scanners are big and noisy and potentially frightening for a child.

If not QCT, what next? Are there other options?

Several investigators have used radiogrammetry. In radiogrammetry, the bone dimensions of finger bones are measured on digital radiographs of the hand. Automated algorithms are used to provide the measurements. In the recent literature, a new pediatric bone index is proposed based on the Exton-Smith index. From the dimensional measurements (bone width and cortical thickness), the cortical area is derived and a correction for the length of the bone is calculated. Because hand radiographs are often made in (diseased) children to assess skeletal age, this is an elegant method because it does not require any additional investigation, just an automated calculation of the bone index. Normal values have been presented for this method.[10] Its clinical value, however, has still to be established.

QUS has been used to investigate bone mineral status. Its lack of radiation dose is attractive in pediatric bone densitometry. In the literature, however, many different QUS machines (with underlying differences in technology and methodology) assessing different skeletal sites (hand, tibia, and heel) with different results on reproducibility, sensitivity to change, and clinical use are presented. None of these techniques currently is completely clinically validated.[11]

Another option could be peripheral QCT (pQCT). Special dedicated pQCT machines have been developed to measure bone density in the forearm. Although initially used in the adult population, there are several published studies on its use in the pediatric population. One of the problems is reliable follow-up forearm measurements because the measurements are done in the growing and, thus, changing skeleton.[12] Normal values have been presented in the recent literature.[13] The measurements are low dose and true volumetric. Its ultimate value still has to be established.

So, there are different methods with different advantages and disadvantages in terms of reproducibility, accuracy, sensitivity to change, ease of use, radiation burden, costs of operation, and clinical validation. The reality is that we currently are more or less stuck with DXA. DXA became a huge commercial success for measuring bone "density" in adults, especially in the field of osteoporosis. It became, therefore, the gold standard in bone densitometry studies, was widely distributed, and sequentially was used in the pediatric population. It is far from ideal but has been used worldwide and many pediatric studies have been published in the field of bone densitometry[5,12] and in the field of body composition studies.[14]

EPILOGUE

If readers are interested in more details about the different techniques, they are referred to review articles that have been published recently.[5,12] The recommendations from the International Society for Clinical Densitometry (ISCD) providing guidelines for assessment, interpretation, and reporting should be noted.[3] The position statement of the ISCD should be used as a guideline and should be standard knowledge for referring and interpreting physicians using bone densitometry in children.

REFERENCES

1. Watts NB. Fundamentals and pitfalls of bone densitometry using dual-energy X-ray absorptiometry (DXA). Osteoporos Int 2004;15:847–54.
2. Bolotin HH. DXA in vivo BMD methodology. An erroneous and misleading research and clinical gauge of bone mineral status, bone fragility, and bone remodelling. Bone 2007;41:138–54.

3. Lewiecki EM, Gordon CM, Baim S, et al. International society for clinical densitometry 2007 adult and pediatric official positions. Bone 2008;43:1115–21.

4. Binkovitz LA, Henwood MJ, Sparke P. Pediatric DXA: technique, interpretation and clinical applications. Pediatr Radiol 2008;38:S227–39.

5. Van Rijn RR, Van Kuijk C. Of small bones and big mistakes; bone densitometry in children revisited. Eur J Radiol 2009;71:432–9.

6. Gilsanz V, Perez FJ, Campbell PP, et al. Quantitative CT reference values for vertebral trabecular bone density in children and young adults. Radiology 2009;250:222–7.

7. Van der Sluis IM, de Ridder MA, Boot AM, et al. Reference data for bone density and body composition measured with dual energy x-ray absorptiometry in white children and young adults. Arch Dis Child 2002;87:341–7.

8. Simpson DE, Dontu VS, Stephens SE, et al. Large variations occur in bone density measurements of children when using different software. Nucl Med Commun 2005;26:483–7.

9. Njeh CF, Fuerst T, Hans D, et al. Radiation exposure in bone mineral density assessment. Appl Radiat Isot 1999;50:215–36.

10. Thodberg HH, Van Rijn RR, Tanaka T, et al. A paediatric bone index derived by automated radiogrammetry. Osteoporos Int 2009. [Epub ahead of print].

11. Baroncelli GI. Quantitative ultrasound methods to assess bone mineral status in children; Technical considerations, performance, and clinical application. Pediatr Res 2008;63:220–8.

12. Binkley TL, Berry R, Specker BL. Methods for measurement of pediatric bone. Rev Endocr Metab Disord 2008;9:95–106.

13. Ashby RL, Ward KA, Roberts SA, et al. A reference database for the Stratec XCT-200 peripheral quantitative computed tomography 9pQCT scanner in healthy children and young adults aged 6–19 years. Osteoporos Int 2009;20:1337–46.

14. Helba M, Binkovitz LA. Pediatric body composition analysis with dual-energy X-ray absortiometry. Pediatr Radiol 2009;39:647–56.

Quality Assurance and Dosimetry in Bone Densitometry

John Damilakis, PhD[a,b,*], Giuseppe Guglielmi, MD[c,d]

KEYWORDS

- Quality assurance • Quality control • Densitometry
- Skeletal status • Radiation dose

Several noninvasive methods have been developed for the assessment of skeletal status. Dual-energy x-ray absorptiometry (DXA) is currently the most widely used method for the measurement of areal bone mineral density (BMD_a) (g/cm^2). Quantitative CT (QCT) is capable of separately assessing the cortical and trabecular bone providing volumetric bone mineral density (BMD) (mg/cm^3). Current research has focused on methods that permit assessment of bone morphology and evaluation of the trabecular bone network properties. Micro-CT and high-resolution (HR) CT techniques developed for assessment of bone status are promising in this respect. Moreover, quantitative ultrasound (QUS) techniques are based on waves influenced by bone structure in addition to bone density.

The practice of bone densitometry involves the integration of several processes, all of which must be controlled. Thus, proper use of the equipment requires a well-trained staff and a program for regular maintenance and quality control (QC). QC consists of a series of standardized periodic tests developed to maintain diagnostic quality. QC of bone densitometers is needed to ensure that these complex systems consistently meet specifications. Radiation exposure levels associated with x-ray methods used for bone status evaluation must also be measured to ensure that the examination is performed with the lowest possible dose to patients consistent with clinical imaging

requirements. Although QC of the equipment used for the assessment of skeletal status is an important component of the management system in a bone densitometry unit, a comprehensive quality assurance (QA) system is required to guarantee that all work is adequately planned and correctly performed. QA in bone densitometry is all those organized actions necessary to (1) maintain adequate equipment performance with minimum exposure and (2) assure that adequate diagnostic information is provided at the lowest possible cost. A QA program should include guidelines, acceptance tests, periodic QC tests, preventive maintenance procedures, education, and training. This review focuses on the QC tests and QA in bone densitometry and discusses issues related to radiation doses from the x-ray methods used for the assessment of bone status.

SPECIFICATIONS OF EQUIPMENT

The technical specifications of new bone densitometry equipment should reflect a facility's clinical requirements. The user should define the equipment, material, and services to be provided by the supplier as well as the required schedule of supply. All clinical applications of the system intended for purchase should be described. For each application, the maximum acceptable in vitro precision should be specified. DXA and QCT should be

a Department of Medical Physics, Faculty of Medicine, University of Crete, PO Box 2208, 71003 Iraklion, Crete, Greece
b Department of Medical Physics, University Hospital of Iraklion, PO Box 2208, 71003 Iraklion, Crete, Greece
c Department of Radiology, University of Foggia, Viale L. Pinto, 71100 Foggia, Italy
d Scientific Institute 'Casa Sollievo della Sofferenza' Hospital, San Giovanni Rotondo 71013, Italy
* Corresponding author. Department of Medical Physics, Faculty of Medicine, University of Crete, PO Box 2208, 71003 Iraklion, Crete, Greece.
E-mail address: damilaki@med.uoc.gr

Radiol Clin N Am 48 (2010) 629–640
doi:10.1016/j.rcl.2010.02.011
0033-8389/10/$ – see front matter © 2010 Elsevier Inc. All rights reserved.

equipped with a reference database to compare patients' measured BMD with that of age- and sex-matched normal subjects and with normal young adults. The printout should include (1) an image of the anatomic area being scanned, (2) a graph that shows patient BMD compared with age- and sex- matched control data, and (3) a table summarizing BMD values for individual regions of interest and Z-score and T-score values. QCT packages should include not only the application-specific software package but also a dedicated calibration phantom scanned simultaneously with the patient to convert the CT numbers into bone equivalent values. All bone densitometry systems should be provided with their own QC phantoms.

INSTALLATION

The installation of a bone densitometer should be followed by procedures developed to insure that the equipment (1) operates properly, (2) meets all current radiation protection requirements, and (3) meets the manufacturer specifications as described in the purchase contract. It is the responsibility of the employer and the installer to make certain that equipment tests and staff training are carried out on new bone densitometry equipment. Machine calibration, accuracy and precision evaluation, and electrical safety checks should be provided by the supplier of the bone densitometry equipment. Radiation safety checks and measurements should be performed in cooperation with the department of medical physics. Clinical applications training should be provided by the supplier of the equipment.

PERIODIC QC TESTS

Most methods developed for noninvasive assessment of bone status provide quantitative information to clinicians and patients as an aid to diagnosis of osteoporosis. The performance of a bone densitometer in terms of accuracy and precision determines its ability to (1) differentiate between healthy and osteoporotic individuals, (2) assess fracture risk, (3) monitor age-related bone density loss, and (4) evaluate the efficacy of therapeutic interventions.

ACCURACY AND PRECISION

Accuracy describes how close the measured BMD value comes to the true value and is expressed in terms of accuracy error. Accuracy error (%) is calculated as follows:

$$\%Accuracy = \frac{(True\ BMD - Measured\ BMD)}{True\ BMD} \cdot 100$$

(1)

The accuracy of a bone densitometry technique determines its ability to differentiate between healthy and diseased individuals or to estimate fracture risk. It is an important characteristic when comparing measurements of the same quantity using 2 different techniques.

To determine the accuracy of a DXA densitometer, a cadaveric bone is scanned to measure the bone mineral content (BMC). The bone is then defatted and ashed. The mass of the ash is considered the real value of bone mineral. The system is calibrated so that the measured BMC results are as similar as possible to the true BMC. The accuracy error of DXA bone densitometers is better than 10%.[1] The accuracy study (described previously) is technically difficult and is not performed when a DXA system is installed. In QA, a phantom containing tissue-mimicking materials of known BMC is scanned daily. Results are entered into the QC database to enable compensation of calibration changes or small drifts. Fig. 1 shows phantoms used for calibration and daily QC scans on bone DXA systems.

DXA units developed by different manufacturers provide different BMD results when used to measure the same skeletal site of a patient. Differences have been found up to 15%.[2,3] This may be attributed to differences in DXA system geometry and design and differences in calibration and image processing software. For this reason, cross-calibration techniques have been developed to reduce differences between DXA systems made by different manufacturers. The term, standardized BMD (sBMD), has been introduced to distinguish interchangeable BMD from manufacturer-specific BMD. The equations used to convert manufacturer-specific BMD to sBMD have been published in the literature.[4,5] Although sBMD values can reduce the differences between equipment made by different manufacturers to less than

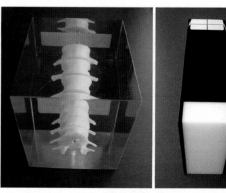

Fig. 1. Calibration phantoms used for daily QC on Hologic (*left*) and GE Lunar (*right*) DXA bone densitometers.

6%, use of different DXA systems to longitudinally monitor the bone status of an individual is not recommended.

QCT examinations are performed using an application-specific software package and a dedicated calibration phantom scanned simultaneously with the patient to convert the CT numbers into bone mineral units. Calibration phantoms contain various concentrations of bone equivalent solid materials. It is emphasized that results from different phantoms are not interchangeable. Phantoms have been developed for cross-calibration and QC, such as the European Spine Phantom.[6] QC phantoms in combination with software packages monitor CT scanners for considerable changes and compensate for uniformity errors and CT scanner fluctuations. The accuracy of QCT bone densitometry is affected by the presence of marrow fat, beam hardening effects, and partial volume averaging. Accuracy errors range between 5% and 15%.[7]

Precision measures the reproducibility of a bone densitometry technique. The precision of a bone densitometry method determines its ability to monitor bone loss and to measure the response to therapy. Precision can be expressed as the SD or in terms of the coefficient of variation (%CV). The SD of BMD measurements in a phantom or in a patient p can be determined as

$$SD_p = \sqrt{\frac{\sum_{i=1}^{n_p}\left(x_{ip} - \overline{x_p}\right)}{n_p - 1}} \qquad (2)$$

where x_{ip} is the value of the ith BMD measurement, $\overline{x_p}$ is the mean BMD, and n_p is the number of BMD measurements.

The %CV is given by

$$\%CV_p = \frac{SD_p}{x_p} \cdot 100 \qquad (3)$$

Precision is influenced by a wide range of parameters, such as fluctuations in the operating characteristics of the bone densitometer over time, skill and training of technical staff performing the scan, inconsistent selection of vertebral levels, site of measurement, and age and clinical status of patients.

At each DXA facility, a precision study should be performed. In vitro short-term precision estimation is possible by scanning manufacturer's QC phantom several times without repositioning. From these measurements, the SD or the %CV is estimated using Equation 1 or Equation 2, respectively. In everyday clinical practice, a phantom scan is performed and the results are entered into the QC software package of the DXA scanner. To verify that the BMD_a of the scanner is within normal limits, the QC plot should be used (Fig. 2). The procedure (described previously) is an essential part of the daily QC. In vivo short-term precision includes errors due to patient repositioning and movement and is determined on a group of volunteers. For a specific skeletal site, multiple BMD_a measurements are performed in several patients. To reduce volunteers' radiation burden, it is recommended to perform 2 BMD_a measurements each for 30 patients. For each individual, measurements should be performed on the same day or within a short period of time (ie. within 2 weeks) to exclude the possibility of a true change in BMD_a. To obtain independent measurements, the individual should be taken off the examination table and repositioned for each subsequent

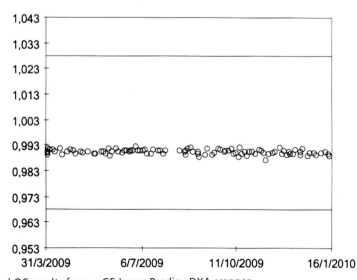

Fig. 2. Longitudinal QC results from a GE Lunar Prodigy DXA scanner.

measurement. The combined precision is given by the root mean square (RMS) SD:

$$SD_{RMS} = \sqrt{\frac{\sum_{p=1}^{q} SD_p^2}{q}} \qquad (4)$$

where q is the number of patients.

The RMS CV is defined as

$$CV_{RMS} = \sqrt{\frac{\sum_{p=1}^{q} CV_p^2}{q}} \qquad (5)$$

The precision error estimated by the manufacturer does not usually represent the error in the clinical setting. For this reason, every facility should determine precision values using in vivo reproducibility data. Participation of subjects is voluntary and each patient must sign an informed consent form prior to the precision study. Although the in vivo determination of precision involves additional radiation dose to a small number of volunteers, the exposure levels associated with bone densitometry are low. Pregnant individuals, children, and radiation workers must be excluded from precision measurements. Precision is dependent on population age and health status and is, therefore, expected to differ between young normal subjects, healthy postmenopausal women, and osteoporotic patients. The short-term in vivo precision of DXA measurements ranges between 1% and 3% at the spine and femur in subjects with normal BMD_a values.[8–10]

Precision errors associated with QCT results arise from parameters, such as staff training, scanner stability, patient positioning, and patient movement. Precision is higher for 3-D multidetector (MD) QCT than for single-slice 2-D QCT. In a recent study, Engelke and colleagues[11] determined interoperator precision errors for 3-D QCT of the spine in postmenopausal women using a variety of whole-body CT scanners. They have found that in vivo precision errors range between 1% and 1.5% for trabecular and 2.5% to 3% for cortical bone measurements.

Precision errors affect the use of bone densitometry when measuring change in BMD in longitudinal studies. It is important to determine whether or not a change in a patient is real or represents a precision error. %CV is used to determine the smallest change in BMD that is statistically significant (least significant change [LSC]) and the minimum time interval for follow-up measurements. A difference in BMD, which exceeds 2.8 times the value of %CV, is considered to be statistically significant at the 95% confidence level:

$$LSC = 2.8 \cdot (\%CV) \qquad (6)$$

As an example, it is assumed that the precision error for a spine DXA scan is 1.5%. In this case, a change in BMD_a of 4.2% or higher is needed for statistical significance. The time interval between 2 measurements in the same individual must be long enough to allow a change greater than LSC. The monitoring time interval (MTI) is given by

$$MTI = \frac{LSC}{\text{median relative response rate}} \qquad (7)$$

Equation 7 shows that MTI is dependent on the reproducibility and the expected rate of bone change. The rate of bone loss varies considerably between individuals. The typical annual bone loss observed in total body BMD after the first few years post menopause is 2% to 3%.[12] Under most circumstances, intervals of 18 to 24 months between scans are required to measure significant changes. Rapid loss of bone mass has been observed, however, in certain cases, for example, in patients who receive corticosteroids. In these cases, the interval between follow-up DXA scans can be much shorter.

Many QUS techniques have been developed for the calculation of broadband ultrasound attenuation (BUA) and speed of sound (SOS). Validated heel QUS systems predict low-energy fractures in postmenopausal women and men over the age of 65 independently of BMD.[13,14] The accuracy and precision of QUS measurements is affected by a wide range of parameters, including method of measurement, surrounding soft tissue composition, bone properties, coupling medium, and patient movement and positioning. To reduce positioning errors, QUS devices have been developed recently. Ultrasound images are used to (1) confirm appropriate positioning of the foot and (2) ensure that the same area of the calcaneus is assessed at repetitive measurements.[15] **Fig. 3** shows a QUS image of the calcaneus produced by the Achilles InSight (GE Lunar, Madison, Wisconsin). To ensure calibration stability and monitor performance, manufacturers of QUS devices provide test objects and phantoms with known acoustic properties (**Fig. 4**). These QA tools can be used to determine in vitro precision of QUS variables. In vivo precision studies of BUA and SOS can be performed with large patient samples and many measurements on each subject because QUS does not use ionizing radiation. The short-term in vivo precision of QUS variables (%CV) ranges from 2.0% to 3.5% for BUA and from 0.3% to 1.5% for SOS depending on the equipment and the skeletal site.[15–19] The %CV value of BUA is not comparable with that for

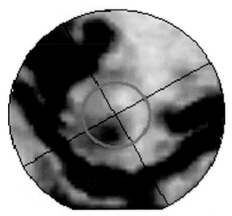

Fig. 3. An ultrasound image of the calcaneus showing the location of a circular region of measurement.

SOS or BMD. A limitation of CV is that precision errors expressed as %CV seem low when the SD value is low and the mean is high (Equation 3). Thus, the precision of a variable, such as SOS associated with high mean and relatively narrow range of values, seems much higher than that of BUA. The 2% to 3% precision of BUA measured at the heel is approximately 6 to 9 times larger than the average annual rate of bone loss in postmenopausal women. The precision error of SOS is 2 to 8 times larger than the annual bone loss rate. Therefore, CV is not appropriate for comparison of different methods. To adjust for differences in

responsiveness to skeletal changes, the standardized CV (SCV) has been defined as

$$SCV = \frac{SD_{RMS}}{Biological\ Range} \cdot 100\% \qquad (8)$$

Several definitions of biologic range have been given by different investigators. For example, Machado and colleagues[20] consider biologic range to be the difference between the mean values in young normal individuals and patients with established osteoporosis. For details on standardized precision, readers are referred to the pertinent literature.[10,21,22]

RADIATION DOSIMETRY
Quantities for Assessing Dose

There are many quantities currently in use for assessing dose from ionizing radiation. Absorbed dose is a measure of the energy per unit of mass deposited in the tissue and organs of the exposed body. The unit for absorbed dose is the gray (Gy). Several investigators have measured entrance surface dose (ESD) from bone densitometry techniques. ESD is the absorbed dose to the skin at the point where the x-ray beam enters the body. Although ESD is easily measured, it does not reflect the true radiogenic risk because the dose to radiosensitive organs differs considerably from skin dose. The International Commission on Radiological Protection (ICRP) has developed the concept of effective dose (ED) to allow estimation of risks from a partial body irradiation.[23] ED is the dose to the whole body that carries the same radiogenic risk as the partial body dose. The ED, expressed in sieverts (Sv), is defined as

$$ED = \sum_{T} w_T D_T \qquad (9)$$

where w_T is a tissue-specific weighting factor for each organ or tissue exposed to radiation and D_T is the absorbed dose to organ/tissue T. ED is best used to compare risks from different sources of ionizing radiation (eg, from DXA and QCT or DXA and natural background radiation). The worldwide average annual level of naturally occurring background radiation is 2.4 mSv.

The main types of dosimetric quantities used in CT are (1) CT dose index (CTDI) and (2) dose-length product (DLP). The CTDI, expressed in mGy, represents the average absorbed dose, along the Z axis, from a series of contiguous x-ray exposures:

$$CTDI = \frac{1}{NT} \cdot \int_{-\infty}^{+\infty} D(z)\ dz \qquad (10)$$

where $D(z)$ is the radiation dose profile along the Z axis and NT is the product of the number of

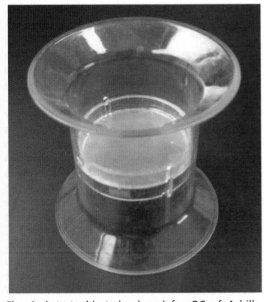

Fig. 4. A test object developed for QC of Achilles InSight QUS device.

independent data channels, N, and the width, along the Z direction at isocenter, imaged by 1 detector channel T (ie, the beam collimation at the isocenter) (eg, 16 × 1.5 mm or 16 × 0.75 mm). Standard CTDI measurements are performed at the periphery $(CTDI_P)$ and at the center $(CTDI_C)$ of cylindrical acrylic phantoms using a 100-mm long, 3-cm^3 active volume pencil ionization chamber. From these measurements, a weighted CTDI $(CTDI_W)$ representing the average dose to a single slice can be derived using the formula

$$CTDI_w = \frac{1}{3} \cdot CTDI_C + \frac{2}{3} \cdot CTDI_P \qquad (11)$$

To take into account the effect of pitch on dose, the use of CTDI volume $(CTDI_V)$ (mGy) has been introduced for scans performed in the spiral mode.

$$CTDI_V = \frac{1}{pitch} \cdot CTDI_w \qquad (12)$$

$CTDI_V$ does not indicate the total energy delivered by a scan protocol because it is not dependent on the scan length. The DLP is a measure of the radiation dose delivered to a patient during a CT scan:

$$DLP = CTDI_V \cdot (scan\ length) \qquad (13)$$

An approximate estimate of ED can be calculated using the formula,

$$ED = DLP \cdot k \qquad (14)$$

where k is body region–specific normalized ED factors $(mSv \cdot mGy^{-1} \cdot cm^{-1})$ published in the literature.[24,25]

The $CTDI_V$ and the DLP are dose quantities displayed in the operator's console of most CT scanners.

Patient Exposure

Patient-effective and organ radiation doses from DXA have been reported in the literature.[26–37] Studies confirm that ED per site scanned is negligible for the first-generation pencil beam scanners (ie, it is well below the ED from the natural background radiation of 7 μSv per day). Radiation doses are higher for the fan beam scanners. A recent study showed that the ED delivered to an adult patient from a spine and hip scan performed on Hologic fan beam DXA scanners (Hologic, Waltham, Massachusetts) ranges from approximately 10 to approximately 20 μSv.[35] Radiation doses to patients undergoing DXA examinations are smaller compared with most diagnostic x-ray examinations. Thus, the ED from a DXA examination is lower than that from x-ray mammography.

There are several parameters that affect the dose to individuals from a DXA examination, such as scanning technique, x-ray tube filtration, efficiency of detection systems, number of scans, exposure parameters, scan speed, scan size, and patient body size. Thus, patient dose from examinations may differ considerably between sites and DXA systems of different manufacturers.

It is important that operators fully appreciate that reducing scan size can decrease radiation dose considerably. The clinical applications of DXA in children and adolescents are exceedingly broad. The use of an adult scan mode leads to unnecessary overexposure of pediatric patients. In children, a lumbar spine or total body scan usually provides enough information pertaining to the bone status. Additional skeletal sites should be scanned only when the radiation dose is justified by the potential clinical benefit to a young individual.

DXA examinations are carried out in pregnant patients unintentionally or because of clinical necessity. Studies confirm that conceptus radiation dose from DXA performed on the mother is low and the risk of abnormality is considered negligible when compared with other risks of pregnancy.[38] Nevertheless, conservative management of pregnant patients is always desirable to keep conceptus radiogenic risks to a minimum. For pregnant patients, DXA examinations should be performed only when BMD_a results are expected to provide important information for clinical decision making. Accidental conceptus irradiation occasionally occurs during diagnostic x-ray examinations performed on pregnant individuals. To avoid inadvertent exposure, the presence of pregnancy should be always evaluated before an x-ray bone densitometry examination.

DXA is frequently used for follow-up studies. Serial spine or hip scans provide longitudinal measurements indicative of osteoporosis progression. Repeated exposure of the same anatomic site increases the radiation burden, however. Referring physicians and radiologists should be aware of the dose consequences of repetitive studies, especially for bone densitometry examinations performed on pediatric patients. Serial DXA scans should be performed only when the expected benefits clearly outweigh the radiogenic risks.

QCT provides a method of separately assessing cortical and trabecular BMD, expressed in mg/cm^3, using general-purpose whole-body CT scanners. A typical single-slice 2-D spine QCT protocol consists of a scout image and 3 slices in the midplane of each of 3 or 4 adjacent vertebrae (T12, L1, L2, and L3). An examination acquired at 80 kVp tube potential and 125 mAs tube load entails a radiation dose to a patient from 60 to approximately 300 µSv, depending on protocol parameters and CT scanner model.[29,32] Recently, 3-D QCT protocols have been developed based on MDCT imaging. MDCT technology with increased resolution has resulted in precise measurements of BMD and bone geometry. MDQCT examinations are associated with high patient doses, however. Carryingout spine or hip 3-D QCT using MD technology incurs a higher radiation dose (1.5 mSv and 2.9 mSv for the spine and the hip scans, respectively) than 2-D QCT.[39,40] QCT is also used for measurements of the appendicular skeleton. Typical parameter settings for acquiring a distal forearm scan are 120 kV, 100 mAs, and pitch 1. Patient ED associated with this scan is negligible (ie, lower than 10 µSv).[41]

Several studies have shown that bone architecture provides information additional to BMD in assessing bone status.[42,43] Clinical whole-body MDCT scanners achieve isotropic spatial resolution in the submillimeter range. Although depiction of individual trabeculae using MDCT is not possible, studies suggest that analysis of MDCT HR image data provides important information about the trabecular bone network.[44,45] Patient doses associated with HR CT are of the order of 3 mSv.[46,47]

Dose reduction from MDCT is possible using reconstruction algorithms that can decrease image noise, providing better image quality at lower radiation burden. Also, proper selection of protocol settings, including the selection of a minimal scan length, results in a considerable reduction of dose. The use of adaptive section collimation, available in new-generation MDCT scanners, allows reduction of exposure due to z overscanning associated with helical scanning.[48,49] An increased contribution to patient dose may be expected due to reduced geometric efficiency of ultrathin (ie, 1.2 and 2 mm) beam collimations. These x-ray beams should be avoided unless ultrathin slice reconstruction is of absolute clinical necessity.[50]

Further research is needed for dose optimization of MDCT bone densitometry methods. Optimizing the x-ray beam spectrum or activating the automatic exposure control (AEC) system of the CT scanner also decreases the radiation dose. Studies are needed to determine the kVp at which a selected signal-to-noise ratio can be reached with the lowest radiation dose. This is very important for pediatric examinations. Also, further experience with new AEC devices is needed.[51] Unfortunately, research experience on patient doses from newly developed techniques, such as 3-D M DQCT and HR MDCT,

is limited. The use of CTDI to ED conversion coefficients may provide an estimate of patient ED from examinations performed on modern MDCT scanners.[52–54] More accurate calculation of patient ED is possible using patient-specific Monte Carlo software packages for CT dosimetry.[55]

Peripheral QCT (pQCT) scanners are dedicated small pQCT scanners capable of assessing bone architecture and BMD at appendicular bones. Using a recently developed HR pQCT scanner, in vivo images have been obtained with an isotropic spatial resolution of 82 µm.[56] The ED from pQCT examinations is on the order on few µSv.[39,41,56]

Occupational Exposure and Shielding

It is the recommendation of the ICRP that the annual ED of occupationally exposed workers should be limited to 20 mSv per year.[23] Larkin and colleagues[36] have found that the annual scatter dose at 1 m from fan beam DXA scanners ranges from 0.5 to 1.5 mSv. Although the annual dose limit is much higher than the expected annual occupational doses from DXA, the use of mobile shielding for staff radiation protection is sometimes necessary to minimize operator ED.

In planning a bone densitometry facility, the main priority is to ensure that persons in the vicinity of the facility are not exposed to dose levels that exceed the current limits for members of the public (ie, 1 mSv/y). Shielding assessment should be done prior to installation of a fan DXA system. The need for shielding mainly depends on patient workload, the size of the installation room, and the type of DXA scanner. In most cases, lead protection in the walls adjacent to DXA is not required.

Dose Measurements

A diagnostic QA program involves periodic checks of the components in a bone densitometry system. **Table 1** shows the minimum acceptable radiation and image quality measurements for a properly managed DXA service.[36,57–59] In addition to dose measurements, a periodic evaluation of the condition of the DXA facility (ie, control of the mechanical and electrical integrity and safety) is needed. The function of features, such as the equipment emergency stop and radiation warning lights, should be checked. The availability and adequacy of patient support devices should also be checked. All test results should be recorded and periodic reviews of the results should be carried out to identify needed changes.

Table 1
Routine radiation and image quality measurements in DXA

Parameter	Equipment	Method	Frequency
Radiation output repeatability	Radiation dosimeter with 180-cm^3 ionization chamber	• Select the AP spine scan protocol • Measure air kerma with a calibrated chamber centered in a 15 × 15-cm^2 field • Perform 5 measurements and calculate precision (%CV). The variation should be no more than 5%	Twice a year or after maintenance
Half value layer	1. Radiation dosimeter with 6-cm^3 ionization chamber 2. Set of aluminum filters	• Measure the output with no attenuator in the beam • Repeat measurements with increasing amounts of attenuator (Al filters) • Plot relative exposure (%) as a function of aluminum thickness	Annually or after maintenance
Dose area product (DAP)	1. Radiation dosimeter with 180-cm^3 ionization chamber 2. A 20-cm thick block of tissue equivalent material	• Measure entrance dose and calculate DAP using the formula DAP = Entrance Dose × Area, where Area is the scan area for each scan mode • Calculate DAP for all scan modes	Annually or after maintenance
Radiation field size	Film cassette or CR plate	• Place the cassette on the examination table surface • Select the AP spine protocol and perform scan • Measure exposed area on film. Compare measurement with nominal value. The difference should not be greater than 1 cm. • Perform measurements for scan modes with different field sizes	Annually or after maintenance

Parameter	Equipment	Procedure	Frequency
Fan angle	Two film cassettes or CR plates	• Place cassette A on the examination table surface and cassette B at 40 cm above cassette A • Perform scan. Measure image width on both films. The fan angle φ is given by $\tan\varphi = $ (image width difference)/40	Annually or after maintenance
Spatial resolution	1. Resolution test pattern 2. A 20-cm thick block of tissue equivalent material	• Place the test pattern on the examination table surface. Place tissue equivalent material over the test pattern. Perform scan. • A line pair grating gives a direct reading of spatial resolution	Annually or after maintenance
Room safety	1. Radiation dosimeter with a large ionization chamber (eg, 1800 cm^3) 2. A 20-cm thick block of tissue equivalent material	• Place tissue equivalent material on the examination table surface. Perform scan • Measure exposure at several locations around the table and behind control panel • Perform measurements for different scan modes • Compare with values specified by the manufacturer	Continuous program

Abbreviations: AP, anterior-posterior; Al, aluminum; CR, computed radiography.

QUALIFICATIONS OF PERSONNEL—EDUCATION AND TRAINING

A bone densitometry unit should have a team of health professionals who have undergone training in osteoporosis. Radiologists should be fully experienced in (1) performance of all radiologic techniques developed for the diagnosis of osteoporosis and (2) bone densitometry diagnostic activity. They should also have knowledge of the treatment options for osteoporosis. Bone densitometry technologists should have sufficient knowledge and experience of the bone densitometry equipment. Duties of the technologists include patient scanning and scan analysis. They should be able to carry out QC procedures and have an understanding of radiation doses in bone densitometry and how to keep them as low as possible. The American Society of Radiologic Technologists recently released the *Bone Densitometry Curriculum* to provide guidelines on the standards for the training of technologists dealing with bone densitometry.[60] Medical physicists should have a profound knowledge of dosimetry techniques in bone densitometry. They should have substantial training in all aspects of the operation and QA of bone densitometry units and associated equipment. The American College of Radiology has published qualifications and responsibilities of personnel working in DXA and QCT facilities.[61] The International Society for Clinical Densitometry provides comprehensive educational courses in bone densitometry and offers certification for radiologists, clinicians, scientists, and radiographers. The periodic renewal of certification is an important step of continuing education because it provides evidence that health professionals involved in bone densitometry continue to expand and maintain knowledge in their certification specialty.

SUMMARY

The importance of QA in bone densitometry facilities has been widely recognized. Bone densitometry service should be characterized by a good QC program and standardization of practice. The primary aim is to ensure reproducible and consistent results at low radiation burden to patients. The establishment of a program of staff continuing education and training is important to maintain or improve the quality of the work.

REFERENCES

1. Kanis JA, Melton LJ III, Christiansen C, et al. The diagnosis of osteoporosis. J Bone Miner Res 1994; 9:1137–41.

2. Gundry CR, Miller CW, Ramos E, et al. Dual-energy radiographic absorptiometry of the lumbar spine: clinical experience with two different systems. Radiology 1990;174:539–41.

3. Pocock NA, Sambrook PN, Nguyen T, et al. Assessment of spinal and femoral bone density by dual X-ray absorptiometry: comparison of Lunar and Hologic instruments. J Bone Miner Res 1992;7:1081–4.

4. Steiger P. Standardization of measurements for assessing BMD by DXA. [letter to the editor]. Calcif Tissue Int 1995;57:469.

5. Hanson J. Standardization of femur BMD. [letter to the editor]. J Bone Miner Res 1997;12:1316–7.

6. Kalender WA, Felsenberg D, Genant HK, et al. The European Spine Phantom—a tool for standardization and quality control in spinal bone mineral measurements by DXA and QCT. Eur J Radiol 1995;20:83–92.

7. Adams JE. Quantitative computed tomography. Eur J Radiol 2009;71:415–24.

8. Adams JE. Dual-energy X-ray absorptiometry. Berlin, Heidelberg. In: Grampp S, editor. Radiology of osteoporosis. 2nd revised edition. New York: Springer; 2008. p. 105–24.

9. Blake G, Fogelman I. The clinical role of dual energy X-ray absorptiometry. Eur J Radiol 2009; 71:406–14.

10. Blake GM, Wahner H, Fogelman I. The evaluation of osteoporosis: dual energy X-ray absorptiometry and ultrasound in clinical practice. London: Dunitz; 1999. 45–71, 147–72.

11. Engelke K, Mastmeyer A, Bousson V, et al. Reanalysis precision of 3D quantitative computed tomography (QCT) of the spine. Bone 2009;44:566–72.

12. Gallagher JC, Goldgar D, Moy A. Total bone calcium in normal women: effect of age and menopause status. J Bone Miner Res 1987;2:491–5.

13. Lewiecki E, Gordon C, Baim S, et al. International Society for Clinical Densitometry 2007 adult and pediatric official positions. Bone 2008;43:1115–21.

14. Damilakis J, Maris T, Karantanas A. An update on the assessment of osteoporosis using radiologic techniques. Eur Radiol 2007;17:1591–602.

15. Damilakis J, Papadokostakis G, Perisinakis K, et al. Hip fracture discrimination by the Achilles insight QUS imaging device. Eur J Radiol 2007; 63:59–62.

16. Guglielmi G, de Terlizzi F. Quantitative ultrasound in the assessment of osteoporosis. Eur J Radiol 2009; 71:425–31.

17. Barkmann R, Laugier P, Moser U, et al. In vivo measurements of ultrasound transmission through the human proximal femur. Ultrasound Med Biol 2008;34:1186–90.

18. Damilakis J, Papadokostakis G, Vrahoriti H, et al. Ultrasound velocity through the cortex of phalanges, radius, and tibia in normal and osteoporotic postmenopausal

women using a new multisite quantitative ultrasound device. Invest Radiol 2003;38:207–11.

19. Guglielmi G, Adams J, Link TM. Quantitative ultrasound in the assessment of skeletal status. Eur Radiol 2009;19:1837–48.

20. Machado A, Hannon R, Henry Y, et al. Standardized coefficient of variation for dual X-ray absorptiometry (DXA), quantitative ultrasound (QUS) and markers of boné turnover [abstract]. J Bone Miner Res 1997; 12(Suppl 1):S258.

21. Lu Y, Gluer CC. Statistical tools in quantitative ultrasound applications. In: Njeh C, Hans D, Fuerst T, et al, editors. Quantitative ultrasound. Assessment of osteoporosis and bone status. London: Dunitz; 1999. p. 77–100.

22. Koo WW, Walters J, Bush AJ, et al. Technical considerations of dual-energy X-ray absorptiometry-based bone mineral measurements for pediatric studies. J Bone Miner Res 1995;10:1998–2004.

23. The 2007 recommendations of the International Commission on Radiological Protection. ICRP publication 103. Ann ICRP 2007;37:1–332.

24. Shrimpton PC, Hillier MC, Lewis MA, et al. National survey of doses in the UK: 2003. Br J Radiol 2006; 79:968–80.

25. Valentin J, International Commission on Radiation Protection. Managing patient dose in multi-detector computed tomography (MDCT). ICRP publication 102. Ann ICRP 2007;37:1–79.

26. Bezakova E, Collins PJ, Beddoe AH. Absorbed dose measurements in dual energy X-ray absorptiometry (DXA). Br J Radiol 1997;70:172–9.

27. Lewis MK, Blake GM, Fogelman I. Patient dose in dual X-ray absorptiometry. Osteoporos Int 1994;4: 11–5.

28. Faulkner RA, Bailey DA, Drinkwater DT, et al. Regional and total body bone mineral content, bone mineral density and total body tissue composition in children 8–16 years of age. Calcif Tissue Int 1993;53:7–12.

29. Huda W, Morin RL. Patient doses in bone mineral densitometry. Br J Radiol 1996;69:422–5.

30. Cawte SA, Pearson D, Green DJ, et al. Cross-calibration, precision and patient dose measurements in preparation for clinical trials using dual energy X-ray absorptiometry of the lumbar spine. Br J Radiol 1999;72:354–62.

31. Njeh CF, Samat SB, Nightingale A, et al. Radiation dose and in vitro precision in bone mineral density measurement using dual X-ray absorptiometry. Br J Radiol 1997;70:719–27.

32. Kalender WA. Effective dose values in bone mineral measurements by photon absorptiometry and computed tomography. Osteoporos Int 1992;2:82–7.

33. Pye DW, Hannan WJ, Hesp R. Effect dose equivalent in dual X-ray absorptiometry [letter]. Br J Radiol 1990;63:746.

34. Steel SA, Baker AJ, Saunderson JR. An assessment of the radiation dose to patients and staff from a Lunar Expert-XL fan beam densitometer. Physiol Meas 1998;19:17–26.

35. Blake G, Naeem M, Boutros M. Comparison of effective dose to children and adults from dual X-ray absorptiometry examinations. Bone 2006; 38:935–42.

36. Larkin A, Sheahan N, O'Connor U, et al. QA/Acceptance testing of DEXA X-ray systems used in bone mineral densitometry. Radiat Prot Dosimetry 2008; 129:279–83.

37. Thomas SR, Kalkwarf HJ, Buckley DD, et al. Effective dose of dual-energy X-ray absorptiometry scans in children as a function of age. J Clin Densitom 2005;8:415–22.

38. Damilakis J, Perisinakis K, Vrahoriti H, et al. Embryo/fetus radiation dose and risk from dual X-ray absorptiometry examinations. Osteoporos Int 2002;13:716–22.

39. Engelke K, Adams JE, Armbrecht G, et al. Clinical use of quantitative computed tomography and peripheral quantitative computed tomography in the management of osteoporosis in adults: the 2007 ISCD Official Positions. J Clin Densitom 2008; 11:123–62.

40. Khoo BC, Brown K, Cann C, et al. Comparison of QCT-derived and DXA-derived areal bone mineral density and T scores. Osteoporos Int 2009;20: 1539–45.

41. Engelke C, Libanati C, Liu Y, et al. Quantitative computed tomography (QCT) of the forearm using general purpose spiral whole-body CT scanners: accuracy, precision and comparison with dual-energy X-ray absorptiometry (DXA). Bone 2009;45: 110–8.

42. Link TM, Vieth V, Matheis J, et al. Bone structure of the distal radius and the calcaneus vs BMD of the spine and proximal femur in the prediction of osteoporotic spine fractures. Eur Radiol 2002;12: 401–8.

43. Stauber M, Rapillard L, van Lenthe GH, et al. Importance of individual rods and plates in the assessment of bone quality and their contribution to bone stiffness. J Bone Miner Res 2006;21:586–95.

44. Issever A, Link T, Kentenich M, et al. Assessment of trabecular bone structure using MDCT: comparison of 64- and 320-slice CT using HR-pQCT as the reference standard. Eur Radiol 2010;20:458–68.

45. Krebs A, Graeff C, Frieling I, et al. High resolution computed tomography of the vertebrae yields accurate information on trabecular distances if processed by 3D fuzzy segmentation approaches. Bone 2009;44:145–52.

46. Ito M, Ikeda K, Nishiguchi M, et al. Multidetector row CT imaging of vertebral microstructure for evaluation of fracture risk. J Bone Miner Res 2005;20:1828–36.

47. Graeff C, Timm W, Nickelsen TN, et al. Monitoring teriparatide-associated changes in vertebral microstructure by high-resolution CT in vivo: results from the EUROFORS study. J Bone Miner Res 2007;22: 1426–33.

48. Tzedakis A, Damilakis J, Perisinakis K, et al. The effect of z overscanning on patient effective dose from multidetector helical computed tomography examinations. Med Phys 2005;32:1621–9.

49. Deak PD, Langner O, Lell M, et al. Effects of adaptive section collimation on patient radiation dose in multisection spiral CT. Radiology 2009; 252:140–7.

50. Perisinakis K, Papadakis A, Damilakis J. The effect of X-ray beam quality and geometry on radiation utilization efficiency in multidetector CT imaging. Med Phys 2009;36:1258–66.

51. Papadakis AE, Perisinakis K, Damilakis J. Automatic exposure control in pediatric and adult multidetector CT examinations: a phantom study on dose reduction and image quality. Med Phys 2008;35:4567–76.

52. Perisinakis K, Tzedakis A, Damilakis J. On the use of Monte Carlo-derived dosimetric data in the estimation of patient dose from CT examinations. Med Phys 2008;35:2018–28.

53. Gregory K, Bibbo G, Pattison J. On the uncertainties in effective dose estimates of adult CT head scans. Med Phys 2008;35:3501–10.

54. Theocharopoulos N, Damilakis J, Perisinakis K, et al. Energy imparted-based estimates of the effect of z overscanning on adult and pediatric patient effective doses from multi-slice computed tomography. Med Phys 2007;34:1139–52.

55. Myronakis M, Perisinakis K, Tzedakis A, et al. Evaluation of a patient-specific Monte Carlo software for CT dosimetry. Radiat Prot Dosimetry 2009;133: 248–55.

56. Bauer JS, Link TM. Advances in osteoporosis imaging. Eur J Radiol 2009;71:440–9.

57. Sheahan NF, Dowling A, O'Reilly G, et al. Commissioning and quality assurance protocol for dual energy X-ray absorptiometry (DEXA) systems. Radiat Prot Dosimetry 2005;117: 288–90.

58. Slavchev A, Avramova-Cholakova S, Vassileva J. National protocol for quality assurance in DXA-bone densitometry. Pol J Med Phys Eng 2008;14: 207–15.

59. Australian and New Zealand Bone and Mineral Society, Australian and New Zealand Association of Physicians in Nuclear Medicine, Royal Australian and New Zealand College of Radiologists, Australasian College of Physical Scientists and Engineers. Accreditation guidelines for bone densitometry. 2004:21–3. Available at: http://www.anzbms.org.au/resources/DXA/guide/index.htm. Accessed February 20, 2010.

60. American Society of Radiologic Technologists. Bone densitometry curriculum. Albuquerque (NM): American Society of Radiologic Technologists; 2009. p. 1–68.

61. American College of Radiology. Practice guidelines for the performance of dual-energy X-ray absorptiometry (DXA). In: Practice guidelines and technical standards. Reston (VA): American College of Radiology; 2008. p. 1–10. Available at: http://www.acr.org/SecondaryMainMenuCategories/quality_safety/guidelines/dx.aspx. Accessed February 20, 2010.

Percutaneous Vertebroplasty or Kyphoplasty

G.C. Anselmetti, MD[a], M. Muto, MD[b],
Giuseppe Guglielmi, MD[c,d], S. Masala, MD[e,f],*

KEYWORDS

• Osteoporosis • Fracture • Kyphosis • Vertebroplasty
• Kyphoplasty • PMMA

Vertebral augmentation techniques are mini-invasive procedures developed in the last 10 years to reduce spine pain owing to their stabilization effect. Percutaneous vertebroplasty (VP), first introduced in 1987 in France by radiologist Harvé Deramond and colleagues[1,2] for symptomatic vertebral angioma and then developed for osteoporotic fracture,[3–5] has gained worldwide acceptance as an effective minimally invasive treatment for back-pain due to osteoporotic vertebral collapses or tumoral vertebral involvement not responding to conservative medical therapy.[6–9] Percutaneous VP consists of the injection of polymethyl methacrylate (PMMA), or other nonacrylic cements, through a relatively large needle (15 to 10 gauge) within the vertebral body under radiological guidance and monitoring.

Kyphoplasty (KP) is also a percutaneous mini-invasive procedure; KP (or balloon-assisted vertebroplasty) can be defined as a development and an evolution of VP. The first KP was performed in California, USA, in 1998,[10] the technique consists in delivering cement—PMMA or other types—into the fractured vertebral body under fluoroscopic guidance after the trabecular bone has been compacted with dedicated balloon tamps.

The rationale of the treatment is to combine the analgesic and vertebral consolidation effect of VP with restoration of the physiologic height of the collapsed vertebral body, reducing the deformity of the vertebral body with resulting normal vertebral statics and biomechanics, and improving respiratory and gastro-intestinal dysfunction.

The main indication for VP is back pain associated with osteoporotic vertebral fractures refractory to medical treatment. Other indications for VP are painful vertebral fractures related to malignant or benign tumors or, less frequently, fractures associated with osteonecrosis.

Recently two randomized trials on osteoporotic vertebral fracture versus sham procedure were published stimulating discussion, criticism, and doubts about this technique.[11,12]

The main indications for KP are osteoporotic vertebral fractures and selected vertebral traumatic fracture types A1 and A3 according to Magerl classification,[13,14] whereas VP is generally preferred in the treatment of primary and secondary vertebral tumors as well as in vertebral hemangioma that can be easily treated in a less invasive way with a thin VP needle.[15]

The origin of the pain in a patient with vertebral benign or malignant collapse or fracture is mostly related to the stretching of the periosteal fibers or nervous structures compression with transmission of the pain to the paravertebral nervous plexus, through the nerve ganglion and spinothalamic-parietal-cortical tract. The techniques have

a Department of Interventional Radiology, Candiolo Hospital Turin, Italy
b Neuroradiology Cardarelli Hospital Naples, Italy
c Department of Radiology, University of Foggia, Viale L. Pinto, 71100 Foggia, Italy
d Scientific Institute 'Casa Sollievo della Sofferenza' Hospital, San Giovanni Rotondo 71013, Italy
e Department of Interventional Radiology, University of Rome Tor Vergata, Italy
f Policlinico Universitario di Tor Vergata Roma, Viale Oxford, 81-00133 Roma, Italy
* Corresponding author. Policlinico Universitario di Tor Vergata Roma, Viale Oxford, 81-00133 Roma, Italy.
E-mail address: salva.masala@tiscali.it

Radiol Clin N Am 48 (2010) 641–649
doi:10.1016/j.rcl.2010.02.020
0033-8389/10/$ – see front matter © 2010 Elsevier Inc. All rights reserved.

major indications for spinal pain refractory to conservative medical and physical treatment.[16–21]

Osteoporosis is certainly the most treated disease with VP or KP, for its high epidemiologic incidence and for the natural history of the disease itself.[22] Currently, in Europe, it is estimated at about 438,750 vertebral collapses per year; that is, 117 out of 100,000 people. In the United States, it is estimated at about 700,000 per year. In women older than 50 years, the incidence of vertebral collapse of osteoporotic nature was estimated to be 26%, with a tendency to increase with age, reaching 40% in women older than 80 years.[23] Moreover, there is evidence that women previously affected by a first osteoporotic vertebral collapse present a risk of developing new fractures in the following year of about 19.2%.[23–26]

INCLUSION CRITERIA

Patients with acute spine thoracic or lumbar pain generally refer to a physician that, after a clinical evaluation, will suggest a medical therapy and a short-term follow-up. If the back pain does not decrease, a second step is represented by radiograph examination that can show normal findings or the presence of an initial vertebral fracture. After at least 4 to 6 weeks from the beginning of clinical symptomatology, a third step is suggested: an MRI examination with sagittal T1, T2, and T2 short tau inversion recovery (STIR)-weighted sequences. T2 STIR sequences are essential in decision-making about the treatment and the number of vertebral body to treat. T2 STIR sequences will show in cases of acute fracture or unhealed fracture the presence of high hyperintensity due to bone marrow edema.

The radiological patterns to distinguish between benign versus malignant are well known, but sometimes differential diagnosis is not simple, especially in cases of vertebral fracture related to multiple myeloma. In these cases, a subsequent CT examination is also suggested to better define lytic lesion and, in patients with metastatic disease, a bone scan is useful for a systemic oncological balance.

The absolute contraindications are the presence of local or systemic infections, the presence of an epidural or foraminal extension associated with neurologic deficit and uncorrectable coagulation disorders. Vertebra plana, mixed secondary lesion, disruption, or epidural extension of the posterior vertebral wall are relative contraindications[21] related to physician's experience in most cases.

The presence of an osteonecrosis (Kummell's disease) is an optimal indication (VP in most cases) as this cystic cavity can be easily filled and vertebral height restored simply with VP procedure.

Multiple myeloma and spine metastases can also be treated with VP or KP.[16]

TECHNIQUE
VP

In most cases, this procedure is performed using a digital C-arm angiographic unit with the patient in the prone position. Treatment of upper thoracic vertebrae (from T2 to T5) and cervical levels can be performed under combined fluoroscopic and CT scan, or in an angiographic flat-panel C-arm with rotational acquisition allowing two-dimensional reconstruction. VP must be performed in sterile conditions and intravenous antibiotics are generally administrated few hours before the procedure. Patient pressure, heart rate, and oxygen saturation are monitored during the whole procedure. In most cases, local anesthesia can be administered by injection (ie, 2 to 3 mL of 2% lidocaine hydrochloride) at the skin level and deeper, to include the periosteum, with a 22-gauge spinal needle. Occasionally, conscious sedation can be useful for uncooperative patients or in poor clinical conditions.

A monolateral parapedicular (thoracic vertebrae), transpedicular (lumbar vertebrae), or anterolateral (cervical) approach with an 11- or 13-gauge bevel needle can be mainly used (**Fig. 1**). A bilateral approach can be employed in selected cases of malignant vertebral involvement to completely fill the disrupted vertebral body (**Fig. 2**). After the needle is advanced into the anterior one-third of the vertebral body in an attempt to reach the midline, the radio-opaque PMMA mixture is injected under continuous fluoroscopic control. The injection needs to be suspended or terminated if venous, disk space, or epidural extravasation is encountered. Postprocedural CT evaluation is useful to assess correct vertebral PMMA injection and to evaluate complications.

Usually, is considered to safe to treat no more than three vertebra each session, but in patients suffering from multiple painful vertebral collapses due to secondary osteoporosis or multiple myeloma, a low-volume, multilevel VP can be performed by experienced interventional radiologists (**Fig. 3**).

After the procedure, the patient remains in strict bed rest for 2 hours and is discharged from the hospital after regaining the ability to perambulate, normally the same procedural day.

KP

For KP, a bilateral transpedicular approach under fluoroscopic guidance is always necessary to obtain an optimal vertebral body filling and height

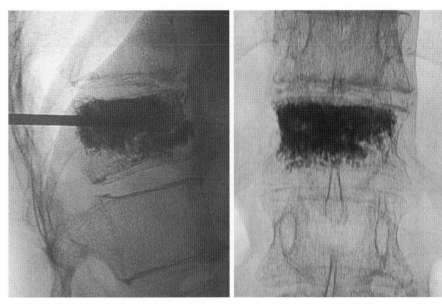

Fig. 1. A monolateral transpedicular approach in latero-lateral and antero-posterior fluoroscopic view.

restoration. High quality fluoroscopy is mandatory to reduce the incidence of side effects and complications, especially in cases of older patients with complex spines disorders, perhaps associated with scoliotic curvature.

Generally, KP requires general anesthesia, especially in cases of more than one level: this is related to the dimension of the cannula that are used in KP (10 gauge) compared with the ones used in VP (13 or 15 gauge). In addition, the time of the procedure is longer with KP than VP.

Once cutaneous, subcutaneous, and periosteal local anesthesia has been administered, the needle will be positioned in the vertebral body through transpedicular approach reaching the posterior wall; the medial margin of the pedicle is an absolute anatomic reference to check before passing the posterior wall of the vertebral body. At this point, a Kirschner wire (K-wire) is inserted. The first cannula is removed, leaving the K-wire on site, and the working cannula is positioned. A metallic drill can also be used to model the trabecular bone such as other osteotomy cannula to lead the insertion of the tamp without problems. The drill is removed and the balloons are inserted; the inflators are connected to the balloon and, under

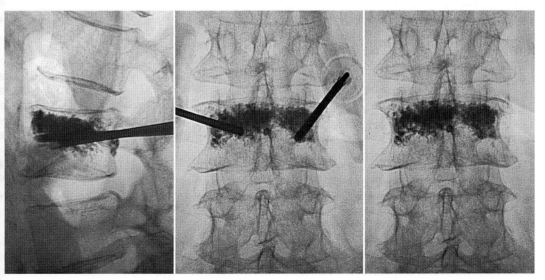

Fig. 2. A bilateral transpedicular approach in latero-lateral and antero-posterior fluoroscopic view.

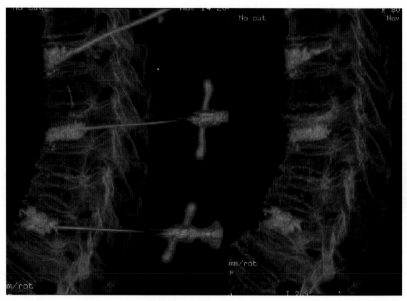

Fig. 3. A CT scan volume rendering postprocessing with biopsy needles positioning and PMMA injection in different vertebral levels during VP.

fluoroscopic control, the inflation of the balloon can be started with the use of diluted contrast media.

The amount of cement injected in the vertebral body is extremely variable—between 2 and 4 mL by each pedicle, depending on the metamer, to treat (thoracic or lumbar) and the degree of the collapsed vertebra (**Fig. 4**).

Owing to the characteristics of restoration of vertebral height and the correction of vertebral kyphosis, KP can be extended for some selected types of traumatic vertebral fracture. Some subtypes of A1 and A3 traumatic vertebral fractures according to the Magerl classification, which generally are treated by conservative treatment with orthosis and bracing for a long time (4–6 months), can be treated with KP leading to optimal bone restoration and healing. In these cases, the timing to perform KP must not be longer than 30 days for young patients (up to 40 years of age) and 60 days for older patients. This is related to different bone activity metabolism.[27]

RESULTS

VP was proven to be safe and effective for pain relief and quality of life improvement in many published series and reviews[14,28,29]—in the osteoporotic patient or in malignancy. Pain, generally evaluated with an 11-point visual analog scale (VAS) where 0 represents no pain and 10 the worst-ever-experienced pain, significantly dropped in around 90% of the osteoporotic patients and 85% of patients with malignancy. Analgesic drug consumption and external brace support decreased after VP. If indications are respected and patients' preprocedure evaluation is correctly performed, an overall quality of life improvement can be achieved with VP. The majority of treated patients report pain relief immediately or within 48 to 72 hours after VP; whereas up to one month is necessary if multilevel treatment was performed. Pain relief is probably obtained by mechanical consolidation of fractured vertebrae as recently demonstrated by an in vivo study[30] pertaining to temperature measurement during PMMA polymerization. The previously proposed mechanism of sensatory nerve thermoablation was ruled out because the temperature in vivo is not long lasting or high enough to determine nerve thermoablation. For that reason, pain relief can be achieved by new bone biologic cements that do not have exothermic reaction during polymerization. Specifically, VP-designed high viscosity bone cements may reduce the risk of leakages and complications and low viscosity may allow a better cancellous bone perfusion with a low-volume injection. The best materials and methods should be considered according to the patient or case.

By re-expanding the vertebra with balloon tamps, KP reduces the pathologic kyphosis, allowing restoration of normal vertebral biomechanics, early mobilization of the patient, and pain relief in 90% of cases.[31–34]

Like VP, KP requires constant fluoroscopic monitoring (angiographic equipment or portable

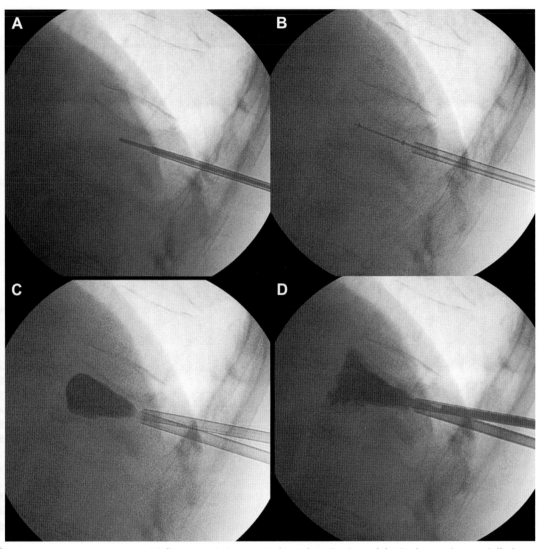

Fig. 4. KP treatment. Sequential fluoroscopic images in lateral projections: (*A*) Kirschner wire coaxially introduced through the 11-G biopsy needles previously positioned with a bilateral transpedicular approach. (*B–C*) Balloon catheter insertion and inflation under continuous fluoroscopic guidance. (*D*) After the balloon catheter has been deflated and removed, the same working cannula is used to inject PMMA into the newly created cavity inside the vertebral body.

C-arm) to ensure correct needle position and general anesthesia.

New cements such as calcium phosphate or tricalcium phosphate/hydroxyapatite or osteoconductive material can be used and associated with KP, extending the indications especially to young patients with recent traumatic fractures (**Fig. 5**).

The characteristics of KP are to create a cavity into the vertebral body by inflating the balloons, leading to a safe injection of PMMA in a low-pressure way, with expectation of low rate of cement leakage—making KP as a safe and important therapeutic option for VCF. In fact, the risk of somatic or venous cement leakage during KP is lower than VP owing to the newly created cavity that has the effect of containing the cement, which is highly viscous and is pushed through the working cannula with a bone-filler device. By PMMA injection into the vertebral body, the vertebral microfractures, responsible for pain, are immobilized, making the vertebral body more compact and resistant. In addition, by inflating the balloon into vertebral body, vertebral kyphosis due to vertebral compression fractures (VCF) can be corrected. However, KP has been shown to restore vertebral height in 20% of cases, with a reduction in wedge angle varying between 6° and 9°.[34–36]

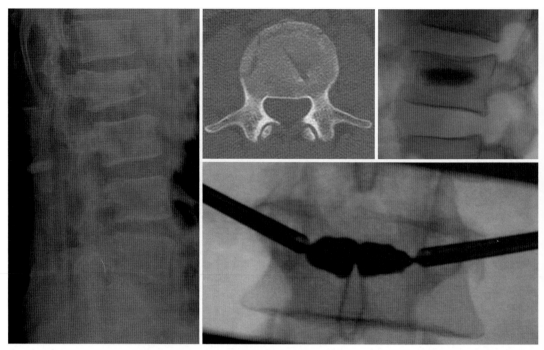

Fig. 5. A KP performed with new bone cement in a traumatic vertebral fracture.

Many studies or trials are performed to analyze the outcome of the technique for pain reduction; kyphosis correction; complications such as cement leakage, disk leakage, and pulmonary embolism; and new vertebral fractures at contiguous or distant vertebral body. The risk of cement leakage is still present (but lower in KP compared with VP), while the incidence rate of a new vertebral fracture to adjacent or distant metamer is similar, mostly related to the osteoporotic disease itself.[14,37]

Recently, a new type of vertebral augmentation technique has been patented using metallic implant to obtain a kyphotic-curve correction, with a balloon tamp and with a stent or with a metallic endovertebral cage to restore the height of the vertebral body (**Fig. 6**). Once this is achieved, the cement or osteoconductive material is injected to obtain vertebral stabilization.

Majd and colleagues[38] performed KP in 360 consecutive osteoporotic cases and reported immediate pain relief in 89% of patients. One patient experienced postoperative pain because of radiculopathy related to bone-filler leakage into the foramen. The remaining patients had persistent pain and were diagnosed with either a new fracture or underlying degenerative disc disease. Greater than or equal to 20% restoration of lost vertebral height (anterior) was observed in 63% of fractures with an overall mean restoration of 30%, and 20% restoration of lost vertebral height (midline) was detected in

69% of fractures with an overall mean restoration of 50%. Only 12% (30 out of 254) of the patients required additional KP procedures to treat 36 symptomatic, new adjacent, and remote fractures. No device-related complications occurred.

Grafe and colleagues[39] compared pain reduction by VAS evaluation in 40 KP-patient groups versus 20 conservative medical treatment patient groups, observing pain scores improved 26.2 to 44.4 in the KP group, and 33.6 to 34.3 in the control group. Significantly, after 12-months, fewer patients with new vertebral fractures of the thoracic and lumbar spine were noted in the KP group than in the control group.

Many studies suggest that VP and KP produce a greater improvement in daily activity, physical function, and pain relief when compared with optimal medical management for osteoporotic VCFs by 6 months after intervention, while there is poor-quality evidence that KP results in greater pain relief for tumor-associated VCFs.[14,37]

By a review of the literature,[40] Eck and colleagues[41] observed that the mean pre- and postoperative VAS scores for KP are 8.06 and 3.46, respectively, with a mean change of 4.60. With KP, the risk of new fracture is 14.1% and the risk of a cement leak is 7.0%.

In a prospective study of stand-alone balloon KP with calcium phosphate cement augmentation in traumatic fractures according to Magerl classification, Maestretti and colleagues[31] reported the

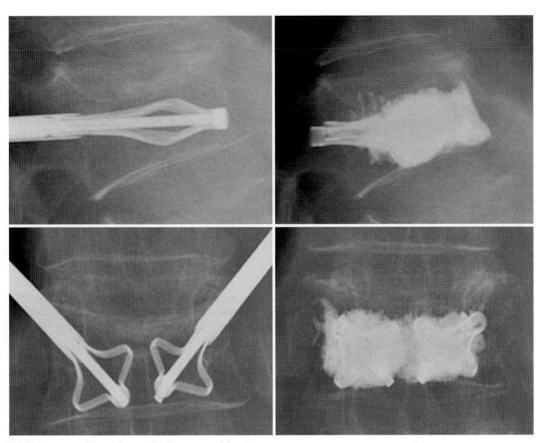

Fig. 6. New metallic endovertebral cage used for KP.

pre- and postoperative and the follow-up results, applying the VAS (0–10) for pain rating, the Roland-Morris (0–24) disability score, with a mean initial vertebral deformity of 17° corrected to a postoperative of 6°. All active patients returned to the same work within 3 months with the same working ability as before. They recommended that, based on its intrinsic characteristics, the biologic cement calcium phosphate for stand-alone reduction and stabilization should only be applied to type A1 and A3 fractures in young patients.

De Falco and colleagues[27] treated eight consecutive patients affected by A1 and A3 Magerl vertebral fractures—using calcium phosphate cement in four cases. They reported pain relief associated with an evident augmentation in the resistance and restoration of the vertebral body's physiology without need of postoperative orthosis shape in all patients. In all the cases, an optimal stabilization in the follow-up minimal to 4 months was noted.

In 39 consecutive patients affected by A1 and A3 Magerl vertebral fractures treated by KP within 3 months of the trauma, Muto and colleagues[42]

achieved pain relief in 90% to 95% of cases—depending on type of fracture—and an increase in vertebral body height sufficient to allow early mobilization of the patient and restoration of the physiologic distribution of postural forces.

COMPLICATIONS

The first step in which it is possible to observe complications is needle (VP) and working cannula (KP) positioning. Three possible approaches are described: transpedicular, parapedicular, and transomatic for lumbar level. At the thoracic level, it is possible to use a costo-trasversal approach. It is very important to perform these procedures with good quality equipment to have always the best anatomic identification. Reviewing the published literature, it is commonly understood that complications are related to abnormal cement distribution with disk, epidural, or vascular leakage. However, more often leakages are completely asymptomatic. Some types of leakages (intraforaminal, radicular vein) can determine transient radicular pain or thecal sac compression, whereas vascular leakage, in most cases asymptomatic, can lead to symptomatic pulmonary emboli, cerebral infarct, or heart and vascular dissection. Disc-bone cement leakage seems to be related to a higher incidence of fracture to the contiguous vertebral body. To avoid complications, two major techniques must be highlighted: use cement with adequate viscosity and inject slowly under constant fluoroscopy monitoring. The posterior wall of the vertebral body is an essential anatomic landmark that should never be passed by cement opacity. This is a key to avoiding diffuse endocanalar cement leakage leading to major complications such as paraplegia or tetraplegia. Generally, major complications can be easily avoided if high-quality imaging systems, proper materials, and correct indications are employed and respected.

SUMMARY

Percutaneous vertebral augmentation techniques performed with VP or KP are safe and effective for the treatment of osteoporotic VCF, primary or secondary spine tumors, and selected traumatic fractures. In most cases, VP alone is sufficient to achieve pain relief and quality of life improvement. The advantages of KP over VP are low-pressure cement injection, the use of high-density cement, and a lower rate of vascular and disk leakage. The disadvantages of KP compared to VP are related to its higher invasiveness, the higher cost (four times higher), the need for deep sedation or general anesthesia, and time required. To the best of the authors' knowledge, the clinical advantages of height restoration that KP can achieve in some cases has to be scientifically proven and it should be considered that most important clinical results (pain relief and quality of life improvement) are the same as shown by the literature. In our opinion, VP should be performed in most cases (older patients with osteoporotic vertebral collapses and palliation in the malignancy) and KP in selected cases only (fresh osteoporotic and traumatic fracture). Both procedures are only intended to cure back-pain. They cannot cure the diseases that caused the fractures (osteoporosis and malignancy). For optimal and lasting long-term results, every patient needs to receive optimal medical therapy before and after VP and KP. The trials of sham procedures recently published by *The New England Journal of Medicine* necessitate an accurate reconsideration concerning the optimal indications of these procedures.[42]

REFERENCES

1. Galibert P, Deramond H, Rosat P, et al. Preliminary note on the treatment of vertebral angioma by percutaneous acrylic vertebroplasty. Neurochirurgie 1987;33(2):166–8.
2. Bostrom MP, Lane JM. Future directions. Augmentation of osteoporotic vertebral bodies. Spine 1997; 22(24 Suppl):38S–42S.
3. Jensen ME, Evans AJ, Mathis JM, et al. Percutaneous polymethylmethacrylate vertebroplasty in the treatment of osteoporotic vertebral body compression fractures: technical aspects. AJNR Am J Neuroradiol 1997;18(10):1897–904.
4. Cortet B, Cotten A, Boutry N, et al. Percutaneous vertebroplasty in the treatment of osteoporotic vertebral compression fractures: an open prospective study. J Rheumatol 1999;26(10):2222–8.
5. Watts NB, Harris ST, Genant HK. Treatment of painful osteoporotic vertebral fractures with percutaneous vertebroplasty or kyphoplasty. Osteoporos Int 2001;12(6):429–37.
6. Ploeg WT, Veldhuizen AG, The B, et al. Percutaneous vertebroplasty as a treatment for osteoporotic vertebral compression fractures: a systematic review. Eur Spine J 2006;15(12):1749–58.
7. Yu SW, Yang SC, Kao YH, et al. Clinical evaluation of vertebroplasty for multiple-level osteoporotic spinal compression fracture in the elderly. Arch Orthop Trauma Surg 2008;128(1):97–101.
8. Anselmetti GC, Corrao G, Monica PD, et al. Pain relief following percutaneous vertebroplasty: results of a series of 283 consecutive patients treated in a single institution. Cardiovasc Intervent Radiol 2007;30(3):441–7.
9. Hierholzer J, Fuchs H, Westphalen K, et al. Incidence of symptomatic vertebral fractures in patients after percutaneous vertebroplasty. Cardiovasc Intervent Radiol 2008;31(6):1178–83.
10. Wong X, Reiley MA, Garfin S. Vertebroplasty/kyphoplasty. J Women's Imaging 2000;2:117–24.
11. Pflugmacher R, Kandziora F, Schroder R, et al. Vertebroplasty and kyphoplasty in osteoporotic fractures of vertebral bodies: a prospective 1-year follow-up analysis. Rofo 2005;177:1670–6.
12. Kallmes DF, Heagerty PJ, Turner JA, et al. A randomized trial of vertebroplasty for osteoporotic spinal fractures. N Engl J Med 2009;361(6):569–79.
13. Buchbinder R, Osborne RH, Murphy B, et al. A randomized trial of vertebroplasty for painful osteoporotic vertebral fractures. N Engl J Med 2009; 361(6):557–68.
14. Mcgirt MJ, Parker SL, Wolinsky JP, et al. Vertebroplasty and kyphoplasty for the treatment of vertebral compression fractures: an evidenced-based review of the literature. Spine J 2009;9(6):501–8.
15. Magerl F, Aebi M, Gertzbein SD, et al. A comprehensive classification of thoracic and lumbar injuries. Eur Spine J 1994;3:184–201.
16. Guarnieri G, Ambrosanio G, Vassallo P, et al. Vertebroplasty as treatment of aggressive and

symptomatic vertebral hemangiomas: up to 4 years of follow-up. Neuroradiology 2009;51(7):471–6.

17. Peh WC, Gilula LA. Percutaneous vertebroplasty: indications, contraindications, and technique. Br J Radiol 2003;76:69–75.

18. Cotten A, Boutry N, Cortet B, et al. Percutaneous vertebroplasty: state of the art. Radiographics 1998;18:311–20.

19. Gangi A, Guth S, Imbert JP, et al. Percutaneous vertebroplasty: indications, technique, and results. Radiographics 2003;23:10–20.

20. Mathis JM, Barr JD, Belkoff SM, et al. Percutaneous vertebroplasty: a developing standard of care for vertebral compression fractures. AJNR Am J Neuroradiol 2001;22:373–81.

21. Ambrosanio G, Lavanga A, Vassallo P, et al. Vertebroplasty in the treatment of spine disease. Interventional Neuroradiology 2005;11:309–23.

22. Uppin AA, Hirsch JA, Centenera LV, et al. Occurrence of new vertebral body fracture after percutaneous vertebroplasty in patients with osteoporosis. Radiology 2003;226:119–24.

23. Bajaj S, Saag KG. Osteoporosis: evaluation and treatment. Curr Womens Health Rep 2003;3:418–24.

24. Lindsay R, Silvermann LS, Seeman E, et al. Risk of new vertebral fracture in the year following a fracture. JAMA 2001;285(3):20–3.

25. Silverman SL. The clinical consequences of vertebral compression fracture. Bone 1992;13:27S–31S.

26. Voormolen MH, Lohle PN, Juttmann JR, et al. The risk of new osteoporotic vertebral compression fractures in the year after percutaneous vertebroplasty. J Vasc Interv Radiol 2006;17:71–6.

27. De Falco R, Scarano E, Guarnieri L, et al. Balloon kyphoplasty in traumatic fractures of the thoracolumbar junction. Preliminary experience in 12 cases. J Neurosurg Sci 2005;49:147–53.

28. Ofluoglu O. Minimally invasive management of spinal metastases. Orthop Clin North Am 2009;40(1):155–68.

29. Masala S, Mammucari M, Angelopoulos G, et al. Percutaneous vertebroplasty in the management of vertebral osteoporotic fractures. Short-term, mid-term and long-term follow-up of 285 patients. Skeletal Radiol 2009;38(9):863–9.

30. Anselmetti GC, Manca A, Kanika K, et al. Temperature measurement during polymerization of bone cement in percutaneous vertebroplasty: an in vivo study in humans. Cardiovasc Intervent Radiol 2009;32(3):491–8.

31. Maestretti G, Cremer C, Otten P, et al. Prospective study of standalone balloon kyphoplasty with calcium phosphate cement augmentation in traumatic fractures. Eur Spine J 2007;16(5):601–10.

32. Fuentes S, Metellus P, Fondop J, et al. Percutaneous pedicle screw fixation and kyphoplasty for management of thoracolumbar burst fractures. Neurochirurgie 2007;53:272–6.

33. Theodoru DJ, Theodorou SJ, Duncan TD, et al. Percutaneous balloon kyphoplasty for the correction of spinal deformity in painful vertebral body compression fractures. Clin Imaging 2002;26:1–5.

34. Deramond H, Salioub G, Aveillana M, et al. Respective contributions of vertebroplasty and kyphoplasty to the management of osteoporotic vertebral fractures. Joint Bone Spine 2006;73:610–3.

35. Voggenreiter G. Balloon kyphoplasty is effective in deformity correction of osteoporotic vertebral compression fractures. Spine 2005;30:2806–12.

36. Hiwatashi A, Moritani T, Numaguchi Y, et al. Increase in vertebral body height after vertebroplasty. AJNR Am J Neuroradiol 2003;24:185–9.

37. Teng MM, Wei CJ, Wei LC, et al. Kyphosis correction and height restoration effects of percutaneous vertebroplasty. AJNR Am J Neuroradiol 2003;24: 1893–900.

38. Majd ME, Farley S, Holt RT, et al. Preliminary outcomes and efficacy of the first 360 consecutive kyphoplasties for the treatment of painful osteoporotic vertebral compression fractures. Spine J 2005;5:244–55.

39. Grafe IA, Da Fonseca K, Hillmeier J, et al. Reduction of pain and fracture incidence after kyphoplasty: 1-year outcomes of a prospective controlled trial of patients with primary osteoporosis. Osteoporos Int 2005;16:2005–12.

40. Frankel BM, Monroe T, Wang C. Percutaneous vertebral augmentation: an elevation in adjacent-level fracture risk in kyphoplasty as compared with vertebroplasty. Spine J 2007;7:575–82.

41. Eck JC, Nachtigall D, Humphreys SC, et al. Comparison of vertebroplasty and balloon kyphoplasty for treatment of vertebral compression fractures: a meta-analysis of the literature. Spine J 2008;8: 488–97.

42. Muto M, Perrotta V, Guarnieri G, et al. Vertebroplasty and kyphoplasty: friends or foes? Radiol Med 2008; 113(8):1171–84.

Index

Note: Page numbers of article titles are in **boldface** type.

Radiol Clin N Am 48 (2010) 651–655
doi:10.1016/S0033-8389(10)00066-7
0033-8389/10/$ – see front matter © 2010 Elsevier Inc. All rights reserved.

Moving?

Make sure your subscription moves with you!

To notify us of your new address, find your **Clinics Account Number** (located on your mailing label above your name), and contact customer service at:

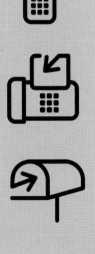

Email: journalscustomerservice-usa@elsevier.com

800-654-2452 (subscribers in the U.S. & Canada)
314-447-8871 (subscribers outside of the U.S. & Canada)

Fax number: 314-447-8029

Elsevier Health Sciences Division
Subscription Customer Service
3251 Riverport Lane
Maryland Heights, MO 63043

*To ensure uninterrupted delivery of your subscription, please notify us at least 4 weeks in advance of move.

ELSEVIER